Clinical Kinesiology

Clinical Kinesiology

Signe Brunnstrom, M.A.

Graduate, Royal Gymnastic Central Institute
Stockholm, Sweden

Instructor in Physical Therapy
College of Physicians and Surgeons
Columbia University, New York City

Third Edition

Revision by

Ruth Dickinson, M.A.

Assistant Professor of Physical Therapy
Columbia University

 F. A. DAVIS COMPANY • PHILADELPHIA

Preface to the Third Edition

In this third edition, those sections of the book which represent the major contributions Miss Brunnstrom has given to our understanding of normal and abnormal kinesiology are unchanged. One of the pertinent changes made in this edition is the revision of the section in Chapter 1 concerned with basic mechanical principles.

Reference is made to recent anatomical, electromyographic and clinical studies and among those included are: scapular and glenohumeral movements (Freedman and Munro, 1966; Doody, Freedman and Waterland, 1970); gastrocnemius and soleus function (Herman and Bragin, 1967); role of leg and foot muscles in normal and flat feet (Gray and Basmajian, 1968, 1969); upper extremity muscular activity during normal gait (Hogue, 1969); intrinsic-extrinsic muscle control of the fingers (Long, 1968); muscles of the thumb, the index and long fingers (Close and Kidd, 1969).

New information and certain details of gait have been provided by Murray and associates, Kinesiology Research Laboratory, Veterans Administration Center, Wood, Wisconsin. Their publications are noted in the text and these are listed among the references primarily to call them to the reader's attention.

The organization of the book, which served so well in the previous editions, remains essentially the same.

RUTH DICKINSON

Preface to the First Edition

Kinesiology—broadly defined as the science of human motion—
has ramifications reaching into many fields of study, such as anatomy, physiology, mechanics, physics, mathematics, orthopedics,
neurology, pathology and psychology. To be of practical value, a
textbook dealing with such a vast subject must be geared to the
specific needs of the groups for which it is intended, in the present
case the members of medical, paramedical and physical education
professions. Because the background requirements and the cur-
ricula for students who prepare to enter these professions include
subjects closely related to kinesiology, the task at hand was to
supplement, not duplicate, the contents of other courses. A certain
amount of overlap between courses in anatomy and kinesiology
was inevitable. However, throughout the preparation of this book
an effort was made to present a minimum of anatomical details
while emphasizing the function of skeletal and neuromuscular
structures. Both the text and the illustrations aim at developing
the student's skill in palpating anatomical structures in the living,
a skill which is invaluable in dealing with patients.

Much of the contents of this book has been used over the years by
the author in teaching kinesiology to students of physical therapy
and occupational therapy. The writing of the book originated with
a teaching grant from the Office of Vocational Rehabilitation
which enabled the author to prepare a mimeographed laboratory
manual to serve as a study aid for students of physical therapy and
occupational therapy at College of Physicians and Surgeons,
Columbia University. The original manual was then revised and
enlarged to include material on certain aspects of pathological
motor behavior. The clinical aspects of kinesiology were given
emphasis to meet the needs of workers in the field of rehabilitation
of the physically handicapped.

Although basic kinesiology is concerned with normal motion of
individuals with intact neuromuscular systems, the inclusion of
selected pathological cases seemed justifiable and desirable. The

effect of loss of specific muscles or muscle groups on movement is particularly well demonstrated in individuals having certain types of peripheral nerve injuries; since the paralysis in this group is specific, illustrations have been drawn mainly from these patients. The motor behavior of patients with upper motoneuron lesions was not included because, to be of value, such a discussion would have to be too lengthy to fit into the framework of this publication.

The section on erect posture, although brief, is intended to present the most important mechanical principles governing the balance of body segments in the upright position. These principles may also serve as a rationale for evaluating the difficulties arising from disorders of the lower extremities, as in persons with paraplegia, lower extremity amputations, poliomyelitis, and the like. By implication, some understanding of the basic principles of bracing and of lower extremity prosthetics should also be derived, although the latter subjects have not been dealt with specifically.

Originally, the author did not intend to discuss human locomotion, but did so at the request of professional personnel who felt that, without a chapter on locomotion, a textbook of kinesiology would be incomplete. ,Justice cannot be done to this subject in one short chapter, hence the locomotion chapter must be looked upon as an introduction only. For the benefit of those who wish to go deeper into the study of locomotion, references to scientific material are given.

In preparing this book, the author was many times tempted to discuss the application of kinesiology to various therapeutic training procedures employed by physical therapists and occupational therapists. Such follow up of the basic material, however, does not belong in this publication—special courses are offered to deal with therapeutic applications.

The book has fulfilled its purpose if the reader gains a basic knowledge and appreciation of human motion and if, to some extent, it opens scientific vistas which call for further exploration and investigation.

SIGNE BRUNNSTROM

Acknowledgments

The author is happy to acknowledge the valuable assistance she has received from colleagues and professional friends in the preparation of this book, and to extend to them her sincere thanks for their efforts and interest:

To Dr. Herbert O. Elftman, Associate Professor of Anatomy, College of Physicians and Surgeons, Columbia University, for reading the manuscript and for giving so generously of his time and effort. Thanks to his constructive criticism, errors have been corrected, questionable statements clarified, and much irrelevant material eliminated. It has been a privilege, indeed, to have Dr. Elftman take an active interest in this publication.

To Dr. Robert E. Darling, Professor of Physical Medicine and Rehabilitation, for his support and encouragement.

To Professor Mary E. Callahan, Director, Courses for Physical Therapy, and to Professor Marie Louise Franciscus, Director, Courses for Occupational Therapy, for their interest and assistance. To Professors Ruth Dickinson, R.P.T., and Martha E. Schnebly, O.T.R., co-instructors in Kinesiology, who have tested and evaluated the material under actual teaching conditions, and who have assisted in numerous ways.

To Dr. T. Campbell Thompson, for the permission to use photographs taken at Hospital for Special Surgery.

The author also wishes to extend her thanks to the young man who patiently served as a model for a great many photographs in this book and to Mr. Crew, of the Crew Photo Studio, Carmel, New York, for his splendid cooperation.

Contents

CHAPTER 1

Mechanical Principles: Application to the Human Body

The subject of mechanics deals with forces acting on bodies and with the result of these forces in terms of equilibrium and movement. The application of mechanics to the living human body is referred to as *biomechanics.*

Mechanics may be subdivided into two main parts, *statics* (Gr. *staticos,* causing to stand) which is concerned with bodies in balance, and *dynamics* (Gr. *dynamis,* force) which treats of bodies in motion. Dynamics is subdivided into *kinematics* (Gr. *kinema,* motion) which is concerned with *geometry of motion,* and *kinetics,* which deals with the *forces* which produce movement.

In biomechanics, equilibrium and motion are so closely interrelated that it becomes rather impractical to discuss statics and dynamics under separate headings. Therefore, certain aspects of statics will be dealt with in conjunction with kinematics and kinetics, as the occasion demands. Equilibrium principles are also discussed in Chapter 10.

KINEMATICS

DEFINITION OF KINEMATICS

Kinematics in its broadest sense may be defined as the science of motion, but, more specifically, it is concerned with the *geometry of motion without regard to the forces acting to produce motion.* The application of kinematics to the living human body involves description, measurement and recording of bodily motion, with due consideration of the characteristics of joints and bony segments involved in such motion.

RECORDING OF POSITIONS AND MOVEMENTS

THREE-DIMENSIONAL SYSTEM OF RECORDING. To record the location in space of specific points on the body surface and inside the body as well as movement paths of such points, a three-dimensional system of coordinates is used. For such purposes, *three planes perpendicular to each other are laid through the center of gravity of the body.* These planes are called the cardinal planes of the body. For the purpose of description, the subject is thought of as standing erect.

The *cardinal sagittal plane* (also called midsagittal) is a vertical plane which divides the body into left and right parts. In Latin, *sagitta* means arrow, the sagittal plane being the plane of the arrow.

The *cardinal frontal plane,* like the sagittal, is a vertical one. It is called frontal because it is parallel to the frontal bone. This plane divides the body into front and back parts.

The *cardinal horizontal plane* (also called transverse plane) divides the body into upper and lower parts.

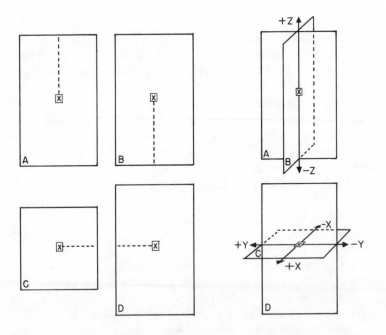

FIG. 1. Model for the establishment of the three cardinal planes of the body. Point ⊠ represents the center of gravity of the body.

For a better visualization of the cardinal planes of the body, it is suggested that a model be made of stiff paper or cardboard, such as 5" x 8" cards. A slit is made in each card, as indicated by the dotted lines in Figures 1A and B, the slit in B being slightly longer than the slit in A. (This is done because, in erect standing, the center of gravity of the body is located somewhat above the halfway mark between the top of the head and the soles of the feet.) The cards are now put together perpendicular to each other thereby establishing the sagittal and the frontal planes. In a similar manner two other cards, C and D, are used to illustrate the relationship between the horizontal and the frontal (or sagittal) planes.

The intersection between the three cardinal planes establishes the X, Y, and Z axes (Fig. 1). The intersection between the sagittal and the horizontal planes, running in an anteroposterior direction, is called the X axis (positive being forward, negative backward); that which is between the horizontal and the frontal planes, which run from side to side, is called the Y axis (positive being on the subject's right, negative on the subject's left); and that between the frontal and sagittal planes, running from the top downward, is called the Z axis (positive upward, negative downward). Fick's (1910) manner of labeling the axes and his use of plus and minus signs have been maintained.

Sagittal, frontal and horizontal planes may be laid through points other than the center of gravity of the body, but these are *secondary planes*. For example, it may be convenient to lay three planes through the center of a joint, such as the hip joint, for determination of body points in relation to such a joint.

TWO-DIMENSIONAL RECORDING. For recording of body points in two dimensions, one plane of reference suffices. When projection is made on the frontal plane, a front or back view of the subject is obtained (Fig. 2A). Projection on a sagittal plane provides a side view (Fig. 2B); projection on a horizontal plane, a view from above or below.

For three-dimensional motions, such as walking, three synchronized motion-picture cameras may be used simultaneously to obtain front, side, and top or bottom views. The data thus obtained may then be reduced, resulting in a three-dimensional record (see also Chapter 11).

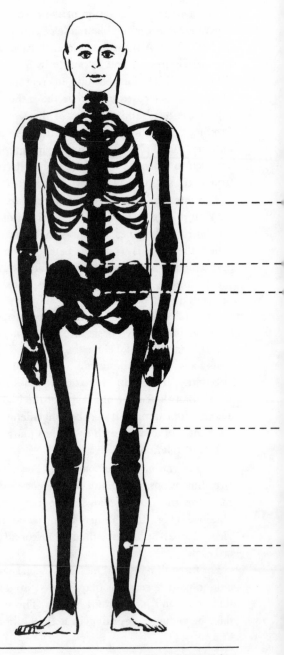

CENTER OF GRAVITY

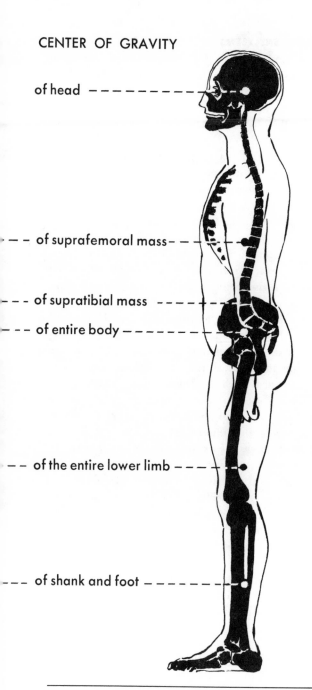

of head – – – – – – – –

– – – of suprafemoral mass – – –

– – – of supratibial mass – – – –

– – – of entire body – – – – – –

– – of the entire lower limb – – –

– – – of shank and foot – – – – – –

ORIENTATION OF MOVEMENT TERMS TO BODY PLANES

Conventionally, anatomical terms for movements of the main joints of the body are oriented to the three planes of the body. The subject is thought of as standing erect, feet symmetrically placed, the nose pointing straight ahead, and the arms at the sides of the body. If the shoulder joint or the hip joint is taken as an example, *flexion-extension* movements take place in a sagittal plane, *abduction-adduction* motions in a frontal plane, and *external-internal rotations* in a horizontal plane. Natural movements seldom, if ever, take place strictly in one of these planes. Oblique planes, the description of which has to be given in terms of degrees of deviation from the sagittal, frontal and horizontal planes, may also be established.

ANATOMICAL POSITION. If in the erect standing position, as described above, the palms are turned forward (i.e., the forearms are supinated) the so-called *anatomical position* is assumed. When the palms are turned forward, the flexor surfaces of forearm and hand face forward, the extensor surfaces backward. In this position, the terms for movements of elbow, wrist, and finger joints, like those of the shoulder joint, may be oriented to the sagittal, frontal and horizontal planes. Flexion-extension motions then take place in the sagittal plane, abduction-adduction in the frontal plane, and pronation-supination of the forearm in the horizontal plane. The anatomical position is frequently used as a starting point in describing motions in order to obtain a certain uniformity of terms. As will be shown presently, the use of the anatomical position proves quite impractical; hence, *in this book the anatomical position will not be used as orientation for movement terms.*

As an example of the confusion arising from orienting all motions to the anatomical position, let us consider the movements at the metacarpophalangeal joint of the little finger. When, in the anatomical position, the little finger is moved away from the other fingers, it moves in a direction toward the body; this motion should be called *adduction,* but it is performed by a muscle called the *abductor digiti minimi.* It certainly seems more appropriate to use the term *abduction* for this movement, regardless of the position of the forearm, and to orient finger abduction-adduction to the center line of the hand, not to the center line of the body.

TERMINOLOGY FOR MOVEMENTS OF JOINTS

It must be emphasized from the onset that either or both of the segments adjacent to a joint may move and, therefore, it is appropriate to speak of movements of *joints* rather than of segments. At most joints and in most activities both segments move simultaneously, although in some instances, the motion of one segment predominates.

Example 1. In *flexion of the elbow,* the forearm may move in relation to the arm, as when the hand is brought to the mouth, or the arm may move in relation to the forearm, as in chinning oneself, or both forearm and arm may move, as in sawing wood. The term *flexion of the forearm* would only apply to the first instance, while *flexion of the elbow* fits all three.

Example 2. *Extension of the knee* may be performed in the sitting position by raising the leg to a horizontal position, by rising from sitting to standing or by squatting and then returning to the upright position. *Extension of the leg* would apply only to the first of these motions, while *extension of the knee* describes all three.

By analyzing a variety of natural movements of the upper and lower extremities it will be seen that proximal segments frequently move in relation to distal segments and that complete stabilization of one of the segments is the exception rather than the rule. It therefore does not seem desirable to assume, as is commonly done, that muscles primarily move distal segments in relation to proximal ones. The muscle has no preference and both types of motions are of equal importance.

Some of the most common terms used in the description of joint movement are as follows:

Flexion, which is employed to indicate that the angle of a joint becomes smaller as the joint is being bent, as, for example, flexion of the elbow, flexion of the knee. *Extension* is the opposite movement.

Abduction is a movement away from a defined line, such as the center line of the body or the center line of the forearm or the hand. Abduction of the hip thus is a movement away from the center line of the body involving either one or both of the segments which participate in hip motions, namely, the pelvis and femur. During abduction, two points situated on the lateral aspects of the two segments approach each other. *Adduction* has the opposite direction to abduction.

Internal rotation (also called medial rotation, inward rotation) is a transverse rotation which is oriented to the anterior side of the body. For example, internal rotation of the hip brings two points on the anterior side of the two segments (pelvis and femur) closer together, regardless of which one of the two segments is moving. *External rotation* (also called lateral rotation, outward rotation) has an opposite direction and is oriented to the posterior side of the body.

Additional terms for joint movements will be defined where they first appear in the text.

DEGREES OF FREEDOM OF MOTION

The expression *degrees of freedom of motion* was originally coined by Reuleaux (1875) for use in engineering and was adapted to biomechanics by Otto Fischer (1907). It has been used extensively by subsequent authors in discussing joint mechanics (Fick, 1910, pp. 77-88; Steindler, 1955, pp. 62-63).

ONE DEGREE OF FREEDOM OF MOTION. Hinge joints, such as the interphalangeal joints of the digits, which permit flexion and extension only, are said to possess one degree of freedom of motion. Move-

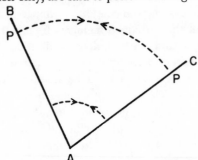

FIG. 3. One degree of freedom of motion characteristic of a hinge joint. Movement takes place about axis A, and either segment or both of the segments may move. Point P is restricted to motion along a line which follows the arc of a circle.

ments take place about *one axis only* which, in the case of the interphalangeal joints, is a transverse one. Any one point on a segment adjacent to the joint is permitted to move along a line only, following a predetermined path (Fig. 3). In the same figure, it can be seen that the segment A-B may move in relation to segment A-C, or segment A-C may move in relation to segment A-B, or both segments may move simultaneously.

The radioulnar connections which permit pronation and supination only, likewise exemplify one degree of freedom, the axis of motion in this case being a longitudinal one (Fig. 30, p. 53). If the hand is free to move while the upper arm is stabilized (as in holding the elbow flexed and close to the body), pronation-supination consists of a movement of the radius in relation to the ulna, and since the hand follows the movement of the radius, the palm is turned alternately up and down. But if the hand has fixation, as in pressing

Clinical Kinesiology

the palm against a firm edge, a pronation-supination motion involves motion of the ulna in relation to the radius. This, of course, can only be accomplished if the shoulder joint is free to permit rotation.

A third example of a joint which possesses one degree of freedom of motion is the joint between the two uppermost cervical vertebrae which permits the first vertebra (and with it the head) to rotate to the right and the left around a vertical axis through the dens (odontoid process) of the second vertebra. If the head is stabilized, the body may of course also rotate in relation to the head.

TWO DEGREES OF FREEDOM OF MOTION. Condyloid joints, such as the metacarpophalangeal joints of the digits which permit flexion-extension and abduction-adduction, are said to possess two degrees of freedom of motion. The saddle joint of the thumb (carpometacarpal joint) and the wrist joint are other examples. The movements take place about *two main axes* perpendicular to each other. In the case of the metacarpophalangeal joints of the digits, one axis is transverse through the center of the head of the metacarpal bone, permitting flexion and extension; the other axis has a dorsopalmar direction, permitting abduction and adduction.

Actually, motions may take place about any number of axes through the center of the metacarpal head which combine various degrees of the two main motions. For example, motion may take place about an oblique axis so that in one direction there is flexion-adduction, and in the opposite direction, extension-abduction. By well-coordinated successive combinations of the movement components, a *circumduction* motion is performed during which the moving segment follows the surface of a cone and the tip of the segment prescribes a circular path. Circumduction is characteristic of joints with two and three degrees of freedom, but cannot take place in joints with one degree of freedom.

THREE DEGREES OF FREEDOM OF MOTION. Ball-and-socket joints, such as the hip joint, which permit flexion-extension, abduction-adduction, and transverse rotation are said to possess three degrees of freedom. Movements take place about three main axes, all of which pass through the center of the joint (in the case of the hip joint, the center of the head of the femur). At the hip, the axis for flexion-extension has a transverse direction (from side to side), the axis for abduction-adduction has a dorsoventral direction, and the axis for transverse rotation courses longitudinally from the center of the hip joint to the center of the knee joint. In the erect standing position, the first two axes are horizontal, the third one vertical. The gleno-humeral joint (shoulder joint) is another example of a joint with three degrees of freedom.

Ball-and-socket joints, as stated above, have three main axes of motion, but movements may take place about an infinite number of *secondary axes* all of which have one thing in common, namely, that they pass through the center of the joint. The variety of motions is much larger than in joints with two degrees of freedom.

Three degrees of freedom of motion are the maximum which a *joint* in the human body can possess. The higher degrees of freedom which are enjoyed by *segments* of the body are obtained by summation of motions of two or more joints. Successively, the more distal segments (if not stabilized distally) have higher degrees of freedom than the proximal ones.

KINEMATIC CHAINS

The term *kinematic chains*, like that of freedom of motion, was introduced by Reuleaux (1875) for use in engineering, and subsequently the term was applied to biomechanics. *A combination of several joints uniting successive segments constitutes a kinematic chain or joint chain.*

OPEN AND CLOSED KINEMATIC CHAINS. In an open kinematic chain the distal segment terminates free in space, while in a closed kinematic chain the end segments are united to form a ring or closed circuit. Closed circuits are commonly used in machines; open chains are more common in the human body, as exemplified by the vertebral column and the limbs. A number of closed chains are also found in the human body, such as: the pelvic girdle where the segments are united by the two sacroiliac joints and the pubic symphysis, and the thorax, where each rib with its vertebral and sternal connections forms a ring.*

FREEDOM OF MOTION OF CHAIN SEGMENTS. Each segment of an open joint chain has a characteristic degree of freedom of motion, the distal segments possessing higher degrees of freedom than the proximal ones. In many instances, the degrees of freedom of a distal segment of an open chain are determined by addition of the free-

*Steindler (1955) gives a different interpretation of a closed kinematic chain (which he calls *kinetic chain*). The term is applied to "all situations in which the peripheral joint of the chain meets with overwhelming external resistance" (p. 63).

doms of the participating joints. In other instances, this may not hold true since one joint may duplicate the freedom of another.

A CHAIN CONSISTING OF TWO HINGE JOINTS WITH PARALLEL AXES has two degrees of freedom of motion, and this is a direct summation of the one degree of freedom possessed by each hinge joint. In Figure 4, two hinge joints, A and D, make up a joint chain. Joint D permits a point P on the end segment to move along a line, following the arc of a circle. But since joint A permits a rotation about its axis of segment A-B, points on the distal segment, such as point P, are no longer restricted to move along a line but are permitted to move over a surface, and have two degrees of freedom.

A CHAIN OF THREE SUCCESSIVE HINGE JOINTS. If the axes of motion of all three joints are parallel, the chain possesses only two degrees of freedom; a point on the end segment can still move only

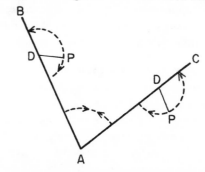

FIG. 4. Summation of free-doms of two hinge joints, A and D, gives two degrees of freedom of motion to point P on the distal segment. Point P is no longer restricted to a motion along a line but can cover a surface.

along a surface, but not away from the surface. In this case, a simple addition of the freedoms of each joint does not give the correct answer for the degrees of freedom of the chain. But if the axis of one of the three hinge joints is not parallel with those of the other two, the chain possesses three degrees of freedom; a point on the end segment is then permitted to move away from the surface to which it was previously limited.

A CHAIN CONSISTING OF A SADDLE JOINT AND A HINGE JOINT. The saddle joint of the thumb possesses two degrees of freedom of motion, that is, points on the metacarpal bone are permitted to move over a surface. If it is first assumed that the metacarpophalangeal and interphalangeal joints of the thumb do not exist, the tip of the thumb can move over a portion of a spherical surface, but cannot move away from this surface. If the interphalangeal joint of the thumb is then incorporated in the system (still disregarding the metacarpophalangeal joint), three degrees of freedom of the distal segment results, that is, the tip of the thumb can now move away from the spherical surface.

HIGHEST DEGREE OF FREEDOM OF MOTION OF A SEGMENT. The highest degree of freedom which a segment can possess is present when the segment is permitted to move freely in space (within certain boundaries), a freedom which is enjoyed by the human hand. Such freedom of motion constitutes the mechanical basis for the performance of skilled manual activities.

The kinematic chain of the upper extremity is composed of many joints, each of which possesses one to three degrees of freedom. The result is that a high degree of freedom is allotted, not only to the end segment in relation to the trunk, but also to various segments in relation to each other. This contributes materially to the versatility of the upper extremity. To a certain extent, such arrangement also minimizes the disabling effect of restriction or elimination of motion of individual joints resulting from injury or disease.

ROTARY AND TRANSLATORY MOTIONS

Rotary motions take place about a fixed or relatively fixed axis. They are called rotary, because every point on a segment adjacent to the joint follows the arc of a circle, the center of which is the joint axis. Thus, in flexion and extension of the elbow, the bones of the forearm (and/or the bone of the upper arm) rotate about the axis of the elbow joint. Individual points on the segment move with different velocities, the velocity of each point being related to its distance from the axis of motion. Thus, if the arm is made to swing forward and backward at the shoulder, the velocity of the hand is greater than that of the elbow and far greater than that of a point on the upper portion of the arm which lies close to the center of rotation.

In mechanics, the term *translatory motion* is applied to a movement of a body during which all parts of the body move in the same direction and with equal velocity. Examples of true translatory motions are: a stone sliding on an icy surface, an object placed on a conveyor belt, passengers riding in a moving train. In walking, the body as a whole moves in a forward direction, but this is not a true translatory motion since body segments move forward with different velocities. The total result, however, is a translation of the body as a whole, achieved by means of rotary motions of various limb segments. That certain combinations of rotary motions may cause a

Clinical Kinesiology

translatory one may be observed also in the upper extremity. Because of rotary motions at several joints, the hand is capable of moving freely in space, that is, take a translatory path.

KINETICS

DEFINITION OF KINETICS

Kinetics, a branch of dynamics, *deals with forces which produce, arrest, or modify motions of bodies*. When producing motions, forces act to disturb the equilibrium of a body; when arresting motions, forces return the body to a state of equilibrium.

EQUILIBRIUM—NEWTON'S FIRST LAW

Stationary bodies and bodies moving with uniform speed are said to be in equilibrium. Newton's first law, the law of inertia, states that *bodies at rest tend to remain at rest; bodies in motion tend to remain in motion*.

EQUILIBRIUM—NEWTON'S THIRD LAW

Bodies in equilibrium are acted upon by forces, but these neutralize each other so that no change in their status occurs. For example, a stationary object on the ground is continuously exposed to the force of gravity, the attraction of the earth, which acts in a vertical direction. The force of gravity produces a ground reaction in accordance with Newton's third law which states that *action and reaction are equal in magnitude but opposite in direction*. Newton's third law applies to all forces, including muscle forces. The reaction forces produced by muscles may not be obvious at first glance but are nevertheless present, contributing importantly to equilibrium and to motion.

FORCE

A simple way to define force is to say that it is a push or a pull. Forces produce or prevent motion or they have a tendency to do so.

In the human body internal forces are produced as a result of muscle contraction and by the internal arrangement of muscles, tendons, and other anatomical structures. In therapy, in exercise and in all activity there are the external forces of gravity and sometimes the manual or mechanical application of an outside force provided by the therapist or by the use of machines, instruments, straps, weights, pulleys or braces.

In order to express the force completely its magnitude and direction must be known. In addition the point of contact between the force and the body to which the force is applied is known. These characteristics, combined, show the line of action of the force.

A force is a vector quantity because it is a quantity which has magnitude and direction. This quantity may be represented graphically by a vector. A vector is a straight line, drawn to scale, with an arrow indicating its direction. A force vector is represented as a push or a pull upon the point where the force acts.

COMPOSITION OF FORCES

RESULTANT FORCE. Usually two or more forces act simultaneously on the same object. A resultant force is the simplest force (or simplest force system) which can produce the same effect as all the forces acting together.

FORCES ACTING IN A LINE. If two or more forces act along a line, the total effect of these forces is obtained by algebraic summation of the forces. For example, if forces A, B and C having a magnitude of 10 lbs., 8 lbs. and 5 lbs. repectively act in the same direction, the resultant force amounts to 23 lbs. (Fig. 5). But if force C pulls in the opposite direction of forces A and B, the resultant force is 13 lbs., the direction of the resultant being that of forces A and B.

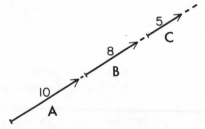

FIG. 5. Algebraic summation of vector forces along a common line of action (see text).

A vector force may be moved along its line of action without causing a change in its effect. For example, force A may exchange place with force C or force B may be moved to a different position along the line of action, but the result is unchanged.

Clinical Kinesiology

FORCES ACTING AT ANGLES. The effect of vector forces acting at an angle to each other cannot be obtained by algebraic summation. The resultant force is found by constructing the parallelogram of forces (Fig. 6). If forces F_1 and F_2 are drawn to scale the resultant R is found by measuring the diagonal of the parallelogram. If two forces, A and B, act at a 90 degree angle to each other, the resultant force may also be calculated by using the right triangle rule: $A^2 + B^2 = H^2$.

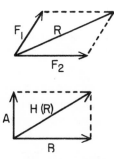

FIG. 6. Composition of forces by constructing parallelogram of forces.

RESOLUTION OF FORCES

The problem in resolution of forces is the converse of a problem in composition of forces. The diagonal of the parallelogram and the angles between the diagonal and each side are given. From this the lengths of the sides are constructed. *Resolution of forces means the separation of a single force into two forces acting in definite directions on the same point.*

Often the action line of muscle pull represents the resultant force and this resultant can be separated into its components. In Figure 7 muscle force M represents the tension produced by the contracting muscle (the brachialis muscle acting over the elbow, for example). Force M may be resolved into two components, f_1 and f_2, the former acting perpendicular to the bony lever, the latter acting in the long axis of the forearm bone. Component f_1 is the rotary component which causes the forearm to rotate about the elbow axis. Component f_2, called the stabilizing component, is ineffective as far as motion of the joint is concerned, but it serves the useful purpose of pressing the joint surfaces firmly together.

Mechanical Principles: Application to the Human Body   15

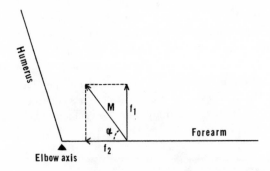

FIG. 7. Resolution of forces. Muscle force M is resolved into forces f_1 and f_2. Force f_1 is the rotary component. Force f_2 is the stabilizing component.

COMPUTATION OF COMPONENTS. The magnitude of these two components can be calculated providing the angle of approach of the muscle to the bone (a) and the contractile force of muscle force M is known. Recall that in a right triangle the sine a is the relationship between the side opposite the angle and the hypotenuse:

$$\text{sine } a = \frac{\text{opposite side}}{\text{hypotenuse}}$$

and that the cosine a is the relationship between the side adjacent to the angle and the hypotenuse:

$$\text{cosine } a = \frac{\text{adjacent side}}{\text{hypotenuse}}$$

The sides of the parallelogram are mutually parallel or perpendicular, thus rotary component f_1 is similar to the side opposite the angle a. Formulae for computing components are then:

$$\text{sine } a = \frac{f_1}{M} \quad \text{and cosine } a = \frac{f_2}{M}$$

CHANGING MAGNITUDE OF ROTARY COMPONENT DURING JOINT MOVEMENT. When joint movement takes place the magnitudes of the two components change continuously. For example, in the case of the brachialis muscle the angle of approach (a) of the muscle is quite small when the elbow is extended, hence the rotary component is also small. As the elbow flexes, the angle of approach becomes larger and the rotary component increases. It reaches its maximum when the angle of approach is 90 degree, that is, when the elbow is flexed to slightly more than a right angle. With further flexion, the magnitude of the rotary component again decreases. Mechanically, therefore, the 90 degree angle of approach of a muscle is the most effective one in producing joint movement.

PARALLEL FORCES AND TORQUE

TORQUE. To understand how parallel forces act to produce rotary motion about a fixed point requires an understanding of torque or moment of force. A parallel force system is one in which the forces act in the same or in opposite directions and they act in one plane.

A rigid bar (Fig. 8A) can pivot about point C.

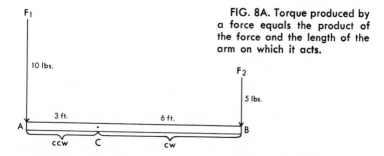

FIG. 8A. Torque produced by a force equals the product of the force and the length of the arm on which it acts.

FIG. 8B. Torque is the product of the force and the perpendicular distance from the point of rotation to the line of action of the force ($F_3 \times d$).

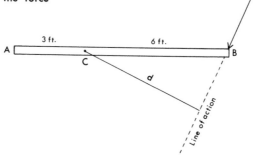

Force F_1 acts downward at the A end of the bar and tends to rotate it in a counterclockwise (ccw) direction. Force F_2, parallel to F_1, acts downward at the B end of the bar and tends to rotate it in a clockwise (cw) direction. The effectiveness with which these forces tend to rotate the bar in either direction depends on the magnitude of the force and the length of the arm on which it acts (CA×10 or CB×6). This tendency of the force to cause the bar to rotate about the pivot point is called torque or moment of force (sometimes referred to as just moment). *Torque is the product of the force times the length of the arm on which it acts.*

Forces may be expressed in pounds or kilograms or some unit thereof; the length of the arm on which the force acts is expressed in feet, centimeters or some unit of these measurements. Foot-pounds is an appropriate unit used to express the moment of force or torque. In Figure 8A the torque in the ccw direction is 30 foot-pounds and it is the same in the cw direction. Here the system is in equilibrium. The ccw torque equals the cw torque, or, expressed another way, the sum of the moments equals zero. Torque in either direction may be altered by changing either the magnitude of the force or the length of the arm on which the force is acting.

In Figure 8A forces act perpendicular to the arm. Should a force (F_3) be applied as illustrated in Figure 8B with a different action line and not perpendicular to the bar, the arm upon which the force acts is no longer CB. The length of the arm upon which the force acts is the perpendicular distance to the line of action of the force, or in Figure 8B it is distance *d*. This perpendicular distance to the line of action of a force is called the lever arm.

THE LEVER. A machine which operates on the principle of a rigid bar being acted upon by forces which tend to rotate the bar about its pivot point is called a lever. A force tends to rotate the bar in one direction. The perpendicular distance from the pivot point (or center of rotation) to the line of action of this force is called the force arm. An opposing force resists this turning effect. The perpendicular distance from the pivot point to the line of action of this resistance or weight is called the resistance arm or the weight arm.

Mechanical advantage (M.A.) of the lever refers to the relation between the length of the force arm and the length of the weight arm and is expressed in this equation:

$$\text{M.A.} = \frac{\text{Force arm}}{\text{Weight arm}} \text{ or } \frac{\text{Force arm}}{\text{Resistance arm}}$$

This equation shows that an increase in the length of the force arm or a decrease in the length of the weight arm (or resistance arm) results in greater mechanical advantage, that is, facilitates the task to be performed.

FIRST CLASS LEVER. This type of leverage is exemplified by the seesaw, where the fulcrum A is located between the weight W and the force F (Fig. 9-I). If the force arm is twice the length of the weight arm, the mechanical advantage of the force is 2. But if the force were applied where the weight is, and vice versa, the mechanical advantage of the force would be ½, and the weight would have the mechanical advantage of 2.

In the human body this type of leverage is found at the atlantooccipital joints, where the head is balanced on top of the spine. Another example is the common hip axis (a transverse line connecting the two femoral heads) which in erect standing serves as the fulcrum or axis of motion for anteroposterior movements of the trunk. In both examples, depending upon the position of the balancing segment, weight or muscle force may balance weight.

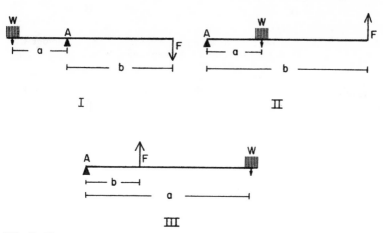

FIG. 9. Three classes of levers. A = axis of motion; W = weight; F = force; a = weight arm; b = force arm.

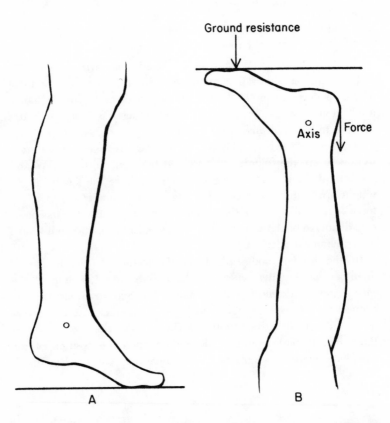

Ground resistance

Axis

Force

FIG. 10. First class leverage. A, Rising on tiptoes. B, Rising on tiptoes visualized in upside-down position.

Equilibration of body parts in the erect position is effected mainly by muscles lying close to the axis of motion, that is, having a short force arm. But since the weight also acts close to the axis of motion comparatively little force is required of the balancing muscles. It appears that these centrally located muscles are the ones responsible for finely graduated postural adjustments needed for the maintenance of the erect position. Gross joint movements which require more force are most efficiently carried out by muscles having longer force arms, that is, better mechanical advantage. In general, it may be stated that the centrally located, deeper muscles are concerned with postural adjustment while the more superficial muscles are utilized for gross movements.

Clinical Kinesiology

SECOND CLASS LEVER. The weight W (or resistance) lies between the fulcrum A and the force F (Fig. 9-II). In this type of leverage the force arm is always longer than the weight arm, and mechanical advantage for the force results. In the illustration, the force arm is three times as long as the weight arm, so that the mechanical advantage is 3. The wheelbarrow is an example of this type of leverage; a crowbar may also be used in this manner.

It is doubtful that second class leverage may be found in the human body. It has been stated, although incorrectly, that this arrangement exists in rising on tiptoes, the toe joints being the fulcrum and the calf muscles, exerting traction on the calcaneus, being the force. It is then assumed that a perpendicular plane through the center of gravity of the body falls between the fulcrum and the force. Although it is true that this body alignment exists *before* one starts rising on tiptoes (as long as the heels are on the ground), it is impossible to start the movement until the body weight has shifted over the ball of the foot, as anyone may demonstrate to himself. A closer examination of the situation indicates that the resistance to be overcome in rising on tiptoes is the floor reaction on the ball of the foot (Newton's third law: Action and reaction are equal in magnitude and opposite in direction). The type of leverage involved becomes clear if one visualizes the foot upside-down (Fig. 10). The ankle joint is the fulcrum of motion, the force (calf muscles) is applied to the calcaneus, and the weight to be overcome is applied to the ball of the foot. This is leverage of the first order.

THIRD CLASS LEVER. The force F is applied between the fulcrum A and the weight W (Fig. 9-III). In this type of leverage the weight arm is always longer than the force arm, so that the weight has mechanical advantage. This arrangement is unsuitable for overcoming heavy resistance but is designed for moving a small weight a long distance and for producing speed of a distal segment. The golf club and the fishing rod are examples.

In the human body this type of leverage is found at all joints of the upper and lower extremities: the deltoid over the shoulder joint, the brachialis over the elbow joint, and the anterior tibialis over the ankle joint.

LEVERS ARE BUILT EITHER FOR FORCE OR SPEED. Second class levers are built for force, since the force always has mechanical advantage; third class levers are built for speed; first class levers may be utilized either to gain force or speed, depending upon the relative lengths of the force arm and weight arm. All three types of levers demonstrate that *what is lost in force is gained in speed* (distance) and, conversely, *what is lost in speed* (distance) *is gained in force.*

COMPUTATION OF TORQUE. The products of muscle forces and the lengths of their lever arms produce torques which cause the bony segments to rotate about their relatively fixed axes at various joints. Moment of force about a joint as it is produced by a contracting muscle may be computed by two methods. In Figure 11 the counterclockwise torque is either the product of the distance (d_1) from the center of joint rotation to the line of action of the muscle force and the magnitude of that force (M) or it is calculated by multiplying the rotary component of the force (f_1) by the distance from the center of joint rotation to the line of action of the rotary component (d_2).

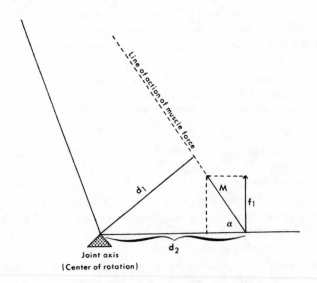

FIG. 11. Two methods of computing torque: $d_1 \times M$ or $d_2 \times f_1$.

If the two right triangles having the common angle (a) are studied it is apparent that:

$$\text{sine } a = \frac{d_1}{d_2}$$

and also

$$\text{sine } a = \frac{f_1}{M}$$

From this results the equation: $d_1 \times M = d_2 \times f_1$.

Total torque, then, may be expressed either by $d_1 \times M$ or $d_2 \times f_1$.

WEIGHT OF LEVER.   In the analysis of body movements the torque produced by the weight of the body part as it is acted upon by the external force of gravity must also be considered. This moment can be determined if the center of gravity of the part in question is known since the weight of a body segment may be concentrated at its center of gravity. Direction of the force of gravity is, of course, always vertical and torque is calculated in the usual manner. (For locations of centers of gravity of body segments and their approximate weights see Chapter 10.)

LINE OF ACTION OF MUSCLES OVER JOINTS.   A first step toward analysis of muscle action is best accomplished by identifying at any single joint all axes about which rotary movement occurs. Following this, the relationship of each muscle action line to each axis can be visualized and the movement capabilities of those muscles will be clarified. If a muscle crosses one joint which permits one degree of freedom of movement and if this muscle runs directly from origin to insertion (i.e., its direction is not changed by protruding bony processes or by other means) its action is comparatively simple to define. Complexity of analysis of muscle action increases where muscles possess widespread origin or insertion and where joints permit increased degrees of freedom of movement. Another important consideration is that lines of muscle action, and hence their relationships to joint axes, change as movements occur. Also muscle *groups,* not isolated individual muscles, act together upon various joints. In addition, total torque is not a result of biomechanical influences alone but rather it depends upon the interaction of mechanical and physiological factors (see Chapter 2).

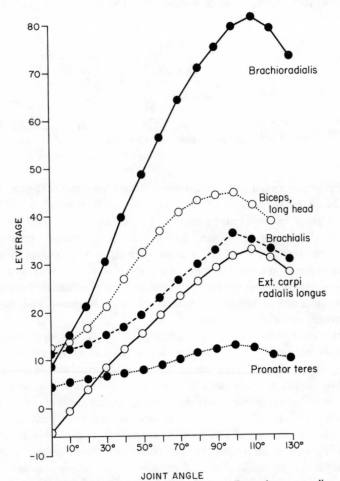

JOINT ANGLE

FIG. 12. Leverage curves of elbow flexors. Zero degrees—elbow extended. (Plotted from figures by Braune and Fischer, 1890, quoted by Fick, 1911, pp. 318-319.)

LEVERAGE CURVES OF ELBOW FLEXORS.   The influence of leverage on moments of force of the elbow flexors at various joint angles was investigated by Braune and Fischer (1890) and the results of this investigation, quoted by Fick (1911, pp. 318-319), is found in Table I in the Appendix. In this table, as in all Fick's tables for *moments of rotation* (Drehungsmomente), the tension of each muscle, regardless of size, is set at one, and the muscle tension is considered constant throughout the joint range. These tables, therefore, show the influence of leverage on torque, not torque itself. To obtain torque, (disregarding length-tension factors) the leverage values must be multiplied by the cross section of the muscle and by the absolute muscle strength of muscle tissue (see Chapter 2).

In Figure 12 the leverage curves for five elbow flexors, plotted from the figures in Table I, are shown. The leverage of each of the muscles in this figure is lowest when the elbow is extended, gradually rises to a maximum at 90 to 110 degrees of flexion, and falls as the joint angle becomes more acute. Note that the curve for the extensor carpi radialis longus has negative values during the first 10 degrees of flexion, indicating that in this joint range it courses on the extensor side of the joint. (These curves are further discussed on page 46.)

MOMENT OF FORCE APPLIED TO TRANSVERSE ROTATION OF BONES. The cross section of a long bone, such as the humerus or the femur, may be compared to a wheel which rotates about a fixed axis (Fig. 13). The moment of force caused by a muscle pulling in a tangential direction is obtained by multiplying the muscle force F by the radius r of the cross section.

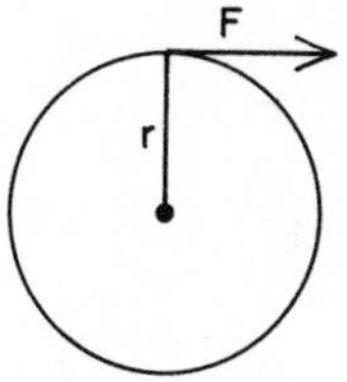

FIG. 13. Torque of wheel-like structure (transverse rotation of bony segments) F × r.

The comparison with the wheel, however, needs qualification. First, muscles seldom, if ever, pull in a strictly tangential direction so that the tangential component must be computed. Second, the circumference of the bone is never a perfect circle and the muscle often inserts into a protruding process. Third, the axis of motion for transverse rotation is not necessarily located at the center of the cross section of the bone. Transverse rotation of the femur, for example, takes place about the mechanical axis of the femur, which is a line connecting the centers of the hip and knee joints, and this axis lies essentially outside the shaft of the femur (see Fig. 111, p. 227).

DIRECTION OF PULL OF MUSCLE FIBERS ON TENDONS. When a muscle is composed of fibers which are arranged as seen in Figure 14A, the entire tension of each fiber is transferred to the tendon of the muscle. Some muscles have this fusiform shape, but more often the muscle fibers approach the tendon of insertion at an angle (Fig. 14B), in which case the effective tension (t) of the fiber is obtained by using the formula: $t = T \times \text{cosine } \alpha$ (T being the tension of the fiber, α being the angle of approach of the fiber to the tendon).

FIG. 14. A, Muscle fibers parallel to tendon. B, Fibers approach tendon at an angle.

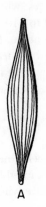

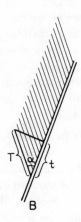

A

B

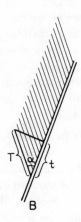

FIG. 15. A force couple. Torque produced by a force couple: F × d.

FORCE COUPLES. In mechanics, a force couple is defined as *two parallel forces, equal in magnitude but opposite in direction, acting on different points of the body a distance apart from each other* (O. Fischer, quoted by Fick, 1911, p. 328).

The action of a force couple is most easily recognized if one considers the forces needed to set a whirligig in motion (Fig. 15). It requires two forces to make the toy whirl around. A force in the direction of arrow a is produced by the right hand while a force in

Clinical Kinesiology

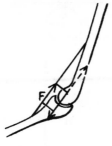

FIG. 16. Force couple acting to produce elbow flexion. Proximal segment stabilized. (Redrawn from Fick, 1910, p. 331.)

the direction of arrow b is produced simultaneously by the left hand, these two forces being parallel but acting a distance apart on different points of the object. The two forces must be equal in magnitude for if one is greater than the other, the whirligig will escape in the direction of the arrow representing the stronger force.

The torque produced by a force couple depends on two factors: the magnitude of the force, and the perpendicular distance between the two forces. The formula $F \times d$ may be used to calculate the torque, F representing one of the forces of the force couple, d being the distance between the two forces. The torque produced by each of the two forces may be computed separately by using d/2 as the lever arm. The sum of the torques produced by the two forces, both acting in a clockwise direction, gives the same result as when the formula $F \times d$ is used.

All rotations about joint axes require the action of a force couple. In elbow flexion, as an example, the force set up by the contraction of the elbow flexors may be represented by a proximally directed arrow F (Fig. 16). This force does not in itself initiate joint movement but produces a pressure at the joint center, represented by the dotted arrow, parallel to arrow F. The resulting counterpressure, equal in magnitude but opposite in direction (distally directed arrow), together with force F, makes up the force couple. The result in this case, when the proximal segment is stabilized, is a motion of the distal segment.

THE PULLEY

SINGLE FIXED PULLEY. The line of action of a force may be changed by means of a pulley (Fig. 17). A force F, acting in a *downward* direction, is utilized to move a weight in an *upward* direction. Such a single fixed pulley does not provide any mechanical advantage to the force, but only changes its direction.

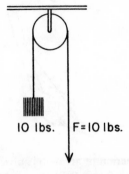

FIG. 17. Fixed pulley. Change of direction of force, but no mechanical advantage.

10 lbs. | F=10 lbs.

DEFLECTION OF TENDON. The tendon of a muscle may be deflected from its straight course by a bony prominence or by other means. Such a pulley arrangement in the human body, unlike the mechanical single pulley, may also provide mechanical advantage to the muscle by lifting the tendon away from the joint axis. The tendon of the quadriceps, for example, not only changes its direction of pull as a result of the interposed patella, but its leverage also improves.

Another type of pulley system involving the tendons of the long finger flexors is found on the flexor side of the finger joints. When the flexor digitorum profundus and superficialis contract, their tendons rise somewhat from the joint axes, excessive rising being prevented by a pulley-like loop. This loop simultaneously causes a deflection of the tendons (Fig. 18). The line of action of the tendon over the joint is represented by a straight line from loop to loop, or from loop to insertion.

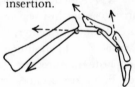

FIG. 18. Pulley-like arrangement, deflecting tendon of flexor digitorum profundus. (Redrawn from Gray's Anatomy.)

MOVABLE PULLEY. If a weight is attached to a movable pulley (Fig. 19), half of the weight is carried by the rope attached to the stationary hook, and half by the rope on the other side of the pulley. Therefore, the mechanical advantage of the force F is 2. What is gained in force, however, is lost in distance. The fixed pulley in the illustration serves only to change the direction of the force but gives no mechanical advantage. The movable pulley is not represented in the body but may be convenient to utilize for exercise equipment.

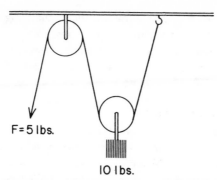

F = 5 lbs.

10 lbs.

FIG. 19. Movable pulley. Mechanical advantage for force.

WORK

UNITS OF WORK. Work is expressed in foot-pounds, kilogrammeters, etc. One foot-pound of work has been performed when one pound has been lifted a vertical distance of one foot.

FORMULA FOR WORK. The formula for work is as follows:

$$\text{Work} = \text{Force} \times \text{Distance}$$

If five pounds are lifted a vertical distance of six feet, the work performed equals 30 foot-pounds. The same amount of work is done if three pounds are lifted a distance of 10 feet.

When an object is raised vertically, the force required equals the weight of the object, but if an object is moved in a horizontal direction, as in sliding it across a horizontal surface, the force required is usually much less than the weight of the object. The amount of force required then depends upon how much friction is encountered. Thus it requires less force to slide an object across a smooth surface, such as a polished floor or ice, than over a rough one. In each case, however, the formula Work = Force × Distance applies.

MUSCLES MAY CONTRACT WITHOUT DOING WORK. If a force is exerted on an object which does not move, a great deal of chemical energy may be expended in maintaining muscle tension, but no physical work has been performed. For example, if one attempts to lift a weight which is too heavy to lift, or push an object which cannot be moved, energy is expended but no work is performed.

Muscles in the human body are often required to contract without doing work. For example, when a weight is held stationary in the hand, no work is performed, nor does the contraction of the muscles result in work if the weight is slowly lowered while the muscles resist to prevent the object from dropping to the floor suddenly. In the first instance, the muscles contract without changing their length and no work is performed; in the latter instance, the muscles are being stretched while resisting the stretching force, and it may be said that *work is being done on the muscles* or that *the muscles do negative work*. (See also page 44.)

WORK CAPACITY OF MUSCLES

The physiological cross section of a muscle is an indication of the muscle's functional capacity: the larger the cross section, the more tension can be produced. The cross section alone, however, does not tell how much work the muscle can produce. To determine the muscle's work capacity, the distance which the muscle can shorten as it functions in the human body must also be known. The product of the muscle's mean tension and its shortening distance gives its work capacity in accordance with the formula Work = Force × Distance.

Rudolph Fick computed the work capacity of individual muscles of the extremities, utilizing, in part, data obtained by previous investigators. (Fick's tables are in the appendix.) By comparing the work capacity of one muscle with that of another, an approximate idea of the relative importance of each muscle for a particular movement is obtained. For example, Fick's tables show that, as an internal rotator of the shoulder, the subscapularis has about five times as much work capacity as the teres major (Table VII); the pronator teres (with elbow at 90 degrees) has about four times as much work capacity in pronation as the pronator quadratus (Table V); and the work capacity of the anterior tibialis in dorsiflexion of the ankle is about eight times as great as its work capacity in inversion or eversion (Tables X and XI).

The work capacity figures given in the last column of each table must not be taken as absolute values, but should be used only for comparison. This is obvious for several reasons: first, individuals vary a great deal in their ability to produce muscular tension and to perform work; not only are there differences between sexes but also between individuals of the same sex. Second, Fick estimated that a muscle could produce a tension of 10 kg. per sq. cm. of physiological cross section (at a length halfway between maximum elongation and maximum shortening), but this figure of absolute muscle strength was proven too high by later investigators; hence the work capacities given in the tables are all too high. (See also page 35.)

POWER

If a pile of bricks is to be loaded on a truck, one individual may do the job in 10 minutes while another needs 15 minutes for the same task. It is obvious that the same amount of work has been done by each individual, but the time required differs. This introduces the term *power* which is defined as the *rate of doing work*. Power is computed by dividing the work performed by the time it takes to do it, or

$$\text{Power} = \frac{\text{Work}}{\text{Time}}$$

The unit of power is expressed in work units per time units, as foot-pounds per second, kilogram-meters per minute, gram-centimeters per second, etc. A common unit is that of *horse power*, one horse power being equal to 550 foot-pounds per second.

Muscles in the human body can produce *tension* and shorten a certain *distance*, and these factors determine their *work capacity*. The *power* of a muscle or muscle group depends upon the rate at which the muscles can do work. A *strong* individual is one who can produce great tension in his muscles, but he can be called *powerful* only if his rate of doing work is high.

CHAPTER 2

Some Aspects of
Muscle Physiology

MOTOR UNIT AND INTERNAL ORGANIZATION
OF MUSCLE

MOTOR UNIT

In the anterior horns of the gray matter of the spinal cord are located the large motor cells which constitute the link to the final pathway of motor response. Such a cell, together with its axon (nerve fiber) and all the muscle fibers which it innervates, is named the *motor unit.* When the threshold of excitation of a nerve cell has been reached, the cell "fires off" and impulses travel along its nerve fiber into its terminal branches causing a contraction of all the muscle fibers supplied by the cell.

Since control of the muscle is exercised through the motor unit, it is theoretically possible to activate a small portion of a muscle without activating the rest of it. In most instances this does not occur because it would not be advantageous for one portion to act alone. However, when a muscle consists of several distinct parts with differing actions, one portion of the muscle may contract without the other. The deltoid is an example of such a muscle: its anterior portion contracts when the arm is raised forward, and its posterior portion contracts when the arm is brought to the rear. Other examples are the upper and lower portions of the pectoralis major, and the upper and lower portions of the trapezius.

INNERVATION RATIOS

Most nerve fibers from motor cells divide profusely and, by means of their terminal branches, innervate numerous muscle fibers. The variation in innervation ratios (the number of nerve fibers to the number of muscle fibers) is extensive. Innervation ratios ranging from 1:100 to 1:2000 have been reported by Clark (1931) and by Feinstein and associates (1955). In some muscles, however, the number of muscle fibers supplied by one nerve cell is much smaller. The eye muscles are known to contain very small units; in the case of the extrinsic eye muscles of sheep, Tergast (1873), quoted by Clark (1931), found a ratio of 1:6 or 1:7.

It would be expected that muscles which are made up of small units would have a greater ability to exercise fine motor control than those consisting of large units. Generally, in muscles which are responsible for gross movements requiring strength, such as the gluteus maximus, the quadriceps, and the gastrocnemius, a large number of muscle fibers are supplied by one nerve fiber. In muscles used for finely coordinated motions, such as the intrinsic muscles of the hand, the innervation ratio is much smaller. In one investigation the innervation ratio of the medial head of the gastrocnemius was found to be 1:1934, while that of the first dorsal interossei muscle was 1:340 and that of the first lumbrical was 1:108 (Feinstein and associates, 1955).

Innervation ratios quoted by the various investigators are mean values. Within muscles with large units, such as the large muscles of the lower extremity, smaller units are also present. These smaller units may be those that are primarily activated when the muscles are called upon for fine adjustments, as in equilibration of body segments in the erect position (Clark, 1931).

FIBERS OF SKELETAL MUSCLE

A large number of muscle fibers go into the formation of a skeletal muscle. The first lumbrical muscle was found to consist of about 10,000 fibers and the first dorsal interosseus muscle consisted of about 40,000 fibers, while the calculated number of fibers of the medial head of the gastrocnemius was about 1,000,000 (Feinstein and associates, 1955).

Our muscles vary not only in size but also in shape, the shape being determined mainly by the space allotted to them. The adjustment to space is accomplished in different ways: by variation in length of the muscle fibers, differences in the angle of approach of the fibers to the tendon, by a rolling or twisting of the muscle, or the like.

PHYSIOLOGICAL CROSS SECTION OF A MUSCLE

The larger the physiological cross section of a muscle, the more tension it can produce. The physiological cross section of a fusiform muscle (all fibers running parallel to the tendon of the muscle) is tantamount to the anatomical cross section of the muscle, which is a section through the thickest portion of the muscle at a right angle to its fibers, the muscle being halfway between complete elongation and complete shortening within the body. The physiological cross section of a muscle with other types of fiber arrangement is obtained by one, two, or more sections at a right angle to the fibers, so that all fibers are included, these sections being added together.

Tables of physiological cross sections of various muscles, compiled by R. Fick, are found in the Appendix. Cross sections vary a great deal in individuals, so that the figures in the tables must not be taken as absolute values. They are useful, however, in *comparing* the cross section of one muscle or muscle group with another, as an indication of the relative strength of each muscle or muscle group.

ABSOLUTE MUSCLE STRENGTH. This term is employed to indicate the maximum tension a muscle is capable of producing per unit physiological cross section. Fick assumed the absolute muscle strength to be 10 kg. per sq. cm. cross section, while von Recklinghausen (1920) gives the figure 3.6 kg. per sq. cm. cross section. Haxton (1944) found the absolute muscle strength of the plantar flexors of the ankle to be 3.9 kg. per sq. cm. cross section. Ramsey and Street (1940) determined the maximum tension of isolated muscle fiber in the frog and found that it varied from 2490 to 4420 grams per sq. cm. cross section, the average being 3534 grams. Generally, 3 to 4 kg. per sq. cm. cross section is accepted as being reasonably correct.

LENGTH-TENSION RELATIONS OF MUSCLE

EXCURSION OF MUSCLE

The functional excursion of a muscle is that distance which the muscle is capable of shortening after it has been elongated as far as the joint or joints over which it passes allows. Weber (1851) determined the excursions of a large number of muscles of the upper and lower extremities and found that, in the muscles investigated, the range varied from 34 to 89 per cent, the mean value being about 50 per cent. The highest excursion requirements were for those muscles which pass more than one joint, such as the hamstrings. The relationship of 2:1 (maximum elongation:maximum shortening of a muscle *in situ*) was originally known as the "Weber law," later as the "Weber-Fick law."

From measurements on cadavers, Haines (1934) concluded that, in the living, straight fibered muscles were capable of shortening to about 57 per cent of their elongated lengths. This percentage also held true for *fibers* of pennate muscles. Exceptions to the rule were found among biarticular muscles, such as the long head of the biceps femoris, the semimembranosus, the rectus femoris, and the gastrocnemius, these muscles being referred to as "muscles of short action."

In most movement combinations, the excursion of a muscle suffices to move the joint full range. But a muscle which passes over two or more joints, if called upon to shorten over all joints simultaneously, may reach a point of shortening at which it can produce no useful tension. It becomes *actively insufficient* and is then unable to complete the range. If the muscles on the opposite side of the joint are also of the pluriarticular type, these muscles become elongated over two or more joints simultaneously and may reach the state of *passive insufficiency,* that is, not allow further elongation. Such restriction by antagonistic muscles is often a contributing factor to incomplete joint range. For example, if in the standing position one foot is lifted off the floor and the knee is flexed *while the hip is held fully extended,* complete range of knee flexion is difficult or becomes impossible; but if the hip is allowed to flex while the knee flexes, complete range of flexion of the knee is obtained without difficulty. In the first case, the hamstring muscles, which pass on the extensor side of the hip joint and the flexor side of the knee joint, are required to shorten over both joints, and the rectus femoris is being elongated simultaneously over both joints. In the latter case, the hamstring muscles are elongated over the hip joint while flexing the knee so that extreme excursion is avoided and no restriction is afforded by the rectus femoris.

Another example of the same principle is seen if a subject attempts to make a firm fist while maintaining the wrist flexed. Under these conditions, the average individual is unable to close the fingers completely or does so with a very weak grip. When the wrist is extended however, the grip becomes firm. This illustrates the principle that a muscle must have a certain amount of elongation in order to produce satisfactory tension.

ISOMETRIC CONTRACTION

When a muscle contracts without being allowed to shorten or lengthen, such contraction is said to be *isometric* (Gr. *isos,* equal, and *metron,* measure). For example, the subject is asked to flex the elbow but the examiner resists the subject's effort and the movement is prevented.

LENGTH-TENSION DIAGRAM (Blix's curve)

If a muscle is detached from its insertion and made to contract isometrically at different lengths, information on the muscle's ability to produce tension at various points of its excursion can be obtained. By plotting the tension produced against the length of the muscle, the so-called *length-tension diagram* is constructed. Blix, a Swedish physiologist, was one of the first scientists to carry out an extensive investigation of length-tension relations of muscle (1892-1895). The length-tension diagram, therefore, is often referred to as Blix's curve. Blix's experiments were undertaken on isolated frog muscle, and tetanic contractions at different lengths were induced by electrical stimulation. Ramsey and Street (1940) further elucidated the principles governing length-tension relations by investigations on isolated fibers of frog muscle. Length-tension studies have also been undertaken on human muscle in arm amputees with cineplastic tunnels,* which offer a unique opportunity for investigations of this kind (Bethe, 1916; Schlesinger, 1920; Inman and Ralston, 1968).

"RESTING LENGTH" OR "NATURAL LENGTH" OF A MUSCLE. When a muscle or muscle fiber is unstimulated and no external forces are acting on it, the muscle or muscle fiber is said to be at resting length (R.L.). At this length no tension is registered in the muscle, and this is the length to which the muscle tends to return when stimulation ceases, provided no external forces act upon it. The resting length of a muscle which has been detached from its insertion is comparatively easy to determine, while that of a muscle attached to skeletal parts can be determined less accurately.

PASSIVE TENSION CURVE. If, starting from resting length, an unstimulated muscle fiber is slowly elongated by an outside force, tension

*Cineplasty (G. *kineo,* I move, and *plasticos,* forming), a surgical procedure in arm amputees to construct a tunnel transversely through a muscle belly into which an ivory or stainless steel pin is inserted. With the pin "harnessed," the contraction of the muscle can activate the terminal device (artificial hand, or hook).

Some Aspects of Muscle Physiology

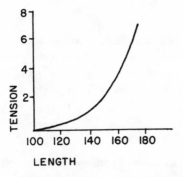

FIG. 20. Passive tension curve of unstimulated muscle fiber. Length in per cent of resting length. Tension in arbitrary units. (Redrawn from Ramsey and Street. 1940.)

is produced in the fiber and rises first very slowly, then more rapidly (Fig. 20). Since the fiber is not stimulated, that is, the contractile elements are inactive, this is a passive tension for which the sarcolemma, not the internal muscle material, is responsible (Ramsey and Street, 1940). This curve is known as the passive tension curve or the passive stretch curve.

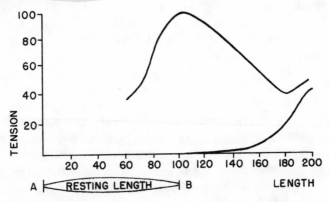

FIG. 21. Length-tension diagram for isometrically stimulated muscle fiber, including fully elongated state of fiber. Length in per cent of resting length. Tension in arbitrary units. (Redrawn from Ramsey and Street, 1940.) Muscle fiber A-B at resting length has been drawn in.

LENGTH-TENSION DIAGRAMS FOR STIMULATED MUSCLE FIBER. These are seen in Figures 21 and 22. The muscle fibers used in this study were obtained from the semitendinosus muscle of frogs. The fiber was first stimulated at resting length and the tension recorded. It was then slowly elongated by small increments and tetanized at each new length until it had been elongated to about 160 per cent

Clinical Kinesiology

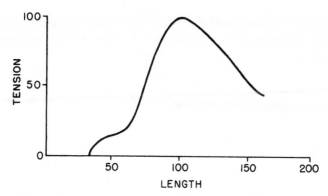

FIG. 22. Length-tension diagram for isometrically stimulated muscle fiber, including extreme shortened state of fiber. (Redrawn from Ramsey and Street, 1940.)

resting length. The same procedure was then repeated at lengths less than resting length. The fiber at these lengths (prior to stimulation) was not taut but hung in a loop which had to be taken up before the fiber could produce tension. In the experiment illustrated in Figure 21, the amount of shortening was not allowed to exceed one-third of resting length, because if carried further the fiber would become damaged and its characteristics would be permanently changed. The tension beyond 160 per cent resting length was then investigated and the curve plotted to the tearing point of the fiber, which in this case occurred at about 200 per cent resting length.

The diagram in Figure 22 shows the result of the investigation of isometric contractions of a fiber at lengths shorter than 66 per cent resting length. The experiment was carried to the point where the fiber, in spite of very strong stimulation, could not produce any tension. This occurred well below 50 per cent resting length.

In the living subject, the joints do not permit extreme shortening or lengthening of a muscle so that the muscle operates within a relatively small portion of the curve and well within safety limits.

The physiologically utilized portion of the length-tension curve has been determined for the gastrocnemius muscle of the frog (Beck, 1921). This portion proved to be from resting length to a few millimeters beyond resting length, a range which corresponds to the ascending portion of the top of the curve in Figures 21 and 22. It should be noted that most investigators have found that maximum isometric tension is obtained when the muscle is elongated slightly beyond its resting length as defined earlier. However, the resting length of a muscle has also been defined as that length at which the muscle can produce maximum tension (Ramsey and Street, 1940). This discrepancy in definition explains why in Figures 21 and 22 the peak of the curve is at 100 per cent resting length.

CONTRACTILE TENSION CURVE. In the diagram shown in Figure 21, the relation of the passive tension curve to the total tension curve is seen. If one were to construct a curve representing the tension produced by the contractile elements of the muscle alone, the left side of the curve would remain unchanged, but beyond resting length the values for passive tension would have to be subtracted from the values for total tension. This curve would therefore fall more rapidly than the total tension curve and would approach zero at the extreme right representing maximum elongation of the muscle.

APPLICATION OF LENGTH-TENSION DIAGRAM TO JOINT MOTION

As previously stated, under normal conditions only the highest, most effective portion of the curve is utilized for producing movement. When a muscle passes only one joint, the excursion of the muscle is limited to the range permitted by the joint. Within this range, the muscle has more physiological advantage when it is elongated than when it is shortened. For optimum effect, therefore, the muscle should be elongated before it is made to contract. This rule is particularly important to remember in the choice of training procedures for weak muscles. A weak muscle may be unable to produce tension in its short range while it may respond if it is somewhat elongated. There need be no fear of damaging a weak one-joint muscle by elongating it, since the joint permits only a moderate amount of stretch to the muscle.

In natural activities elongation of a muscle occurs almost without exception when a sudden burst of tension of the muscle is needed. Athletic activities provide ample examples of such elongation prior to shortening: the swing of a golf club or tennis racket, the crouch before the start of a dash, the forward reach of the oarsman. etc. Nature utilizes the beneficial effect of stretch of a muscle to save energy in many daily activities. In walking, for example, the hip flexors are elongated just before the start of the forward swing of the limb, so that only a small amount of effort is needed to start the movement.

Muscles passing more than one joint have potential excursions far beyond the range allowed for one-joint muscles. This, under certain circumstances, may be an advantage, but may also expose the muscle to undue stretch beyond safe limits.

TENDON ACTION OF MUSCLE

Passive tension without accompanying muscular contraction may produce movements of joints if a muscle is elongated over two or more joints simultaneously, and this is referred to as *tendon action* of a muscle. For example, if the wrist is allowed to flex by the weight of the hand, the digits will automatically extend without contraction of the finger extensors. By reversing the wrist movement, the fingers will partially flex. The first mentioned tendon action may be used to advantage by an individual who has lost his ability to extend the fingers while retaining control of finger flexion. Such an individual can hold an object in the hand, and release of grip is accomplished by letting the wrist drop. The second movement, wrist extension causing finger flexion, may enable an individual to keep a light object of proper size in the hand, even with little or no strength left in the finger flexors.

DAMAGE OF TWO-JOINT MUSCLES BY PASSIVE STRETCH

The hamstring muscles, if weakened by paralysis, might become damaged if forcibly stretched over hip and knee simultaneously. This might occur in complete trunk flexion forward in sitting on the floor with the knees extended, or supine if hip flexion were forced while the knees were kept extended.

When normal nonparalytic hamstrings are stretched beyond a certain point they offer resistance to the movement. Discomfort or pain accompanies such stretching so that it is not likely that an individual will permit stretching to the point of damage. Weakened or paralyzed muscles, however, must be handled with care and overstretching avoided.

FUNCTIONAL ADVANTAGE OF MUSCLES PASSING TWO OR MORE JOINTS

When muscles, such as the hamstrings, are utilized for movements, they are mostly activated in movement combinations which call for elongation of the muscle over one joint while joint movement is produced at the other joint. Under these circumstances,

---

Some Aspects of Muscle Physiology   **41**

two-joint muscles are more efficient than one-joint muscles because they retain a favorable length through a larger range and their rate of shortening is less than that of one-joint muscles.

ISOTONIC CONTRACTION

The word *isotonic* is derived from the Greek *isos,* equal, and *tonus,* tension. During isotonic contraction, therefore, the muscle maintains constant tension. In the laboratory when the muscle is detached from its insertion, isotonic contraction may be investigated, but such contraction seldom, if ever, occurs under conditions of ordinary activity.

The term, isotonic contraction, has been employed, although incorrectly, when a movement is performed against a resistance of constant magnitude, as in flexing the elbow while holding a weight in the hand. Even though the weight remains the same throughout the movement, the tension requirements of the muscle change continuously with changing leverage. Furthermore, the rotary force exerted by the weight also changes with changing joint angles. It is, therefore, inaccurate to speak about true isotonic contraction in dealing with joint movement. The term should be avoided and other expressions, such as *shortening contraction* and *lengthening contraction,* should be employed. The former term indicates that the origin and the insertion of the muscle are moving in the direction toward each other as the muscle contracts, the latter that the muscle becomes longer while contracting as it resists a stretching force.

INFLUENCE OF SPEED OF CONTRACTION ON TENSION

The speed of contraction, or rate of shortening, substantially influences the tension which a muscle can produce. The relationship between the maximum force developed by the muscle and the velocity of shortening is seen in Figure 23 where velocity is plotted against force. When the muscle contracts isometrically (velocity zero) it develops a certain tension P_0. As the velocity of shortening increases ($+V_1, +V_2$), the tension (P_1, P_2) developed by the muscle decreases (solid line). When the muscle is being stretched while resisting the stretching force, tension first rises with increasing velocity of stretch, then levels off (dotted line). The rules governing velocity of shortening (or lengthening) and maximum tension produced by a muscle or muscle fiber may be stated as follows:

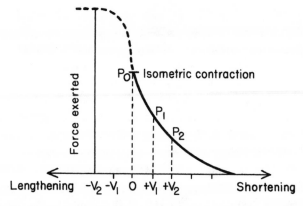

FIG. 23. Force-velocity curve of human muscle. Solid line: data obtained from human subjects (elbow flexion). Dotted line: constructed by extrapolating curve backwards. (Redrawn from Wilkie, 1950, and from Abbott and associates, 1952.)

1. Isometric contractions have higher tension values than shortening contractions.
2. As velocity of shortening increases, tension decreases.
3. During a lengthening contraction more tension can be produced than during isometric or shortening contractions.
4. Up to a certain point, as velocity of stretch of the muscle increases, the tension rises.

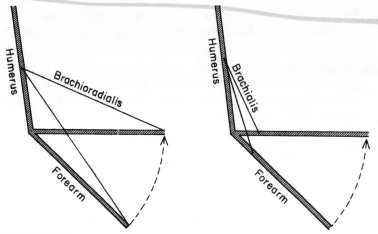

FIG. 24. Illustrating rate of shortening of brachioradialis as compared to brachialis in flexion of the elbow. For brachioradialis, high velocity of shortening; for brachialis, low velocity of shortening.

Some Aspects of Muscle Physiology

It is thus seen that for producing tension it is favorable for a muscle to be passively stretched or to shorten at a low velocity. When a joint movement takes place due to muscle shortening, such as when the elbow is flexed in the upright position, a number of muscles participate, but these muscles have to shorten with different velocities in accordance with their anatomical position. Owing to their insertions relatively close to the axis of the elbow joint, the biceps and the brachialis shorten only a small distance to produce a large displacement of the hand, while the brachioradialis which inserts more distally has to shorten a longer distance to produce an equal joint motion (Figure 24). The rate of shortening of the brachioradialis, therefore, is higher than that of the other two elbow flexors. Although the brachioradialis possesses a mechanical advantage far beyond that of the biceps and the brachialis, the effect of such excellent leverage is considerably lessened by its high rate of shortening.

Similar conditions exist at the hip. The sartorius, which has the best leverage of the hip flexors, requires a high rate of shortening, while the iliopsoas, having less good leverage, can move through an identical joint range with lesser rate of shortening.

POSITIVE AND NEGATIVE WORK

If a weight is lifted, the muscles do *positive work* in accordance with the formula: Work = Force × Distance. But if the weight is lowered while the muscles contract to slow down the motion, *no work* is being done by the muscles. In the latter instance, the muscles are being stretched while resisting the stretching force (gravity), and it may be said that *work is being done on the muscles* or that the *muscles do negative work.*

It is common experience that positive work is more demanding than negative work. For example, it is more fatiguing to walk uphill than downhill, a fact which becomes even more apparent if a burden is carried.

Since chemical energy is expended whenever a muscle contracts, oxygen is consumed both during positive and negative work. The cost of negative as compared to positive work was investigated by Abbott and associates (1952) who measured the oxygen consumption of two cyclists on bicycle ergometers placed back to back and coupled by a chain. One cyclist was doing positive work (pedaling forward) while the other one was resisting the movement with the same force. The experiment was set up in such a fashion that the two subjects employed approximately the same muscles although their muscles were utilized in different ways: the muscles of the forward pedaling subject shortened while those of the other subject were being stretched.

The data obtained from this investigation show that positive work is far more costly in terms of oxygen consumption than the same amount of negative work, and that the faster the speed, the greater the difference. For speeds of 25 revs./min. the forward pedaling cyclist used 2.4 times as much oxygen as the resisting cyclist. The ratio rose to 3.7 at a speed of 35.4 revs./min. and to 5.2 at a speed of 52 revs./min.

It has long been known that when a muscle maximally resists a stretching force (the so-called *brake test*), it can produce a force which is greater than the isometric value (Bethe, 1925). To produce an equal force, less effort is needed for the brake test than for an isometric contraction, and it may be assumed that fewer muscle fibers are activated and/or less frequency of discharge of the fibers occurs when the muscle resists a stretching force than when it contracts isometrically. Abbott and associates (1952) conclude that, at least in part, this is the explanation for the difference in oxygen consumption during positive and negative work.

The principle of the brake test may be employed clinically in the training of weak muscles. A patient may be capable of resisting a passive stretch of the muscle but be unable to produce an isometric or shortening contraction of the same muscle. The success that the patient experiences in resisting the movement encourages him to further effort, while an attempt at using a shortening contraction which does not result in movement is most discouraging.

The economy of muscle activity under conditions of resistance to stretch is frequently utilized in daily activities. Walking is a good example. Most of the muscles called upon to act in walking are activated while they are being elongated: the dorsiflexors of the ankle, following heel contact; the quadriceps, as the body weight tends to flex the knee in early stance; and the hamstrings, as they decelerate hip flexion and the forward swing of the leg prior to heel contact.

INTERACTION OF MECHANICAL AND PHYSIOLOGICAL FACTORS DURING JOINT MOVEMENT

At each position of a joint, the result of maximal isometric muscle contraction in terms of torque depends in part upon mechanical conditions (the leverage of the muscle at that particular joint angle), and in part upon the relative length of the muscle in accordance with the length-tension diagram. During joint movement, furthermore, the *speed of contraction* must be taken into consideration, since the tension which a muscle can develop decreases with increasing rate of shortening of the muscle.

LEVERAGE CURVES

The leverage factor for the elbow flexors at various joint angles is seen in Figure 12. The curves are plotted from figures given by Braune and Fischer (1890) as quoted by R. Fick (see Table I). These curves show that all elbow flexors have extremely poor leverage at the beginning of flexion, and that the leverage increases rapidly to reach a peak at 100 to 110 degrees of flexion from which point it again falls as the elbow angle becomes more acute.

The leverage curves of the biceps and the brachialis are very similar in shape, both reaching their peaks at 100 degrees of flexion. Throughout the joint range, the curve for the biceps is higher than that of the brachialis, that is, the tendon of the biceps lies further away from the joint axis than that of the brachialis. The pronator teres is characterized by a very low curve, indicating that it courses quite close to the axis of motion and that, consequently, its importance as an elbow flexor is negligible, even though its cross section is considerable.

The steep rise and the high peak of the curve for the brachioradialis indicates that this muscle has by far the best leverage of all the elbow flexors. This can be observed easily in the living subject if resistance is given to elbow flexion at a joint angle of approximately 90 degrees. The muscle belly of the brachioradialis is then plainly visible as it rises from the underlying structures, and its long distance from the joint axis may well be appreciated. It would be erroneous, however, to conclude that, because of its excellent leverage, the brachioradialis is the most effective of the elbow flexors. It must be kept in mind, first, that the brachioradialis has a comparatively small cross section (which furthermore is quite variable in individuals) and, second, that during joint motion its rate of short-ening is much higher than that of the biceps and the brachialis, owing to its insertion on the distal end of the radius (compare Fig. 24). These two factors both have an unfavorable influence on the effectiveness of the brachioradialis as an elbow flexor.

The leverage curve for the extensor carpi radialis longus as an elbow flexor is included in Figure 12. During the first ten degrees of elbow flexion, the curve has negative values, that is, in this range the muscle lies on the extensor side of the elbow joint. The curve then rises rapidly so that its leverage soon becomes comparable to that of the brachialis. However, the extensor carpi radialis longus does not, under all circumstances, contribute to elbow flexion. It is primarily a wrist extensor and, unless it acts simultaneously in this capacity, it may not be called upon to act in elbow flexion. But, when a firm fist is made, the extensor carpi radialis longus springs into action to stabilize the wrist in extension and it will then also have effect on elbow flexion.

TORQUE CURVES

If the maximal torque, which a muscle or muscle group can pro-duce by isometric contraction at various positions of the joint, is plotted against the joint angle, one has a *torque curve.* Torque curves may be constructed either from data obtained from the ca-daver (anatomical-mathematical method), or by direct measure-ment of torque in the living subject. Each of these methods has advantages and disadvantages, which will be discussed below.

ANATOMICAL-MATHEMATICAL METHOD. The maximal force which a muscle can produce is computed from its cross section and the absolute muscle strength, and it is assumed that the muscle force is constant throughout the range. The force arm of the muscle (the perpendicular distance from the axis of motion to the line of action of the muscle) is measured at consecutive positions of the joint. The torque is then computed, using the formula: Torque = Force × Force arm. This method has one advantage: the torque produced by *individual* muscles can be determined so that the relative im-portance of the various muscles acting over a joint may be appre-ciated. But since length-tension relations of muscle are not taken into consideration and other variables exist which data from a cadaver cannot yield, these curves cannot without reservation be applied to the living subject.

Torque curves for each of the elbow flexors whose leverage curves are seen in Figure 12 may be constructed by multiplying the leverage value at each joint angle with the cross section of the muscle in question. These torque curves would of course present shapes and heights very different from those of the leverage curves, as the reader may ascertain by undertaking to plot them.

TORQUE CURVES FROM DETERMINATIONS ON THE LIVING. The maximal torque which a muscle group can produce over a joint may be determined directly by having a subject make a maximal effort against a stationary resistance, the resistance being applied at a 90-degree angle to the bony lever at all positions of the joint. The magnitude of the resistance is read on a dynamometer or tensiometer and the joint angle on a goniometer. This method was employed by Bethe and Franke (1919) and more recently by Williams and Stutzman (1959). Torque curves obtained in this manner have more meaning than those plotted by the anatomical-mathematical method, since they show the actual torque produced rather than a theoretical one derived from calculations. However, no information can be obtained concerning the part played by individual muscles.

Torque curves constructed by Bethe and Franke are reproduced in Figures 25 to 28. These curves show that the relative importance of the two determining factors, the mechanical and the physiological, varies from joint to joint. In flexion of the elbow, for example, the mechanical influence predominates so that maximal torque obtains at an elbow angle of about 90 degrees in spite of the fact that the elbow flexors at this angle are relatively short. The benefit derived from elongation of the elbow flexors when the elbow is extended or nearing extension does not outweigh the effect of the poor mechanical conditions then existing, hence flexor torque is much less in the extended position of the joint.

At many joints the physiological factor predominates and maximal torque is obtained when the muscle group being tested is elongated. Pronation and supination of the forearm, for instance, follow this rule so that maximal pronator torque is obtained when the forearm is fully supinated, and, conversely, maximal supinator torque is obtained when the forearm is fully pronated (Fig. 26). This rule applies also to flexion and extension of the shoulder (Fig. 27).

Since the physiological influence appears to predominate in most of the torque curves investigated, it may be stated that a typical torque curve shows maximal torque at a position of the joint where

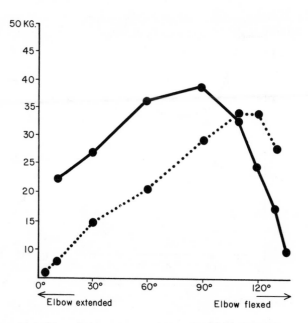

FIG. 25. Torque curves for flexion and extension of right elbow, derived from determinations on four male subjects. Solid curve: elbow flexion. Dotted curve: elbow extension. (Redrawn from Bethe and Franke, 1919.)

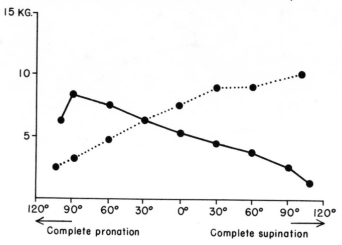

FIG. 26. Torque curves for pronation and supination of right forearm, derived from determinations on four male subjects. Elbow at 90 degrees of flexion. Solid curve: supination. Dotted curve: pronation. Zero position: thumb upward. (Redrawn from Bethe and Franke, 1919.)

Some Aspects of Muscle Physiology

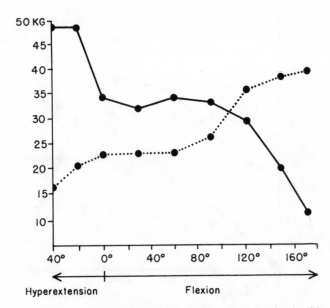

FIG. 27. Torque curves for flexion and extension of right shoulder, derived from determinations on four male subjects. Solid curve: flexion. Dotted curve: extension. (Redrawn from Bethe and Franke, 1919.)

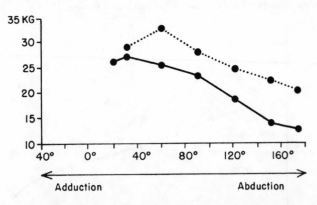

FIG. 28. Torque curve for abduction and adduction of right shoulder, derived from determinations on ten male subjects. Solid curve: abduction. Dotted curve: adduction. Zero position: arm at side of body. (Redrawn from Bethe and Franke, 1919.)

the muscles are elongated and that curves, such as produced by the elbow flexors, are exceptions.

The curves for the abductors and adductors of the shoulder (Fig.

Clinical Kinesiology

28) run almost parallel. Maximal abduction torque is registered when the arm is close to the body, that is, when the abductors are elongated, as would be expected. But the adductors show maximal torque when the shoulder is abducted only about 60 degrees, at which joint angle these muscles have already shortened considerably. Bethe and Franke suggest that the atypical shape of this curve is more apparent than real and that, if the curve were continued toward the left, it would fall rapidly and its shape would become more typical. Data for that portion of the curve, however, cannot be obtained since contact of the arm with the side of the body prevents further adduction. To these remarks by Bethe and Franke it may be added that the relatively low torque of the adductors when these muscles are elongated (arm over head) may be explained by the poor mechanical conditions at this joint range.

It is of interest to compare the shapes of the curves for two antagonistic muscle groups and to note at what angle the curves cross each other (Figs. 26 and 27). Such curves, even when "typical," are never the exact mirror images of each other, and the curves do not cross at the halfway mark of the joint range, as may be seen in the illustrations.

In comparing torque curves for the preferred and nonpreferred upper extremities, Bethe and Franke found a considerable difference not only in the height of the curves, but also in their shapes. Torque curves for women were found to be lower and less steep than for men, but, in general, the curves had similar shapes.

Later investigators (Williams and Stutzman, 1959; Williams and associates, 1965), in spite of differences in testing conditions and instrumentation, obtained results which compared favorably with those of Bethe and Franke. Some of the curves obtained by the two groups of investigators were strikingly alike, as for example the curves for shoulder flexors and extensors. Curves for pronation and supination of the forearm, as plotted by Bethe and Franke (1919), by Salter and Darcus (1952) and by Williams and associates (1965), were also very much alike. While Bethe and Franke were concerned with torque curves for the upper extremity only, Williams and Stutzman also plotted curves for joints of the lower extremity and demonstrated, among other things, the effect of positioning of the hip in flexion or extension when testing knee flexion. As would be expected from a consideration of length-tension relations, the curves for the knee flexors had lower values throughout the range when the hip was extended.

Classification of Muscles According to Their Interaction in Joint Movement

For the classification of muscles as they act in joint movement many different terms are found in professional literature, such as agonists, antagonists, assistant movers, true synergists, assistant synergists, fixators, neutralizers, and stabilizers. While some of these terms are descriptive, they are often used loosely and have come to have different meanings to different writers. Therefore, when encountering such terms in the literature, the reader must ascertain in what specific sense the terms are used. For the sake of simplicity, this author has chosen to use three terms only, namely, *agonist, antagonist* and *synergist.*

AGONIST AND ANTAGONIST

A muscle which is considered to be the principal one in producing a specific movement is referred to as an *agonist* (Gr. *agon,* contest) ; the *antagonist* (Gr. *anti,* against) acts on the joint in the opposite direction. For example, in extension of the elbow, the triceps is the agonist, the brachialis the antagonist; in flexion of the elbow, the brachialis is the agonist, the triceps the antagonist.

SYNERGIST

Generally speaking, a muscle may be called a *synergist* (Gr. *syn,* with, together, and *ergon,* work) whenever it contracts together with another muscle. In the sense that the term is used by this author, the action of a synergist may be identical, or nearly identical, with that of the agonist, as when the brachioradialis as a synergist aids the brachialis in flexing the elbow; or a synergist may act at a different joint, as when the wrist extensors act together (synergically) with the finger flexors in closing the fist.

In the chapters which follow, it will be pointed out repeatedly that two muscles may act as synergists in one movement and as antagonists in another movement—they do not have an absolute status with respect to each other. Thus the biceps and the triceps are antagonists with respect to flexion and extension of the elbow, but are synergists in an activity such as using a screwdriver.

CHAPTER 3

Elbow and Forearm

BONES

PALPABLE STRUCTURES

EPICONDYLES. The epicondyles are bony prominences on the distal enlargements (condyles) of the humerus and since they are readily identified they serve as landmarks in this region. When the shoulder is externally rotated, the *medial epicondyle* lies close to the body, the *lateral epicondyle* away from the body. But when the humerus is internally rotated, the medial epicondyle points to the rear, the lateral epicondyle to the front. The medial epicondyle is known as the *flexor epicondyle* because it serves as the origin of many flexor muscles of the wrist and digits. For similar reasons, the lateral epicondyle is referred to as the *extensor epicondyle.*

OLECRANON PROCESS. When the tip of the elbow is placed on the table with the forearm vertical, the prominent olecranon process of the ulna hits the table. This process is quite large and by following it distally, the *dorsal margin of the ulna* may be palpated all the way down to the *styloid process* of the ulna at the wrist. If the palpating fingers move medially from the olecranon process into the groove between it and the medial epicondyle, the ulnar nerve may be felt as a round cord. Friction across the nerve at this point or slightly more proximal produces a prickling sensation in the little finger; hence, the area where the ulnar nerve can be pressed against the bone is popularly known as the "funny bone."

HEAD OF RADIUS. The head of the radius is identified at a point just distal to the lateral epicondyle. When the elbow is fully extended, the circumference of the head of the radius may be felt rolling under the skin as pronation and supination are carried out. Once the head of the radius has been identified with the elbow extended, it should be easy to palpate it when the elbow is flexed and the forearm is either supinated or pronated. The location of the head of the radius with the forearm pronated is seen in Figures 32 and 37.

NONPALPABLE STRUCTURES

Bony structures which lie too deep to be palpated should be studied on the skeleton. Some of these are the *olecranon fossa*, the *trochlea* and the *capitulum of the humerus*, the *trochlear notch* and the *coronoid process of the ulna*, the *neck of the radius* and the *radial tuberosity*.

ELBOW JOINT (ARTICULATIO CUBITI)

TYPE OF JOINT

The elbow is a uniaxial joint of the hinge type (ginglymus) permitting flexion and extension by means of mixed gliding and rolling (one degree of freedom of motion). The trochlea of the humerus articulates with the trochlear notch of the ulna, while the capitulum of the humerus apposes the radius. The joint thus has ulnotrochlear and radiocapitular components which work in unison in flexion and extension.

AXIS OF MOTION

The axis for flexion and extension of the elbow is represented by a line through the centers of the trochlea and the capitulum (Fig. 29A). The approximate location of this axis in the living may be found by grasping the elbow from side to side slightly distal to the lateral and medial epicondyles of the humerus which are easily palpated through the skin.

CARRYING ANGLE

Since the trochlea extends more distally than the capitulum, the axis for flexion and extension of the elbow is not fully perpendicular to the shaft of the humerus; therefore, when the elbow is extended and the forearm supinated, the forearm deviates laterally in relation to the humerus, which accounts for the *carrying angle* or cubital angle (Fig. 29B). This angle varies somewhat in individuals, the angle usually being more pronounced in women than in men. Excessive lateral angulation of the forearm with respect to the humerus is known as *cubitus valgus*.

Clinical Kinesiology

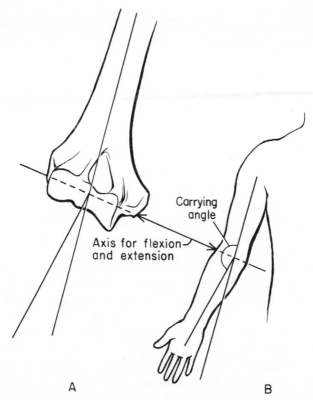

Carrying
angle

Axis for flexion
and extension

A   B

FIG. 29. A, Axis for flexion and extension of elbow courses through trochlea and capitulum. One degree of freedom of motion. B, Carrying angle of elbow when forearm is supinated.

It has been claimed that the carrying angle serves the purpose of keeping objects carried in the hand away from the body. However, the natural and common way of carrying an object in the hand is with the forearm pronated, or partly pronated, and in these positions when the radius lies across the ulna, the carrying angle is obliterated. Clearance is gained by abduction or internal rotation of the humerus at the shoulder or both or by lateral bending of the trunk.

RADIOULNAR ARTICULATION

TYPE OF JOINT

The connections between the radius and the ulna allow the radius to rotate in relation to the ulna so that in one position the two bones lie parallel (supination), and in another position the radius crosses over the ulna (pronation). The hand that is attached to the radius at the radiocarpal articulation follows the movement of the radius so that during supination the palm turns up, and during pronation the palm turns down. The movements of supination and pronation are made possible because there are two separate articulations between the radius and the ulna, one proximal, the other distal. The two joints acting together form a *uniaxial joint* (one degree of freedom) allowing pronation and supination only.

The elbow joint and the radioulnar joints thus both are uniaxial; in the elbow joint the axis of motion is nearly transverse to the shaft of the bones, while in the radioulnar articulation the axis of motion is almost parallel to the shafts of the participating bony segments.

AXIS OF MOTION

The axis of motion of the radioulnar articulation is represented by a line through the center of the head of the radius proximally and through the center of the head of the ulna distally (Fig. 30). In order to locate the direction of this line in the living subject, the forearm is held supinated and the circumference of the head of the radius is identified as previously described. The head of the ulna is then palpated near the wrist on the side of the little finger. The location of the center of the heads of the two bones must then be visualized and an imaginary line passing through these centers must be established.

PROXIMAL RADIOULNAR JOINT

The proximal radioulnar joint lies within the capsule of the elbow joint and may be described as a trochoid or pivot joint. The side of the head of the radius articulates with the radial notch of the ulna. The fibrous *annular ligament* forms a ring around the head of the radius. The annular ligament has firm fibrous connections with the ulna and is anchored to the neck of the radius by a broad ligament. The radial head thus rotates within a firm ring which permits transverse rotation while preventing movements in other directions.

DISTAL RADIOULNAR JOINT

The articular surface of the radius (ulnar notch) is concave so that the radius (with wrist and hand) can pivot around the head of the

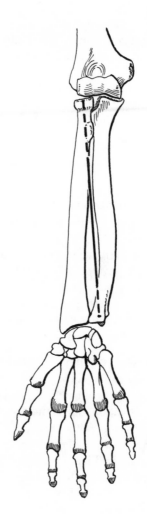

FIG. 30. Axis for pronation and supination of forearm courses through head of radius proximally and head of ulna distally. One degree of freedom of motion. (Redrawn from Grant: An Atlas of Anatomy.)

ulna while staying in close proximity to it. An articular disk is interposed between the head of the ulna and the adjacent carpal bones.

ISOLATION OF PRONATION AND SUPINATION
FROM SHOULDER ROTATION

When observing or testing range of pronation-supination, the elbow is held flexed and in contact with the side of the body. This prevents the shoulder from participating. The entire range of pronation, starting from the fully supinated position, is less than 180 degrees. In turning the palm up and down, slight movements at the

---

radiocarpal and intercarpal joints may also occur, particularly if the motion is performed passively, so that the range of motion as indicated by the palm is approximately 180 degrees.

If pronation and supination are carried out with the elbow extended, internal and external rotation of the shoulder occurs simultaneously, and in that case the palm can be turned through a much larger range.

GENERAL MUSCLE DISTRIBUTION IN ARM AND FOREARM

TWO MUSCLE GROUPS ABOVE THE ELBOW

By manipulating the soft tissue of the arm as seen in Figure 31, the biceps and the brachialis, flexors of the elbow, may be separated from the triceps, which muscle extends the elbow. Anatomically, these muscle groups are separated both medially and laterally by intermuscular septa of the fascia. The biceps, originating above the shoulder joint and inserting below the elbow joint, has no direct connection with the humerus and can, therefore, be moved about more easily than muscles which take their origin on the humerus.

THREE MUSCLE GROUPS IN FOREARM

GROUP ON RADIAL SIDE. The radial group of muscles is best manipulated when the elbow is flexed and the forearm is in midposition between pronation and supination. The group can then be partially separated from the other groups. The bulging shape of this group is seen in Figure 33 as the subject grasps around the adjacent dorsoulnar group. In Figure 32, a pencil has been placed between the radial and the dorsoulnar group. As may be judged from the illustrations (Figs. 32 and 33), when the elbow is flexed, the muscle mass of the radial group lies on the flexor side of the axis of the elbow joint.

The radial group consists of three muscles: brachioradialis, extensor carpi radialis longus and extensor carpi radialis brevis, all three originating from the region of the lateral epicondyle. They receive their innervation from the radial nerve and act in flexion of the elbow and (the latter two) in extension of the wrist. On the volar side of the forearm this group lies close to the antecubital fossa where the tendon of the biceps is palpated.

GROUP ON DORSOULNAR SIDE. This group comprises muscles located on the dorsum of the forearm which are concerned with ex-

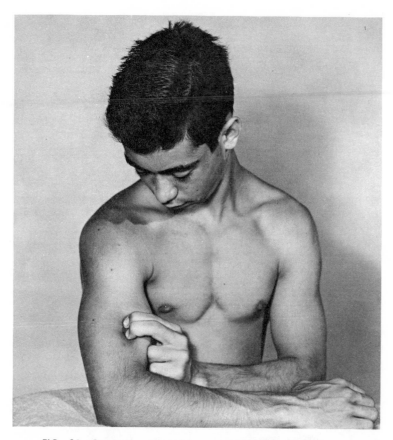

FIG. 31. Grasp to separate biceps and brachialis from triceps.

tension of wrist and digits and with supination of the forearm. They are innervated by the radial nerve. The subject in Figure 33 grasps around this group which on palpation feels rather flat and which adheres more firmly to underlying structures than do the other groups. The approximate boundary between this group and the radial group is seen in Figure 32. The dorsal margin of the ulna separates it from the next group. Some of the muscles of this area have a close relation to those of the radial group, being partly covered by them.

GROUP ON VOLAR-ULNAR SIDE. Muscles belonging to this group originate in the region of the medial (flexor) epicondyle of the humerus. Proximally, they are covered by the bicipital aponeurosis.

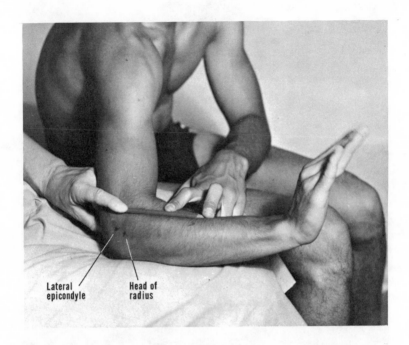

Lateral
epicondyle

Head of
radius

FIG. 32. Separating radial group of forearm (brachioradialis, extensor carpi radialis longus and extensor carpi radialis brevis) from the dorsoulnar group. Proximal cross-mark: lateral epicondyle. Distal cross-mark: head of radius.

Figure 34 illustrates how this group may be identified. The thumb is placed in the antecubital fossa and grasps around the pronator teres. The other digits are close to the dorsal margin of the ulna. Most of the muscles of this group are innervated by the median nerve and act in pronation of the forearm and in flexion of the wrist and digits.

MUSCLE DISTRIBUTION IN RELATION TO AXIS OF ELBOW JOINT

By grasping the elbow from side to side just distally to the epicondyles the approximate axis of motion is located and a general idea of the muscle distribution relative to the axis is obtained. A muscle which passes anterior to this axis is a flexor or potential flexor, and one which passes posteriorly is an extensor or potential extensor.

Clinical Kinesiology

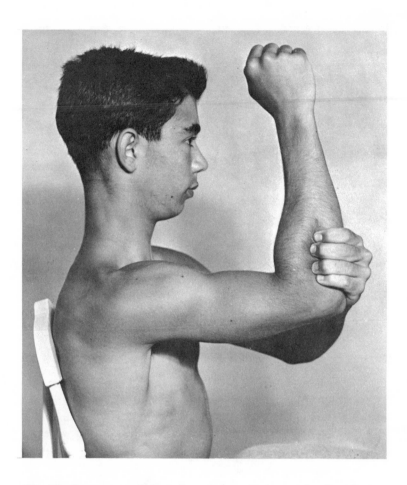

FIG. 33. Grasp around dorsoulnar group, simultaneously showing area of palpation for supinator. The radial group is being pushed aside.

MUSCLES PERFORMING FLEXION

The muscles which, according to Fick (1911, p. 320), pass anterior to the axis of the elbow joint when this joint is flexed to a right angle are: *brachialis, biceps, brachioradialis, pronator teres, extensor carpi radialis longus, extensor carpi radialis brevis, flexor carpi radialis* and *palmaris longus*. (See also Table II, Appendix.)

Which of the above muscles will be called upon to flex the elbow depends upon the particular movement combination desired. The first four muscles are the principal flexors of the elbow, while the

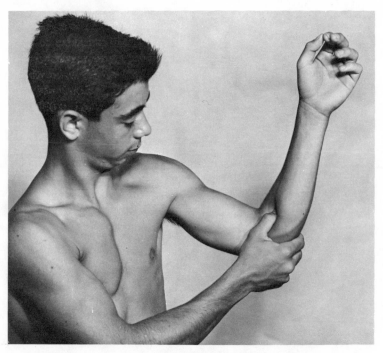

FIG. 34. Grasping around volar-ulnar (pronator) group.

last four exert their action mainly at the wrist; the latter are likely
to lie idle in elbow flexion unless wrist action is required simultaneously, as when an object grasped in the hand resists elbow flexion.

Briefly, the actions of the four principal elbow flexors are as follows:

Biceps brachii —Flexor of elbow, supinator of forearm (See
Chapter 5 for biceps action at the shoulder.)

Brachialis —Pure flexor of elbow

Brachioradialis —Flexor of elbow, has negligible action on
forearm

Pronator teres —Flexor of elbow, pronator of forearm

The elbow may be flexed with the forearm in pronation or supination, and in any desired position between pronation and supination. This is accomplished by activation of the various muscles in
proper proportions, taking advantage of the action of the biceps
as a supinator and the action of the pronator teres as a pronator.

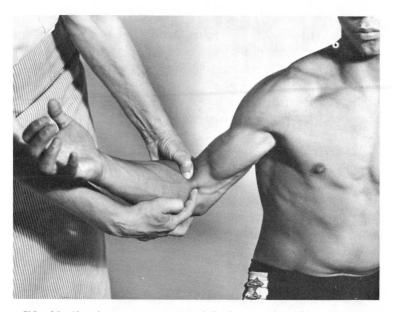

FIG. 35. The characteristic contour of the biceps is brought out by flexion of the elbow and supination of the forearm. The examiner grasps around tendon of biceps in the "fold" of the elbow.

BICEPS BRACHII. The muscular portion of the biceps is located above the elbow. *Origin:* By two heads from above the shoulder joint. The *long head* arises by a long tendon from the supraglenoid tubercle of the scapula. The tendon courses within the capsule of the shoulder joint and in the intertubercular groove of the humerus. The *short head* arises, also by a long tendon, from the coracoid process of the scapula. The two heads have separate bellies in the proximal portion of the arm, and these fuse to form one belly in the middle of the arm. The muscle fibers belonging to the short head make up the medial portion of the common belly while those of the long head make up the lateral portion. *Insertion:* Tuberosity of the radius and, in part, spreading out to form the bicipital aponeurosis (lacertus fibrosus). *Innervation:* Musculocutaneous nerve.

Inspection and palpation: The biceps brachii is one of the easiest muscles to identify, and to the layman, "making a muscle" means tightening the biceps. The contour of the biceps in a muscular individual is seen in many of the photographs in this book. A maximum shortening of the muscle is effected by simultaneous flexion of the elbow and supination of the forearm (Fig. 35). With this movement combination the muscular portion retracts considerably so that in the illustration the tendon appears to be quite long.

The tendon of the biceps is best identified in the "fold" of the elbow when the forearm is supinated. In a muscular subject the tendon is rather broad, as shown by the examiner's grasp. The examiner's thumb indicates the location of that part of the tendon which dips into the antecubital fossa on its way to the tuberosity of the radius. The examiner's index finger is seen palpating the bicipital aponeurosis which spreads out to cover the pronator teres and other muscles of this region.

The biceps and its tendon should next be palpated when the muscle is relaxed as when the forearm rests on the table or in the lap. It is then possible to grasp around the muscle, lift it from underlying structures and move it from side to side, a maneuver which is useful in separating it from the more deeply located brachialis muscle.

Finally, it should be observed that the biceps contracts strongly when a fist is made, as in sqeezing an object in the hand, and that this contraction is automatic and cannot be inhibited by the will. The strength of the contraction is in direct proportion to the firmness of the grip. Note that the triceps contracts simultaneously.

BRACHIALIS. This muscle takes its *origin* from halfway up the shaft of the humerus, and is *inserted* into the coronoid process of the ulna and adjacent areas of the ulna. *Innervation:* Musculocutaneous nerve.

Palpation: The muscular portion of the brachialis is located in the lower half of the arm, where it is largely covered by the biceps. The palpating fingers are placed laterally and medially to the biceps, an inch or two higher than the grasp seen in Figure 35. The subject's forearm should be pronated and resting in the lap or on a pillow, as seen in Figure 31, which secures relaxation of the biceps. If now the elbow is flexed with as little effort as possible, the contraction of the brachialis may be felt. Under the above conditions, the brachialis flexes the elbow with little or no participation by the biceps. Once the palpating fingers are properly placed, a quick flexion in small range may be performed, resulting in stronger contraction of the brachialis.

Clinical Kinesiology

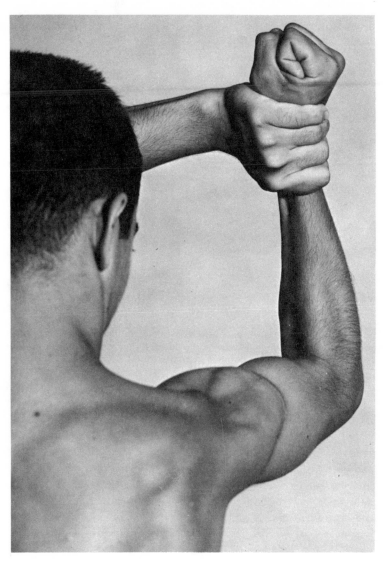

FIG. 36. Brachioradialis is brought out by resistance to flexion of the elbow with the forearm in midposition between pronation and supination.

BRACHIORADIALIS. The most prominent and the largest of the three muscles of the radial group of the forearm, the brachioradialis varies considerably in size in individuals. *Origin:* From a ridge on the hu-

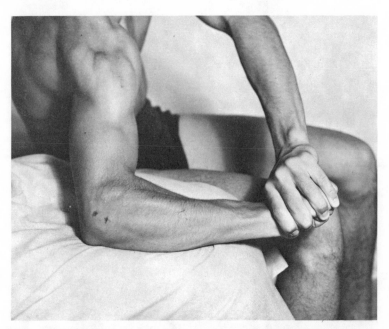

FIG. 37. Resistance to wrist extension brings out the wrist extensors and also the brachioradialis. Cross-marks identify lateral epicondyle of the humerus (proximal mark) and head of radius (distal mark).

merus above the lateral epicondyle. *Insertion:* Near the styloid process of the radius. *Innervation:* Radial nerve. Note that this muscle is a flexor of the elbow but as far as innervation is concerned it is associated with the extensors.

Inspection and palpation: The brachioradialis is best observed and palpated when resistance is given to flexion of the elbow while the elbow angle is about 90 degrees and the forearm is in midposition between pronation and supination (Fig. 36). Figure 37 shows the contour of this muscle and its relation to the extensor carpi radialis longus and brevis. The muscle is superficial and can readily be palpated along most of its course. Above the elbow it lies between the triceps and the brachialis. At and below the elbow it forms the lateral border of the antecubital fossa. Its muscular part may be followed halfway down the forearm, but its point of insertion is less readily palpated because its tendon of insertion is flat and partially covered by tendons of muscles passing over the wrist to the hand and because these tendons are held down by ligamentous structures which cross obliquely from the ulnar to the radial side of the wrist. When the muscle contracts, its upper portion rises from the underlying structures so that its perpendicular distance to the elbow joint increases, which enhances its function.

PRONATOR TERES. The bulk of this muscle is located below the elbow. It courses rather close to the axis of the elbow joint so that it has comparatively poor leverage for elbow flexion. *Origin:* Medial epicondyle of humerus and a smaller portion from the coronoid process of the ulna. The muscle fibers cross obliquely from medial to lateral on the volar aspect of the forearm. *Insertion:* Lateral side of the radius, about halfway down the forearm. *Innervation:* Median nerve.

Palpation: The muscle is superficial and may be palpated in the fold of the elbow and below. It forms the medial margin of the antecubital fossa and its fibers are easily identified in this region when the forearm is pronated while the elbow is flexed or semiflexed. Resistance to elbow flexion with the forearm pronated also makes for easy identification.

In Figure 34, the subject's thumb grasps around the edge of the pronator teres. If, from the position shown, the forearm is further pronated or resistance is given to pronation or flexion, the muscle hardens markedly.

The pronator teres lies close to the flexor carpi radialis and both these muscles are covered by the bicipital aponeurosis. More distally, as it crosses over toward the radial side, the pronator teres is covered by the brachioradialis, and if the pronator teres is to be palpated close to its insertion, the brachioradialis must be relaxed. This is accomplished by resting the forearm in the lap or on the table. The forearm is then pronated which activates the pronator while the brachioradialis remains essentially relaxed. The movement of pronation should be performed with little effort, or additional muscles in the region will become tense.

MUSCLES PERFORMING EXTENSION

The principal extensor of the elbow is the triceps brachii, with the small anconeus adding only insignificantly to the total strength of elbow extension.

TRICEPS BRACHII. This makes up the entire muscle mass on the posterior aspect of the arm. *Origin:* By three heads: the *long head,* the *medial head,* and the *lateral head.* The long head arises from

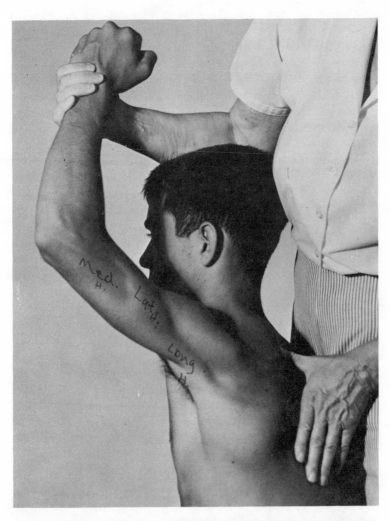

FIG. 38. Triceps brachii and other muscles brought out by examiner's resistance to extension of elbow. Long head of triceps is responsible for contour at lower margin of arm. Note its relation to teres major and latissimus near the axilla. Lateral head appears separated from the deltoid by a groove. The flat area between the lateral and the long heads identifies the broad common tendon of insertion.

the infraglenoid tubercle of the scapula by a broad tendon which has a close relation to the capsule of the shoulder joint. The medial head takes its origin distally on the humerus and has a fleshy origin.

       Clinical Kinesiology

The lateral head arises from the lateral aspect of the humerus, a short distance below the shoulder joint. *Insertion:* The three heads join a sturdy broad tendon which attaches to the olecranon process of the ulna and which also sends an expansion spreading out over the anconeus muscle into the dorsal fascia of the forearm. *Innervation:* Radial (musculospiral) nerve.

Inspection and palpation: The *long head* is identified in its proximal portion as it emerges from underneath the lowest fibers of the posterior deltoid (Figs. 38 and 39). It may be followed distally halfway down the arm. The muscular portion of the *lateral head,* which is the strongest of the three heads, is palpated distal to the posterior deltoid. It is well recognizable in Figure 38. The long head and the lateral head join the common tendon of insertion from opposite sides, much like the two heads of the gastrocnemius approach the Achilles' tendon. Note in the illustration the flat area between the lateral and the long heads. This is the broad superficial portion of the triceps tendon into which the two heads insert, partially from underneath and partially from the sides. The *medial head* is covered, in part, by the long head and is best palpated in its distal por-

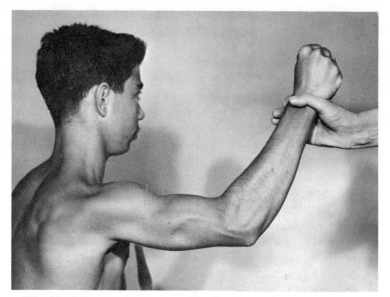

FIG. 39. Triceps cnd anconeus. Elbow extension is resisted. The short triangular-shaped anconeus lies close to the tip of the elbow and near the upper portion of extensor carpi ulnaris.

tion, near the medial epicondyle. For palpation of the medial head it is suggested that the dorsum of the wrist be placed on the edge of a table and pressure be applied in a downward direction, the table supplying resistance to elbow extension. The medial head may then be felt contracting.

ANCONEUS. This muscle *originates* from the region of the lateral epicondyle of the humerus and *inserts* into the ulna, partly into the olecranon process, partly below this process. *Innervation:* Radial nerve.

Palpation: If one finger tip is placed on the lateral epicondyle and one on the olecranon process, the muscular portion of the anconeus is palpated distally at a point which forms a triangle with the other two points. The anconeus may be identified in Figure 39, but should not be confused with the extensor carpi ulnaris which lies close to it. In the illustration, the two muscles appear almost as one, but by keeping in mind that the direction of the two muscles differs and that the anconeus lies more proximal and is very short, while the extensor carpi ulnaris runs down the forearm, each muscle may be identified.

MUSCLE DISTRIBUTION IN RELATION TO AXIS OF PRONATION-SUPINATION

MUSCLES PERFORMING SUPINATION

In general, muscles capable of supination originate from the lateral (extensor) epicondyle of the humerus and adjacent structures, and cross the axis of pronation-supination posterior to the interosseous membrane which unites the two bones of the forearm and which divides the forearm in posterior and anterior parts. The muscles are associated with the extensors of the wrist and the digits, in regard to anatomical position and innervation (radial nerve). The biceps brachii undertakes the task of supination in a different manner by exerting a pull on the tuberosity of the radius.

The muscles which, according to Fick (1911, pp. 348, 349), are in a position that enables them to supinate the forearm are the *biceps brachii, supinator, brachioradialis* (extremely short range), *abductor pollicis longus, extensor pollicis brevis* and *extensor indicis proprius.* (See also Table IV, Appendix.) The first two muscles are the most important supinators. The brachioradialis can be disregarded as a supinator (see p. 71). The last four are mechanically capable of aiding in supination but are primarily concerned with movements of the thumb and index finger and will be discussed in Chapter 4.

Origin, insertion and palpation of the biceps brachii have already been discussed.

SUPINATOR. The supinator is a deep muscle, located on the dorsal side of the interosseous membrane between the two bones of the forearm. It is covered by the anconeus, the extensor carpi radialis longus and the brachioradialis. *Origin:* Lateral epicondyle of humerus and adjacent areas of the ulna. It is a fairly short and rather flat muscle, triangular in shape, which winds around the proximal portion of the radius close to the bone to be *inserted* into the radius. *Innervation:* A branch of the radial nerve.

Palpation: The area where the supinator, although deeply located, may be palpated is shown in Figure 33. The fingertips are pushing the muscles of the radial group in a radial direction so that there will be no interference with palpation. The best position for palpation is perhaps to sit with the pronated forearm resting in the lap and to grasp the radial muscle group from the radial side, pulling it out of the way as much as it will permit. As the forearm is supinated through short range, the supinator may be felt under the palpating fingers.

MUSCLES PERFORMING PRONATION

All muscles capable of pronation are located in the forearm. In general, they arise from the region of the medial epicondyle of the humerus and/or adjacent areas of the ulna and cross the axis of pronation-supination on the anterior (palmar) side of the interosseous membrane. These muscles are closely related to the flexors of the wrist and digits in regard to both location and innervation (median nerve). One of the pronators, the pronator quadratus, is located more distally but, like the other pronators, crosses the axis of motion on the anterior side.

The muscles which, according to Fick (1911, p. 351), are capable of pronating the forearm when the elbow is flexed at 90 degrees are the *pronator teres, flexor carpi radialis, palmaris longus, brachioradialis* (range of pronation is short, but longer than that of supination), *extensor carpi radialis longus* and *pronator quadratus.* (See also Table V, Appendix.)

The pronator teres and pronator quadratus are the most important pronators. The brachioradialis may be disregarded as a pronator

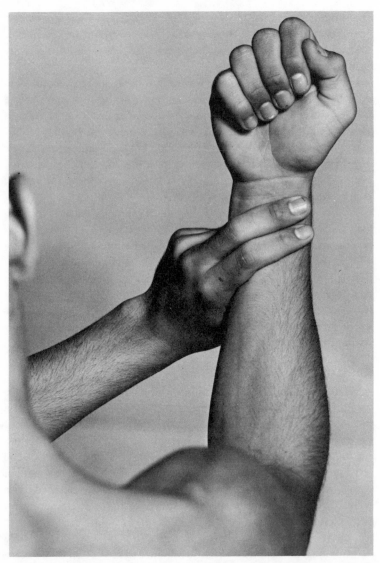

FIG. 40. Demonstrating line of action of deeply situated pronator quadratus.

because it is mainly concerned with flexion of the elbow. The other muscles are concerned with wrist movements and will be discussed in Chapter 4. The pronator teres has been discussed previously in this chapter.

PRONATOR QUADRATUS. This muscle crosses transversely over the ulna and the radius in the distal region of the forearm near the wrist. It is deeply situated on the palmar side, lying directly over the bones and the interosseous membrane, and is covered by the flexors of wrist and digits. *Origin:* Ulna. *Insertion:* Radius. *Innervation:* A branch of the median nerve. *Palpation* is difficult or impossible, but the approximate length and direction of its fibers is indicated in Figure 40.

DISCUSSION OF FUNCTIONS OF MUSCLES ACTING ON ELBOW AND FOREARM

CROSS SECTION OF FLEXORS AS COMPARED TO EXTENSORS

In the subject, investigated by Fick, the total cross section of all the flexor muscles was 26.5 sq. cm., and of the extensors, 20.3 sq. cm. Since the tension which a muscle can produce has a direct relationship to its physiological cross section, it is obvious that the flexors surpass considerably the extensors in their ability to produce tension, an indication of the greater demands placed on the flexors.

A total paralysis of the flexors is far more disabling than a total paralysis of the extensors. For example, a hand-to-mouth movement is not affected by an extensor paralysis since the hand is lowered by the force of gravity, but a total flexor paralysis makes a hand-to-mouth movement impossible. A fraction of the total strength of the flexors suffices for light tasks, so that a partial paralysis does not prove disastrous. Nature has also provided a safety measure in the manner in which the flexors are innervated, namely by three different peripheral nerves (musculocutaneous, radial and median), while the extensors are innervated by the radial nerve only.

By comparing the physiological cross section of the various flexor muscles, an approximate idea of the contribution of each muscle to elbow flexion is obtained. In the subject investigated (Table II, Appendix), the biceps had the largest cross section, the brachialis only slightly less, the pronator teres about half that of the biceps, and the brachioradialis considerably less.

For proper appreciation of the relative importance of the individual muscles in elbow flexion, however, the leverage of each muscle at various elbow angles must also be considered, as discussed in Chapters 1 and 2. Table I in the Appendix gives leverage values for individual muscles passing anterior to the axis of the elbow joint at angles from 0 to 130 degrees of flexion.

Elbow and Forearm   73

CROSS SECTION OF PRONATORS AS COMPARED TO SUPINATORS

According to Fick, the combined cross section of the pronator teres and pronator quadratus was 58.2 sq. cm. and of the biceps and the supinator, 87.5 sq. cm. If the total cross section of all the muscles mechanically capable of participating in pronation is determined, the figure would be 139 sq. cm.; the corresponding figure for the supinators is 152 sq. cm. The supinators thus have a larger cross section and surpass the pronators in their ability of producing tension. Yet, torque curves for pronation have higher values than those for supination when determined in the living subject (Bethe and Franke, 1919; Salter and Darcus, 1952).

SELECTION OF MUSCLES IN MOVEMENT

In general, it may be stated that those muscles which best serve a particular purpose with the least amount of expenditure of energy are the ones selected by the nervous system. For any movement combination, however, a perfect selection of muscles is only achieved by highly skilled individuals. Unskilled movements are wasteful of energy since muscles not necessarily needed for the movement contract together with those needed. As skill increases, the selection improves and gradation of contraction becomes more refined, resulting in smoother movements which are less fatiguing and, from the esthetic standpoint, are more pleasing to the eye.

The number of muscles involved in movements also is determined by the effort needed for a particular task. Thus, if great resistance is encountered, more muscles are recruited not only at the joint or joints where the movements take place, but also at joints far away from the scene of action. A typical example is that of making a fist, which involves primarily the flexors of the digits and the extensors of the wrist. When the effort increases, as in testing grip strength on a manometer, not only do the finger flexors and the wrist extensors increase their tension, but there is a successive recruitment of muscles at the elbow, the shoulder, and even the trunk until with greatest effort practically all muscles of the body appear to participate.

Many muscles act over more than one joint and they are the ones usually selected for a task involving these joints. For example, the biceps brachii is a flexor of the elbow and a supinator of the forearm, and when both these movements are wanted simultaneously, the biceps is the logical selection. This movement combination, of course, could also be performed by the brachioradialis and the supinator, as is indeed the case in musculocutaneous nerve injuries when the biceps and the brachialis are paralyzed. Ordinarily, for light tasks, Nature prefers to have one muscle do the job of two when such a muscle is available.

The brachialis, a one-joint muscle, is the perfect selection for flexion of the elbow if neither supination nor pronation is willed. For such motion, it would be wasteful to use the biceps since supination would have to be depressed by the pronators, and it would be equally wasteful to use the pronator teres, since pronation would have to be prevented by the supinators.

Often it becomes economical to use a two-joint muscle to produce movement over one joint only, in which case synergic muscle action (or gravitational forces) stabilizes the other joint or moves that joint in the opposite direction. This latter arrangement enables a muscle to do work in a relatively elongated state through a large range of motion, thus utilizing a favorable portion of the length-tension diagram (see Chapter 2).

The foregoing discussion emphasizes that muscles may team up in many different ways and that synergism among muscles is ever changing depending upon requirements. Consequently, it can never be stated that two specific muscles are always synergists or antagonists, but the muscles may be so labeled for specific movement combinations only.

The manner in which the individual muscles team up to flex the elbow has been the subject of much discussion and a considerable amount of dissension mainly because the variety of requirements and individual variations in skill have not been sufficiently appreciated. Recent electromyographic studies indicate that, as would be expected, there are considerable variations of muscle action among individuals, both in the selection of muscles and in the sequence of recruitment of the muscles.

BRACHIALIS. The brachialis is the least controversial of the flexors of the elbow. It is uninfluenced by the position of the forearm, being as effective when the forearm is pronated as when it is supinated. Studies by Basmajian and Latif (1957) show that flexion of the elbow, whether fast or slow and with or without a load, as well as the maintenance of a flexed position against gravity, brings it into action.

BRACHIORADIALIS. It is universally agreed upon that this muscle is a flexor of the elbow, but actions of supination and pronation have also been ascribed to it. It was named the supinator longus by the early anatomists. Fick states that, mechanically, it is capable of performing a limited range of pronation from the fully supinated position and a still more limited range of supination from the fully pronated position. Beevor (1903) considers the brachioradialis to be a pure flexor of the elbow. His observations have been substantiated by electromyographic studies (Basmajian and Latif, 1957) which showed that, with the elbow extended, no electrical activity appeared in the muscle when the forearm was pronated from the fully supinated position or supinated from the fully pronated position, unless the motions were resisted. In that case, the brachioradialis may act for stabilization purposes rather than for pronation and supination. Functionally, therefore, the brachioradialis may be considered a pure flexor of the elbow.

BICEPS BRACHII. An isolated unopposed contraction of the biceps would produce simultaneous flexion of the elbow and supination of the forearm. Either of these actions can be suppressed by synergic action of other muscles.

Electromyographic studies by the above authors show that the biceps takes little or no part in slow flexion of the elbow when the forearm is pronated, even when a load of two pounds, held loosely in the hand, is lifted or lowered. But when the forearm is supinated, the biceps acts in flexion of the elbow both with and without a load, in slow as well as in fast movements, and regardless of whether it acts in a shortening or lengthening capacity. With increasing speed and increasing load, however, the biceps acts also when the forearm is pronated.

COMPARISON BETWEEN ACTIONS OF THE BICEPS BRACHII AND THE SUPINATOR. The biceps acts most effectively as a supinator when the elbow is flexed at an angle of about 90 degrees, a conclusion gained from observing the angle of approach of its tendon to the long axis of the radius. As the elbow extends, the effectiveness of the muscle as a supinator lessens; the effectiveness of the supinator muscle is not influenced by the elbow angle. Fick calculated that, at an angle of 90 degrees, the biceps is almost four times as effective as the supinator. When the elbow is extended, however, the effectiveness of the biceps is only twice that of the supinator.

Since the supinator's sole action is supination while the biceps is also a flexor of the elbow, it is logical to conclude that the supinator would be called upon to contract when supination without elbow flexion is willed, provided that the movement is performed slowly and without resistance. Clinically, this assumption may be confirmed as follows:

The subject is seated with the forearm resting in the lap. The palpating fingers are placed on the tendon of the biceps in the fold of the elbow. If supination is performed slowly and the forearm remains in the lap, the tendon of the biceps remains relaxed, and it may be concluded that the movement is performed by the supinator. But, if a quick supination is performed, the biceps immediately springs into action and its tendon stands out markedly.

The above procedure is employed for isolated testing of the supinator, although in normal individuals no information about the *strength* of the supinator is obtained. The test is also useful in patients with radial nerve injuries to determine when regeneration of the nerve has progressed to the supinator. As long as the supinator is denervated, a slow supination of the forearm in the position described causes the biceps tendon to become prominent. When the supinator has been re-innervated, this is no longer the case.

The ability of the supinator to perform supination without the aid of the biceps has been verified by Basmajian and Latif (1957). In most subjects investigated, no electrical activity was registered in either head of the biceps when the forearm was supinated while the elbow was in extension. But if resistance was applied to supination, the biceps became active also when the elbow was extended.

COMPARISON BETWEEN ACTIONS OF THE PRONATOR TERES AND THE PRONATOR QUADRATUS. The pronator teres is the strongest of the pronators and since it is superficial its contraction can be ascertained by palpation. The role played by the pronator quadratus is difficult to assess since it cannot be palpated readily. Its cross section is almost two-thirds of that of the pronator teres and compares favorably with that of the supinator. Its shortening distance, however, is small. One may assume that the pronator quadratus pronates the forearm unaided by other muscles if pronation is performed slowly without resistance and without active elbow flexion. These conditions are met if the subject lies prone with the forearm hanging vertically over the edge of the table and if little effort is used in pronation.

COMPARISON BETWEEN ACTIONS OF THE TRICEPS AND THE ANCONEUS. Both the triceps and the anconeus are extensors of the elbow, the triceps being by far the more powerful of the two. The triceps has a cross section about five times, and a shortening range about twice that of the anconeus (Table III, Appendix). The fascia over the triceps tendon continues over the anconeus which muscle has a close relation to the elbow joint and the proximal radioular joint. Both muscles, therefore, contribute to the protection of these joints.

TWO-JOINT MUSCLES OF THE ELBOW AND SHOULDER

The two heads of the biceps and the long head of the triceps originate above the shoulder joint so that the lengths of these muscles are influenced by the position of the shoulder as well as that of the elbow joint.

BICEPS. The tendons of origin of both heads of the biceps are elongated when the shoulder is extended or hyperextended. Therefore, *elbow flexion combined with shoulder extension enhances the action of the biceps.* By means of this two-joint mechanism the muscle maintains favorable tension while flexing the elbow through a large range. This combination—elbow flexion and shoulder hyperextension—is utilized in "pulling" activities and contributes materially to the strength of elbow flexion.

TRICEPS. The long head of the triceps, because of its posterior origin on the scapula, is elongated when the shoulder is flexed. Therefore, *elbow extension combined with shoulder flexion enhances the activity of the triceps.* This two-joint mechanism is the reverse of the flexion combination and is used to advantage in "pushing" activities. The flexion and extension combinations are used alternately in scores of functional activities, such as sanding, polishing, pulling the beater of a loom, using a carpet sweeper, sawing wood, throwing a ball, etc. Examples of such two-joint mechanisms are numerous throughout the body.

BICEPS AND TRICEPS ACTING AS SYNERGISTS. In flexion and extension of the elbow, the biceps and triceps act antagonistically, but frequently they are called upon to contract simultaneously, such as when using a screw driver. To force the screw in, the triceps extends or stabilizes the elbow in the position desired while the biceps supinates the forearm. This action can be confirmed by palpation. It should be noted that, when using a screw driver, one tends to keep the elbow at an angle of approximately 90 degrees, at which angle the biceps has its highest efficiency for supination. In this activity then, the two muscles work together, and thus act as synergists. Simultaneous contraction of the biceps and the triceps also occurs when a firm fist is made, in which case the two muscles act together to stabilize the elbow.

PECTORALIS MAJOR IN EXTENSION OF THE ELBOW

When the hand is in contact with an object in front of the body, the pectoralis major, by exerting its pull on the humerus, contributes significantly to elbow extension. This is demonstrated when a heavy object is pushed away from the body and when push-ups are performed on horizontal bars or on the floor. The triceps and the pectoralis major then act in unison. In certain pathological cases, when the elbow is nearly in complete extension, the pectoralis major may, under above conditions, perform elbow extension without the aid of the triceps.

PERIPHERAL NERVE INJURIES AFFECTING MUSCLES
OF THE ELBOW AND FOREARM

If the *radial nerve* is severed in the axilla all the muscles supplied by this nerve will be paralyzed: the triceps, brachioradialis, supinator, wrist extensors and long extensors of the digits. The nerve, however, may be injured distally to the branches supplying the triceps, as often occurs in fractures of the humerus, in which case the triceps is spared while the more distally innervated muscles are paralyzed.

In radial nerve injuries, in spite of the loss of the brachioradialis, elbow flexion is affected but little since the other flexors remain intact. Supination can be performed satisfactorily by the biceps without the supinator, but some strength in supination is lost.

A *musculocutaneous nerve injury* affects the biceps and the brachialis, causing a marked weakness of elbow flexion. Elbow flexion, however, can still be performed even against some resistance, since the brachioradialis and the pronator teres remain intact (Brunnstrom, 1946). With the loss of the biceps, supination is much weakened but can be carried out by the supinator alone; however, only a small amount of resistance can be overcome (Brunnstrom, 1946).

A *median nerve injury* affects elbow flexion very little for, although the pronator teres is paralyzed, the main flexors are intact. Pronation is severely affected since both the pronator teres and the pronator quadratus are innervated by the median nerve.

Elbow and Forearm 79

CHAPTER 4

Wrist and Hand

BONES

PALPABLE STRUCTURES OF THE WRIST

HEAD OF THE ULNA. If the wrist is grasped from side to side at its narrowest portion, as seen in Figure 41A, the bony eminence proximal to the examiner's index finger on the dorsum of the wrist is identified as the head of the ulna. In the pronated position of the forearm this eminence is seen beneath the skin. If one fingertip is placed on the highest part of this bony eminence and the forearm is slowly supinated, this portion of the bone recedes and can no longer be palpated, because during supination the distal portion of the radius rotates around the head of the ulna, thus partially hiding the head of the ulna from palpation.

STYLOID PROCESS OF THE ULNA. The position of the examiner's index finger in Figure 41A indicates the approximate location of this process. The tendon of the extensor carpi ulnaris, however, courses in this region and interferes with palpation. By sliding the index finger over this tendon in a palmar direction, the styloid process becomes more accessible for palpation. This process is smaller and feels sharper than the head of the ulna and it may be palpated both in the pronated and in the supinated position of the forearm.

STYLOID PROCESS OF THE RADIUS. The position of the examiner's thumb in Figure 41A indicates the point where the styloid process of the radius may be palpated. This process extends somewhat more distally than the corresponding process of the ulna.

The styloid processes serve as attachments to the ulnar and radial carpal collateral ligaments, respectively.

Wrist and Hand

GROOVES AND PROMINENCES ON DISTAL END OF RADIUS. On the dorsal aspect of the broad distal end of the radius are found a number of grooves for tendons passing to the hand, these grooves being separated by prominences. The *tubercle of the radius,* sometimes referred to as Lister's tubercle, may be palpated about level with the head of the ulna (Fig. 41A). The tendon of the extensor pollicis longus lies in a groove on the ulnar side of this tubercle and, on palpation, appears to be hooked around it. The tubercle serves as landmark for locating several other tendons in this region: the deeply situated tendon of the extensor carpi radialis brevis; the tendon of the extensor indicis proprius which crosses over the tendon of the extensor carpi radialis brevis; and the tendon of the extensor digitorum communis to the index finger which is superficial and visible under the skin. The deep tendons, however, are difficult to identify with certainty by palpation.

CAPITATE BONE (os magnum). Occupying a central position at the wrist (in line with the middle finger), the capitate bone is best approached from the dorsum where a slight depression indicates its location (Fig. 41A). The axis of motion for ulnar and radial abduction goes through this bone in a dorsal-palmar direction (41B).

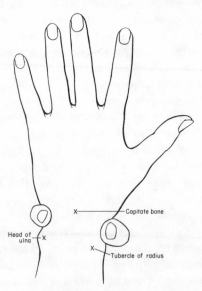

FIG. 41A. Grip around wrist indicates approximate location of transverse axis for flexion and extension of wrist.

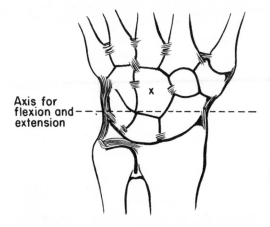

Axis for
flexion and
extension

FIG. 41B. Axis for
flexion and extension
of wrist in relation to
carpal bones. Cross-
mark (x) on capitate
bone indicates loca-
tion of the dorsal-pal-
mar axis for radial
and ulnar abduction.

SCAPHOID (navicular) BONE. This bone is palpated distal to the styloid process of the radius. The scaphoid bone and the *trapezium* (greater multangular) make up the floor of the "anatomical snuff box" (fovea radialis), the depression seen between the tendons of the thumb extensor muscles (extensor pollicis longus and brevis) when these muscles are tensed. It should be remembered that the scaphoid belongs to the proximal row and the trapezium to the distal row of carpal bones.

PISIFORM BONE (shape of a pea). Palpated on the palmar side of the wrist near the ulnar border, the pisiform bone can be grasped and moved from side to side. It serves as the attachment to the tendon of the flexor carpi ulnaris.

OTHER CARPAL BONES. These bones are somewhat more difficult to identify by palpation than those just mentioned. The proximal row of bones, starting on the radial side and proceeding toward the ulnar side, is made up of the *scaphoid* (navicular), *lunate* (semilunar), *triquetrum* (triangular), and *pisiform* bones. The distal row consists of the *trapezium* (greater multangular), *trapezoid* (lesser multangular), *capitate* (os magnum) and *hamate* (unciform) bones. The approximate location of each bone may be determined by its relation to those carpal bones which are most easily palpated.

PALPABLE STRUCTURES OF THE DIGITS

FIVE METACARPALS. Each metacarpal has a *base* which articulates proximally with one or more carpal bones and with adjacent metacarpals, a *shaft* which is slightly curved, and a *head* which articulates with the base of a proximal phalanx. Each metacarpal can be palpated throughout its length on the dorsum of the hand. Note the *tubercle at the base of the fifth metacarpal* which is located just distal to the examiner's index finger in Figure 41A, and which serves as the insertion for the extensor carpi ulnaris. At the base of the second metacarpal bone (dorsally), an eminence may be felt which serves as the insertion for the extensor carpi radialis longus. The palmar surface of the base of the second metacarpal also presents a rough area which serves as the insertion for the flexor carpi radialis, but this lies in a position that is too deep for palpation. The head of each metacarpal bone presents a convex articular surface which becomes part of the metacarpophalangeal joint, and which may, in part, be palpated when the joint is flexed.

PHALANGES. The two phalanges of the thumb and the three phalanges of each of the other digits may be palpated without difficulty. To differentiate the phalanges of the thumb, the terms *proximal* and *distal* are used; for the other digits, *proximal, middle* and *distal*. These terms are preferred to first and second, and to first, second and third, respectively.

JOINTS

RADIOCARPAL JOINT

TYPE OF JOINT. This is a condyloid joint. The articular surface of the radius is *concave,* and the concave surface includes an articular disk located toward the ulnar side. The articular surface of the carpal bones (scaphoid, lunate, triquetrum) is convex to correspond with the concavity of the radius. Note that the ulna is not part of this joint and that the joint is separated from the distal radioulnar joint by an articular disk.

CAPSULE AND LIGAMENTS. The capsule of the radiocarpal joint is loose and allows extensive wrist movements. An elaborate ligamentous apparatus binds the osseous structures together and reinforces the capsule. The strong *ulnar collateral ligament* extends from the styloid process of the ulna proximally to the carpal bones distally. In its upper portion it blends with the articular disk of the radiocarpal joint. One part of this ligament attaches to the pisiform bone and is in close relation to the tendon of the flexor carpi ulnaris muscle. The *radial collateral ligament* originates from the styloid process of the radius and attaches to several of the carpal bones. It is in close relation to the tendons of the abductor pollicis longus and the extensor pollicis brevis muscles.

INTERCARPAL JOINTS

The joints between the first and second row of carpal bones and between the bones in each row participate to some extent in wrist movements. The greatest part of wrist movement, however, takes place at the radiocarpal joint. The intercarpal joints communicate with each other but usually not with the radiocarpal joint. Functionally, the radiocarpal and intercarpal joints, although separate entities anatomically, may be considered as one joint, the "wrist joint."

WRIST JOINT

AXIS OF MOTION OF WRIST JOINT. The approximate location of the axis for *flexion and extension* of the wrist is found if the wrist is gripped from side to side as seen in Figure 41A. The location of this axis in relation to the bones of the wrist is seen in Figure 41B. In order to obtain maximum range of motion about this axis the fist should be closed for extension and open for flexion (Fig. 42).

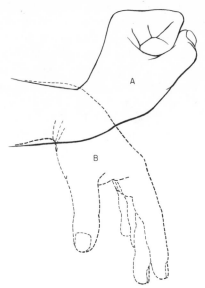

FIG. 42. For maximum range of motion at wrist, the fist should be closed in extension (A) and open in flexion (B).

The *axis for radial and ulnar abduction* is perpendicular to the former axis and passes in a dorsal-palmar direction through the capitate bone (Fig. 41A and B). By placing a pencil perpendicular to the dorsum of the wrist at the point indicated in the illustration, the direction of this axis is demonstrated. Note that more range is permitted in ulnar than in radial abduction if, at the onset, the hand is held in line with the forearm.

CARPOMETACARPAL JOINTS OF DIGITS II TO V

The trapezoid, capitate and hamate bones of the distal row of carpal bones articulate with metacarpals II to V in a rather irregular fashion. These joints may be described as modified saddle joints. Movements, however, are quite limited. The fourth and fifth metacarpal bones demonstrate more range of motion than do the others. If the fist is tightly closed, it may be observed that these bones, particularly the fifth, move in a palmar direction, that is, they flex at their carpometacarpal joints. When the little finger is opposed to the thumb, movements at these joints also take place.

CARPOMETACARPAL JOINT OF THE THUMB

The base of the metacarpal bone of the thumb articulates with the trapezium, and this joint has a true saddle shape (Fig. 41B). The joint capsule is thick but loose, thus permitting great freedom of motion. The joint allows the thumb to move into *opposition* so that the palmar surface of the tip of the thumb is directed toward the palmar surface of the other digits. Anatomically, the term *opposition* refers to the carpometacarpal joint of the thumb only, but clinically, *opposition of the thumb* has come to mean the entire movement of bringing the palmar surface of the thumb in contact with one or more of the other digits. *Reposition* is the reverse of opposition.

The saddle joint of the thumb also permits movements of *abduction* and *adduction,* and these movements take place about an axis which is perpendicular to the axis of opposition and reposition.

METACARPOPHALANGEAL JOINTS OF DIGITS II TO V

The metacarpophalangeal joints of digits II to V are of the condyloid type, the rounded surfaces of the heads of the metacarpals articulating with the shallow concave surfaces on the bases of the proximal phalanges. The articular surfaces of the heads of the metacarpals extend more toward the palmar than toward the dorsal side to permit closing of the fist.

At their bases the metacarpal bones lie side by side, connected by firm joints, but they spread apart distally so that their heads do not contact each other. An extensive ligamentous apparatus, however, binds them together. The *deep transverse metacarpal* (transverse capitular) *ligament* on the palmar side of the metacarpal heads limits the distance by which the heads may be separated.

The metacarpal bones have different lengths, so that when a fist is made the knuckles do not form a straight line. The metacarpals belonging to the index and middle fingers are approximately the same length, while those of the ring and little fingers are shorter.

AXES OF MOTION. The axes for *flexion and extension* and for *abduction* and *adduction* both pass through the head of the metacarpal bone, the former being a transverse axis, the latter having a dorsal-palmar direction. The joint surfaces also allow a circumduction movement which can be performed actively. Passively, a small amount of rotation about a longitudinal axis is permitted.

METACARPOPHALANGEAL JOINT OF THE THUMB

This joint is usually described as a hinge joint, but functionally, it possesses all the characteristics of the other metacarpophalangeal joints, even though range of motion is more limited. Two small sesamoid bones, interconnected by a ligament, are found on the palmar side of the joint. The tendon of the long flexor of the thumb passes in a groove between the sesamoid bones.

AXES OF MOTION. Movements permitted in this joint are flexion and extension and a small amount of abduction and adduction. The axis for flexion-extension passes transversely, that for abduction-adduction in a dorsal-palmar direction through the head of the metacarpal bone. Both axes are oriented to the plane of the thumb. The relation to the plane of the palm varies in accordance with the position of the carpometacarpal joint.

Range of motion in flexion-extension is quite variable in individuals. In some subjects, flexion is less than 45 degrees, in others as much as 90 degrees. Abduction-adduction of the metacarpophalangeal joint of the thumb is of smaller range than at the corresponding joints of the other digits. To observe the presence of this motion in the thumb, the metacarpal bone must be stabilized firmly, or the carpometacarpal joint will participate.

INTERPHALANGEAL JOINTS

Each of the digits II to V has two interphalangeal joints, while the thumb has only one. These joints are hinge joints, permitting flexion and extension only. Range of motion is larger at the proximal than at the distal joints of digits II to V. The interphalangeal joint of the thumb has a range of approximately 90 degrees.

MUSCLES OF THE WRIST AND HAND

The muscles listed below should be studied on the skeleton, on the cadaver and in the living subject. For an understanding of the actions of these muscles it is important to consider: (1) over which joint or joints each muscle passes; (2) the line of action of the muscle; (3) the distance of the muscle to the axis of motion of the joint at various positions of the joint; (4) the relative length of the muscle; and (5) the functional unit to which the muscle belongs. Memorizing the exact origins and insertions of the muscles is of little help in the general understanding of their functions.

LIST OF MUSCLES ACTING ON THE WRIST AND DIGITS

Muscles Acting on Wrist Only
Extensor carpi radialis longus
Extensor carpi radialis brevis
Extensor carpi ulnaris
Flexor carpi radialis
Palmaris longus
Flexor carpi ulnaris

Muscles Acting on Wrist and Digits
Extensor digitorum communis
Extensor indicis proprius
Extensor digiti minimi proprius
Extensor pollicis longus
Extensor pollicis brevis
Abductor pollicis longus
Flexor digitorum superficialis
Flexor digitorum profundus
Flexor pollicis longus

Muscles Acting on Digits Only
Four lumbricals
Three (four) palmar interossei*

---

*The deep portion of flexor pollicis brevis is sometimes described as the first palmar interosseus. In that case, the palmar interossei are four in number.

Four dorsal interossei
Thenar muscles
    Opponens pollicis
    Abductor pollicis brevis
    Adductor pollicis
    Flexor pollicis brevis
Hypothenar muscles
    Opponens digiti minimi
    Abductor digiti minimi
    Flexor digiti minimi brevis
Palmaris brevis

The innervation of muscles acting on wrist and digits is as follows:

Radial Nerve

Extensor carpi radialis longus
Extensor carpi radialis brevis
Extensor carpi ulnaris
Extensor digitorum communis
Extensor indicis proprius
Extensor digiti minimi proprius
Extensor pollicis longus
Extensor pollicis brevis
Abductor pollicis longus

Median Nerve

Flexor carpi radialis
Palmaris longus
Flexor digitorum superficialis
Radial half of flexor digitorum profundus
    and the two radial lumbricals
Flexor pollicis longus
Superficial portion of flexor pollicis brevis
Opponens pollicis
Abductor pollicis brevis

Ulnar Nerve

Flexor carpi ulnaris
Ulnar half of flexor digitorum profundus
    and the two ulnar lumbricals
All interossei muscles
All hypothenar muscles
Palmaris brevis
Deep portion of flexor pollicis brevis
Adductor pollicis

It is suggested that the muscles be thought of in groups, innervated as follows: The *radial nerve* supplies all the extensors of wrist

---

and digits originating in the forearm and in the region of the lateral epicondyle. The *median nerve* supplies most of the flexors of the wrist and digits originating in the forearm and in the region of the medial epicondyle. The *ulnar nerve* supplies most of the small muscles in the hand. Exceptions are: "half-half" supply of flexor digitorum profundus and lumbricals (median and ulnar); ulnar nerve supply to flexor carpi ulnaris; and median nerve supply to thenar muscles.

WRIST MOVEMENTS

Movements of the hand in relation to the forearm, without consideration of simultaneous finger movements, will be considered here. Synergic action of wrist and finger muscles will be discussed under Hand Function, page 96. Cross sections and work capacities of muscles passing the wrist are given in Table VI in the Appendix.

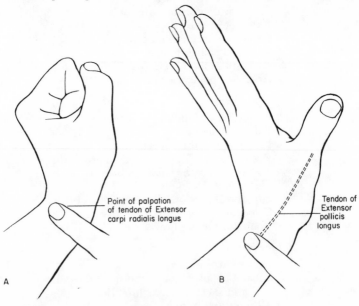

Point of palpation
of tendon of Extensor
carpi radialis longus

Tendon of
Extensor
pollicis
longus

A

B

FIG. 43. A, Palpation of tendon of extensor carpi radialis longus when fist is closed. B, When fingers are extended, extensor digitorum communis takes over task of extending wrist. Note that tendon of extensor pollicis longus also courses on extensor side of wrist, not far from the tendon of extensor carpi radialis longus.

NOMENCLATURE

Movements of the wrist are described as *flexion and extension* and as *radial and ulnar abduction*. By combining these motions the complex movement of *circumduction* may be performed, during which the hand executes a circling movement. Orientation for radial and ulnar abduction is a line drawn longitudinally through the forearm and the middle finger.

PALPATION OF MUSCLES ACTING IN EXTENSION OF THE WRIST

If the wrist is extended with the fist closed, the *tendon of the extensor carpi radialis longus* becomes prominent and is palpated as seen in Figure 43. The tendon lies on the radial side of the capitate bone but on the ulnar side of the tubercle of the radius, and courses toward the base of the metacarpal bone of the index finger, into which it is inserted. The *extensor carpi radialis brevis* is inserted into the base of the metacarpal bone of the middle finger and is therefore more centrally located at its point of insertion. It is crossed over by the tendon of the extensor of the index finger and, therefore, may be somewhat more difficult to identify. Its tendon can usually be felt rising somewhat if the thumb is moved in a palmar direction, in a plane perpendicular to the palm of the hand (see also p. 121).

The muscular parts of the two wrist extensors, together with the brachioradialis, make up the radial muscle group at the elbow. By manipulating the muscle tissue, this group may be separated from the other extensors on the dorsum of the forearm and from the flexor group on the palmar side of the forearm. To locate the radial extensors of the wrist, the brachioradialis is first identified by resistance to elbow flexion with the forearm halfway between pronation and supination (Fig. 36). The muscular portion of the extensor carpi radialis longus is then located close to the brachioradialis, toward the dorsal side of the forearm. It is a superficial muscle and may readily be identified when resistance is given to extension of the wrist (Fig. 37). The extensor carpi radialis brevis is found somewhat more distally.

The *extensor digitorum communis* participates in extension of the wrist only when the fingers are simultaneously extended; in fact, the finger extensors then appear to take over the task of wrist extension altogether. To feel the shift from wrist extensors to finger extensors, the wrist should first be extended with the fist closed, and the prominent tendon of extensor carpi radialis longus palpated (Fig. 43A). While maintaining the wrist in this position, the fingers are extended (Fig. 43B). It will then be noted that the prominent tendon being palpated "disappears," a sign that the muscle "lets go" or diminishes its contraction. This shift is regulated entirely automatically. For a more detailed analysis of the relationships between the wrist extensors and the finger extensors, the reader is referred to Beevor's Croonian Lecture (1903).

The tendon of the *extensor carpi ulnaris* is palpated between the head of the ulna and a prominent tubercle on the base of the fifth metacarpal bone, the latter serving as its point of insertion. The tendon becomes prominent if the wrist is extended with the fist closed, and even more prominent if the wrist is simultaneously ulnar abducted (Fig. 44). The tendon is also easily palpable when the thumb is extended and abducted as seen in Figure 63.

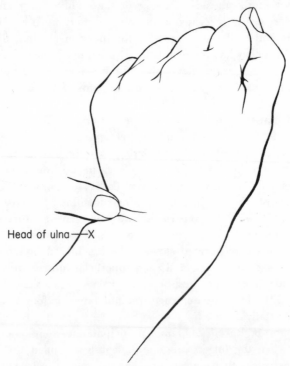

Head of ulna

FIG. 44. Palpation of extensor carpi ulnaris in fist closure.

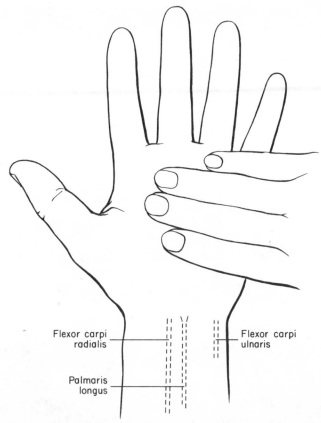

Flexor carpi
radialis

Flexor carpi
ulnaris

Palmaris
longus

FIG. 45. Resistance to wrist flexion applied in palm of hand brings out
tendons of wrist flexors.

The muscular portion of the extensor carpi ulnaris is best palpated about two inches below the lateral epicondyle of the humerus,
where it lies between the anconeus and the extensor digitorum communis (Fig. 39). From this point on, it may be followed distally
along the dorsal-ulnar aspect of the forearm in a direction toward
the head of the ulna.

PALPATION OF MUSCLES ACTING IN FLEXION OF THE WRIST

The three tendons of the wrist flexors become prominent if resistance is given to flexion of the wrist (Fig. 45). The most centrally
located tendon is that of the *palmaris longus;* it varies in size in different individuals, or it may be missing altogether. Radial to it,

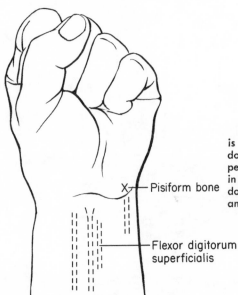

X — Pisiform bone

Flexor digitorum
superficialis

FIG. 46. When a tight fist
is made, one or more ten-
dons of flexor digitorum superficialis may be observed
in the space between the tendons of the palmaris longus
and the flexor carpi ulnaris.

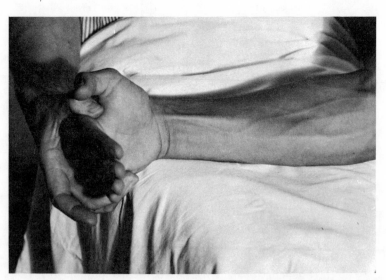

FIG. 47. Absence of palmaris longus. The prominent tendon is that of the
flexor carpi radialis. When this subject moves the digits, the play of the
flexor tendons can be observed well. Ordinarily, the palmaris longus partially
obstructs the view.

the strong tendon of the *flexor carpi radialis* is identified. This tendon lies in a superficial position in the lower part of the forearm, is held down by the transverse carpal ligament at the wrist, and disappears into a groove in the trapezium bone. It cannot be followed to its insertion into the base of the second metacarpal bone. The tendon of the *flexor carpi ulnaris* lies close to the ulnar border of the forearm and may be palpated between the styloid process of the ulna and the pisiform bone, into which it is inserted.

If the fist is tightly closed and the wrist simultaneously somewhat flexed (Fig. 46), it may be observed that the pisiform bone is pulled distally by the hypothenar muscles which permits easier palpation of the tendon of the flexor carpi ulnaris. With the fist tightly closed, one or more tendons of the *flexor digitorum superficialis* become prominent in the space between the palmaris longus and flexor carpi ulnaris (Fig. 45). It appears to be the tendon of the fourth finger which rises to the surface. In individuals lacking the palmaris longus, a more complete play of the tendons of the long finger flexors may be observed if flexion of the wrist is resisted and the subject then flexes one finger after the other or all fingers simultaneously (Fig. 47).

MUSCLES ACTING IN RADIAL AND ULNAR
ABDUCTION OF THE WRIST

The palmaris longus and the extensor carpi radialis brevis have a central location at the wrist; the other wrist flexors and extensors are situated either toward the radial or toward the ulnar side of the wrist. They are therefore capable of producing movements from side to side as well as flexion and extension.

When the extensor carpi ulnaris and flexor carpi ulnaris combine their actions, ulnar abduction of the wrist results. The extensor carpi radialis longus and the flexor carpi radialis, aided by the abductor pollicis longus and the extensor pollicis brevis, produce radial abduction. The latter two muscles have a favorable line of action for performing radial abduction, and they do so regardless of the position of the thumb, whether flexed, extended, abducted or adducted.

The wrist furnishes typical examples of how muscles may act either as synergists or antagonists. For instance, in flexion and extension of the wrist, the flexor carpi ulnaris and the extensor carpi ulnaris are antagonists, but in ulnar abduction of the wrist these two muscles act as synergists.

HAND FUNCTION

The function of the hand depends upon the team work of many muscles, of those acting on the wrist as well as on the digits. The wrist muscles are an integral part of hand function, since they prevent undesired wrist movements and keep the finger muscles at a length that is favorable for producing tension. An extensive ligamentous apparatus, particularly well developed on the dorsum of the digits (here variably named *extensor sleeve, aponeurotic sleeve* or *extensor hood*), is admirably designed to enhance and regulate the function of the muscles moving the digits.

Many of the muscles participating in hand function are pluriarticular muscles, that is, they pass over several joints before reaching their point of insertion. A pluriarticular muscle, if contracting in an isolated fashion, tends to produce movements in all the joints over which it passes. Such movements, however, do not usually materialize, since synergic muscles spring into action to stabilize one or more joints where movements are undesirable.

In studying the function of the hand, close attention must be paid to the manner in which various muscles combine their actions as the hand is used for grasp and release and for various skilled movements. The muscles which make up such a "team," or movement synergy, are so strongly linked together neurophysiologically that the individual is unable voluntarily to omit a muscle from the combination to which it belongs (Beevor, 1903).

Closing the Fist

ROLE OF THE WRIST EXTENSORS IN GRASPING

When the fist closes, the fingers fold into the palm of the hand or close around an object by the action of the long finger flexors (profundus and superficialis), probably aided by some of the intrinsic muscles of the hand. Since these long finger flexors originate in the forearm and their tendons pass on the flexor side of the wrist, these muscles, if unopposed, would cause the wrist to flex during grasp. Such action is prevented by the stabilizing action of the wrist extensors. The strength of contraction of the wrist extensors is in direct proportion to the effort of the grip—the harder the grip, the stronger the contraction of the wrist extensors.

If the wrist is allowed to drop during finger flexion, the grip is markedly weakened; in fact, it then becomes almost impossible to

Clinical Kinesiology

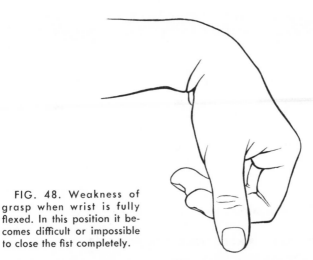

FIG. 48. Weakness of grasp when wrist is fully flexed. In this position it becomes difficult or impossible to close the fist completely.

close the fist completely (Fig. 48). This difficulty arises partly because the finger extension apparatus may not permit further elongation, and partly because of the marked approximation of the origin and the insertion of the finger flexors, which weakens their contraction so that they may attain a length at which they are unable to produce effective tension (compare the length-tension curve on page 34).

PALPATION OF THE WRIST EXTENSORS IN GRASPING

For palpation of the *extensor carpi radialis longus,* the subject places his lightly closed fist on the table or in the lap, forearm pronated, and the examiner palpates on the radiodorsal aspect of the wrist, as explained previously. By having the subject alternately close the fist firmly and relax the grip, the rise and fall of the tendon of the extensor carpi radialis longus may be felt and its contracting muscle belly identified in the forearm close to the brachioradialis. To eliminate the possibility of palpating the wrong tendon, the tendon of the extensor pollicis longus should first be identified. This poses no difficulty because the tendon is visible under the skin when the thumb is held in extension.

The *extensor carpi radialis brevis* also participates in wrist fixation for grasp, but its tendon protrudes less than that of the extensor carpi radialis longus and is therefore somewhat more difficult to identify. Its tendon may be palpated on the dorsum of the wrist, in line with the third metacarpal bone, when the fist is firmly closed.

Another, perhaps even better, method of identifying the tendon of the extensor carpi radialis brevis is to have the subject place his lightly closed fist in the lap, ulnar side down, and then move the thumb in a horizontal plane and in a palmar direction. This thumb movement involves the action of the palmaris longus muscle, the tendon of which passes down the middle of the palmar aspect of the wrist. The extensor carpi radialis brevis, the tendon of which occupies a similar position on the dorsum of the wrist, is the logical muscle to use for wrist fixation so that wrist flexion by the palmaris longus is prevented.

The *extensor carpi ulnaris* also participates in wrist fixation for grasp. When a fist is made, its tendon and muscle belly may be palpated in the location previously described (Fig. 44).

ROLE OF THE LONG FINGER FLEXORS IN GRASPING

Flexor digitorum superficialis and profundus serve the second to fifth digits for flexion at the interphalangeal joints. Since the tendons of these muscles pass on the palmar side of the wrist and of the metacarpophalangeal joints, they also tend to produce flexion of these joints. In using the hand for grasping, flexion of the meta-carpophalangeal joints is necessary for proper shape of the hand, while flexion at the wrist is undesirable because it decreases the force exerted by the flexors by shortening them. Fortunately, the latter is prevented by synergic contraction of the wrist extensors.

The superficialis, inserting into the base of the middle phalanx, flexes the proximal interphalangeal joint. The profundus tendon, after perforating the superficialis tendon, inserts into the base of the distal phalanx and acts as a flexor of the distal as well as the proximal interphalangeal joint. The profundus is the only muscle capable of flexing the distal joint.

PALPATION AND TESTING OF THE LONG FINGER FLEXORS

The *flexor digitorum superficialis* is located underneath the flexor carpi radialis and the palmaris longus, and the general direction of the muscle is from the flexor (medial) epicondyle to the center of the palmar side of the wrist. It is difficult or impossible to palpate the muscle at its origin since this is widespread and in part tendinous, or to distinguish the separate muscle bellies serving the four fingers, but the movement of the tendons may be observed in the forearm and at the wrist beneath the tendons of the flexor carpi radialis and palmaris longus, and particularly in the space between the tendons of the flexor carpi ulnaris and the palmaris longus. In this region, as previously mentioned, the tendon serving the fourth finger usually stands out prominently if a firm fist is made while the wrist is somewhat flexed. In subjects lacking the palmaris longus, observation is considerably easier.

Isolated action of the flexor digitorum superficialis is obtained if the proximal interphalangeal joint is flexed while the distal one remains inactive, a movement which is best performed with one finger at a time (Fig. 49). The coordination needed for this movement can be mastered by most individuals; if some difficulty arises, the examiner should stabilize the proximal phalanx.

Another way in which the superficialis of one digit may be tested without participation by the profundus is for the examiner to maintain the other digits in full extension at all joints (Fig. 50). This throws the profundus out of action so that the subject is unable to flex the distal joint.

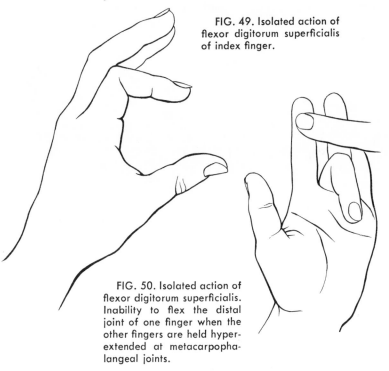

FIG. 49. Isolated action of flexor digitorum superficialis of index finger.

FIG. 50. Isolated action of flexor digitorum superficialis. Inability to flex the distal joint of one finger when the other fingers are held hyperextended at metacarpophalangeal joints.

The *flexor digitorum profundus* is deeply located, being covered by the superficialis, flexor carpi ulnaris, palmaris longus, flexor carpi radialis and pronator teres. It is muscular only in the upper half of the forearm. The muscle bellies serving the individual fingers are not nearly as well separated as those of the superficialis.

In spite of the deep location of the profundus, its contracting muscle belly may be palpated, provided that tension is minimal in the more superficial muscles. To achieve relative relaxation of the overlying muscles, the subject is seated with his forearm supinated and resting in the lap while the wrist is extended by the weight of the hand (protruding over the lap). When the arm is in this position and the subject closes his fist fully but with moderate effort, the profundus may be felt rising under the examiner's fingers which are placed in the region between the pronator teres and the flexor carpi ulnaris, about two inches below the medial epicondyle of the humerus.

In testing the profundus, one finger at a time is stabilized over the middle phalanx, as seen in Figure 51. During this test, it may be observed that the index finger is able to move well without drawing the other fingers into action, and the middle finger comparatively well, while isolated flexion of the fourth and the fifth fingers is difficult or impossible.

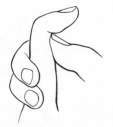

FIG. 51. Testing flexor digitorum profundus of index finger.

Ordinarily, a subject is unable to move the distal interphalangeal joint separately when no fixation of the middle phalanx is given. This is understandable, because the tendon of the profundus acts on the two interphalangeal joints simultaneously. Under normal circumstances, there is no extensor mechanism capable of extending the proximal joint separately. There are subjects, however, whose proximal interphalangeal joints allow hyperextension, and these persons will succeed in flexing the distal joints in an isolated fashion (Fig. 52). The middle band of the extensor mechanism then "locks" the proximal joint in hyperextension, preventing the profundus

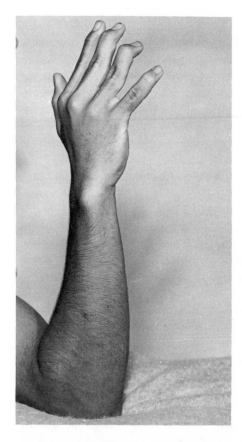

FIG. 52. A subject who is capable of stabilizing the proximal interphalangeal joint in hyperextension can flex the distal joint in an isolated fashion by flexor digitorum profundus. Ordinarily, the profundus acts on both joints.

from flexing it. When the proximal joint is hyperextended, the lateral bands become slack and therefore can exert no action on the distal joint.

Differential action of the two long finger flexors in grasping has been revealed by electromyography. Studies by Long and Brown (1964) and reiterated by Long (1968) indicate that the flexor digitorum profundus is the most important muscle for unresisted flexion of the fingers. When each subject closed his hand until the fingertips lightly touched the palm, this muscle showed consistent and strong electrical activity. The flexor digitorum superficialis was found to be less consistent in its action, and its activity appeared to be related to the position of the wrist. When the wrist was extended, little or no activity was registered. Activity increased progressively as the wrist was flexed.

Wrist and Hand   101

It has been stated previously that ordinarily, for light tasks, Nature prefers to have one muscle do the job of two when such a muscle is available. Evidence that this rule applies to fist closure is now available. When the wrist is extended, length-tension relations of flexor digitorum profundus are favorable for producing tensions, a tension which suffices for light closure of the fist. With progressive flexion of the wrist, however, length-tension relations of the profundus become less favorable and the flexor digitorum superficialis is recruited to aid in fist closure.

The cross sections of the two long finger flexors are about equal in size (see Appendix); therefore, the two muscles would be capable of producing approximately equal tension. It would be expected that the superficial flexor would contract strongly in forceful fist closure, such as that needed for firm grasping of tools. Close and Kidd (1969), in recording synchronous hand motion and action potentials in the muscles, did observe simultaneous activity in flexors digitorum profundus and superficialis. They graded the activity from medium to full and they described the hand motions as pinch or grip or grasp, activities which seem to imply the need for added force.

DISCUSSION OF THE ROLE OF THE INTRINSIC MUSCLES IN GRASPING

ANATOMICAL AND MECHANICAL CONSIDERATIONS. The location of the dorsal interosseous muscles would indicate that these muscles are essentially neutral with respect to flexion and extension of the metacarpophalangeal joints. But the palmar interossei and the lumbrical muscles course definitely on the palmar side of the axis for flexion and extension of these joints and are therefore mechanically capable of producing flexion. The leverage of the lumbrical muscles for flexion is more favorable than that of the palmar interossei— the former course on the palmar, the latter on the dorsal side of the transverse metacarpal ligament.

When a lumbrical is stimulated by a high intensity electrical current, the result is strong extension of the interphalangeal joints and flexion of the metacarpophalangeal joint to about 80 degrees. But when a low current is used (minimal to produce response), the interphalangeal joints extend but the metacarpophalangeal joint flexes very little or not at all (Backhouse and Catton, 1954). This suggests that the leverage of a lumbrical muscle for extension of the interphalangeal joints is far better than its leverage for flexion of the metacarpophalangeal joint. The high-current experiment also demonstrates that a lumbrical muscle when contracting maximally is capable of shortening effectively through a long range. Such long effective excursion is remarkable when one considers that, under the above experimental conditions, the origin of the lumbrical muscle must be poorly stabilized since the flexor digitorum profundus muscle is inactive.

ELECTROMYOGRAPHIC FINDINGS. When the fist is slowly and lightly closed, the lumbrical muscles have been found electrically silent (Backhouse and Catton, 1954; Long and Brown, 1964). Inactivity of the lumbrical muscles was also demonstrated when resistance was applied to simultaneous flexion of all three finger joints (Backhouse and Catton, 1954). The common conception that the lumbrical muscles actively aid the long finger flexors in closure of the hand must therefore be questioned. A different role for the lumbricals has been suggested by Landsmeer and Long (1965) and again by Long (1968), that these muscles may contribute to metacarpophalangeal flexion by their passive tension. It is pointed out that a contraction of the flexor digitorum profundus exerts traction on the lumbrical muscles in a proximal direction and that, simultaneously, as the interphalangeal joints flex, these muscles are

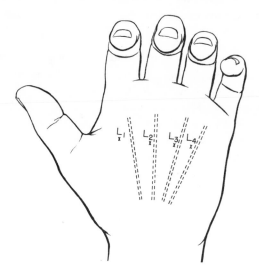

FIG. 53. The muscular portions of the lumbricals are located on the radial side of the tendons of the long finger flexors.

put on a stretch distally. It may well be that under these circumstances the passive tension curve could be used. This contention, for the time being, however, must be looked upon as a hypothesis only. The electromyographic study of Close and Kidd (1969) does not support this theory for they did observe simultaneous lumbrical and deep flexor activity in motions they describe as pinch and grasp. Perhaps the differences noted can be attributed in part to the total force requirement of the hand activity.

PALPATION OF THE INTRINSIC MUSCLES

The muscular portions of the lumbricals are located on the radial side of the tendons of the long finger flexors. In most hands, these tendons are best visible in the clawhand position, that is, when the metacarpophalangeal joints are hyperextended and the interphalangeal joints are flexed (Fig. 53). Identification of the lumbrical muscles by palpation is difficult since these muscles are small and covered by fascia and skin.

The palmar interossei are located deep in the palm of the hand beneath the lumbricals and between the metacarpal bones. They are even less accessible to palpation than the lumbricals. The dorsal interosseous muscles may be palpated from the dorsal side (see p. 111).

COORDINATED ACTION OF THE THREE FINGER JOINTS IN GRASPING

In normal hand closure, all three finger joints flex simultaneously, which enables the palm of the hand to make proper contact with an object grasped. As stated above, the flexor digitorum profundus is the principal muscle employed in light hand closure, apparently acting effectively over all three finger joints simultaneously. However, subjects with long-standing paralysis of the intrinsic muscles, even though the flexor digitorum profundus and superficialis are intact, have an ineffective grasp. Such a subject is still capable of making a fist, but the interphalangeal joints flex first and the metacarpophalangeal joints a fraction of a second later (Fig. 54). Without the intrinsic muscles, some difficulty arises when the subject attempts an activity which requires quick closure of the hand, as in catching a ball. Disturbance of the extrinsic-intrinsic muscle balance eventually results in a "claw" posture of the hand. Changes in capsules and ligaments and atrophy and loss of elastic properties of the intrinsic muscles are part of the picture.

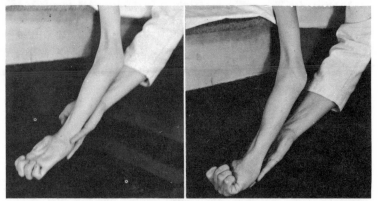

FIG. 54. Manner of closure of fist when intrinsic muscles of hand are para-lyzed. The interphalangeal joints are first flexed by the long finger flexors. Then, in continued action, these muscles flex also the metacarpophalangeal joints, so that the fingers "roll" into the palm. Simultaneous flexion of all finger joints, such as needed in catching a ball, cannot be accomplished.

Opening the Fist

ROLE OF THE WRIST FLEXORS IN EXTENSION OF THE FINGERS

The long extensor muscles of the fingers originate in the forearm and pass over the wrist and then over the metacarpophalangeal joints. If these muscles were to contract in an isolated fashion, they would extend not only the joints of the fingers, but also the wrist. To prevent them from moving the wrist, the wrist flexors contract synergically, keeping the wrist in a neutral position or flexing it. The association between finger extensors and wrist flexors is strong, and it takes concentrated effort to interrupt the linkage.

If complete finger extension is alternated with grasp in rapid succession, it will be observed that the wrist as well as the fingers are in constant motion: flexion of the wrist accompanies finger extension; extension of the wrist occurs when the fist is closed. These combinations are automatic, and the less attention paid to the details of the performance, the more obvious they will be. Note that the wrist movements which take place are in a direction opposite to the finger motions, so that an alternate elongation of the finger extensors and the finger flexors over the wrist is obtained. Such elongation adds to the efficiency of these muscles in extending and flexing the fingers.

PALPATION OF THE WRIST FLEXORS IN EXTENSION OF THE FINGERS

When the fingers are extended, the tendons of the wrist flexors are palpated on the palmar side of the wrist: the flexor carpi radialis and the palmaris longus in the center, the flexor carpi ulnaris near the pisiform bone—all three muscles spring into action. With increased forcefulness of finger extension, increased tension can be felt in the wrist flexors.

THE EXTENSOR ASSEMBLY

The finger joints may be extended in many ways, such as extension of all finger joints simultaneously; extension of the interphalangeal joints with metacarpophalangeal joint flexed (Fig. 55); extension of the metacarpophalangeal joints while the interphalangeal joints are flexed (Fig. 53), and in many in-between positions. For such variations of motion, the extensor digitorum communis is aided by the intrinsic muscles of the hand, the long finger flexors, and by muscles acting upon the wrist. The effect obtained when these muscles combine their actions in different manners is regulated in part by the dorsal aponeurosis, particularly by its proximal portion, which forms the main part of the so-called *aponeurotic sleeve.*

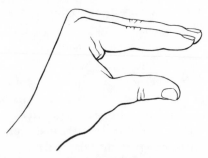

FIG. 55. Flexion of metacarpophalangeal joints, extension of interphalangeal joints.

The muscles which insert into the dorsal aponeurosis are the extensor digitorum communis, extensor indicis proprius, extensor digiti minimi proprius, lumbricals and interossei.

The tendon of the *long extensor* of each finger passes on the dorsum of its respective metacarpophalangeal joint. Having passed this joint, the tendon not only gives off a "central deep ribbon" from its undersurface which acts to extend the joint (Bunnell, 1956), but is also bound to the capsule of the joint. The extensor tendon then continues distally and spreads into a broad aponeurosis which covers the dorsum and partially covers the sides of the proximal phalanx. Three more or less distinct tendon slips, incorporated in the dorsal aponeurosis, may be seen: the central one coursing dorsally to be inserted into the base of the middle phalanx and serving to extend the proximal interphalangeal joint; and the two lateral ones passing on the sides of the phalanx and forming the lateral bands.

The *four lumbrical muscles* pass on the flexor side of the metacarpophalangeal joints and join the dorsal aponeurosis on the radial side of each finger. By means of their attachment to the dorsal aponeurosis the lumbricals are instrumental in extending the two interphalangeal joints.

The *interosseous muscles,* except for the dorsal components of the dorsal interossei, would be expected to flex the metacarpophalangeal joints and, by their insertion into the dorsal aponeurosis, to extend the two interphalangeal joints.

The tendons of the lumbricals and the interossei spread into the extensor aponeurosis by means of transverse and longitudinal fibers, the latter forming part of the lateral bands. Somewhat more distally, the lateral bands on each side of the finger divide as follows: The more central portions course dorsally joining the central portion of the tendon of the extensor digitorum communis to extend the proximal interphalangeal joint; and the lateral portions bypass the proximal interphalangeal joint and then turn dorsally to extend the distal interphalangeal joint.

INTEGRATED ACTION OF EXTRINSIC AND INTRINSIC MUSCLES

Various theories have arisen with respect to interaction of intrinsic and extrinsic muscles in flexion and extension of the digits. Beevor (1903) observed that extension and hyperextension of the metacarpophalangeal joint is carried out by the extensor digitorum communis, but that this muscle has little or no effect on interphalangeal extension, an observation also made by Duchenne (1867). For extension of the interphalangeal joints, both Duchenne and Beevor held that intrinsic muscle action is required. Subjects with paralysis of the intrinsic muscles develop a clawhand and are incapable of extending the interphalangeal joints. In these subjects, an effort to extend all three finger joints simultaneously only results in extreme hyperextension of the metacarpophalangeal joints while the interphalangeal joints remain flexed. Beevor further observed that in paralysis of the intrinsic mucles, if the metacarpophalangeal joints were kept passively flexed, the subjects could then use the extensor digitorum communis to extend the interphalangeal joints. He concluded that "it seems probable that in the clawhand the inability of the extensor digitorum communis to extend the terminal phalanges is due to its energy being expended on the first phalanges, which are not prevented from overextending by the interossei and lumbricales, as these are paralysed."

A widely accepted theory of the interaction of extrinsic and intrinsic muscles in the hand was formulated by Sterling Bunnell, whose extensive experience as a hand surgeon made him well qualified to discuss hand function (1938, 1942, 1956). He stressed in particular the function of the aponeurotic sleeve in coordinating the actions of the extrinsic and intrinsic muscles. The quotations which follow are from Chapter 10 of Bunnell's book *Surgery of the Hand* (1956).

"*Shift of aponeurotic sleeve.* At the base of the finger there is a remarkable mechanism which allows the conjoined tendons of the interossei and lumbricales either to flex the proximal finger joint or to extend the distal two finger joints according to whether the aponeurotic sleeve shifts distalward or proximalward, respectively . . . The dorsal part of the sleeve, in company with the extensor tendon, can be passively made to shift on the phalanx longitudinally 15 mm., but the ventral portion only 3 mm. The dorsal portion, when in ordinary use, shifts on the phalanx about 7 mm., just enough for its thickened portion to lie across the phalanx or over the joint.

"When the sleeve is distalward down the back of the phalanx, the intrinsic muscles can flex the proximal joints, but when the sleeve is drawn proximalward by the action of the long extensor tendon, the sleeve is over the proximal joint itself, thus robbing the intrinsic muscles of their leverage on the phalanx for use in flexion. It is like the shifting of gear . . . When the long extensor stabilizes the proximal joint in extension, the intrinsic muscles extend the two distal joints. They flex the proximal joint only when the long extensor is relaxed.

* * *

"Extension of the distal two finger joints by the interossei and lumbricales is strong when the proximal finger joints are straight or hyperextended but, as they flex to near 45 degrees, the action of the interossei and lumbricales becomes less, and beyond 45 degrees it becomes negligible. During flexion of the proximal joints, the long extensor takes on more and more duty of extending the distal two joints and its maximum action is reached when the proximal joint is three-fourths flexed . . . The gradation between the action of the intrinsic muscles and long extensor is gradual, with the balance of power changing when the proximal joints are at about 45 degrees of flexion."

The theory that the extensor digitorum is instrumental in extending the interphalangeal joints when the metacarpophalangeal joints are flexed appears to be substantiated by observations on patients with paralysis of the intrinsic muscles. However, conclusions drawn from observations on pathological cases cannot necessarily be applied to subjects with normal functioning of the neuromuscular system—this has been convincingly demonstrated by electromyography. A brief review of some of the pertinent electromyographic findings follows (Backhouse and Catton, 1954; Long and Brown, 1964; Landsmeer and Long, 1965; Long, 1968).

The lumbrical muscles do not associate themselves with the flexor digitorum profundus in closure of the fist as has been assumed in the past; they are consistently silent in this activity. In opening of the fist, there is synchronous activity of the extensor digitorum communis and the lumbricals, and the latter muscles exhibit maximal activity. The contraction of the lumbrical muscles extends the interphalangeal joints but simultaneously might draw the tendons of the flexor digitorum profundus distally. This latter muscle has been found electrically silent when the hand is opened, and therefore would offer poor fixation to the origins of the lumbricals. With the tendons of the flexor digitorum profundus drawn distally, digital extension is facilitated as the passive resistance of the profundus is overcome. That such passive resistance is present may be concluded from the semiflexed position of the fingers when the arm hangs relaxed at the side of the body. Earlier investigators (Poore, 1881; Sunderland, 1945; Kaplan, 1953) already suggested this function of the lumbrical muscles but the theory was not universally accepted.

Anatomists have assumed that the interosseous muscles contribute to interphalangeal extension in opening the hand, but this has not been confirmed by electromyography. While in this activity (opening the hand fully but without great force) the lumbrical muscles show high level electrical activity, the interossei show little or no activity.

In performing metacarpophalangeal extension and interphalangeal flexion (Fig. 53) high level activity was registered in the extensor digitorum communis and the flexor digitorum profundus while the flexor digitorum superficialis showed little or no activity. The lumbrical and interosseous muscles were essentially silent. Performance of the opposite motion—metacarpophalangeal flexion with interphalangeal extension (Fig. 55)—was accompanied by high level activity of the lumbricals and the interossei, which muscles thus appear to be the principal ones in this motion. The electrical activity in the extensor digitorum communis varied in individuals from zero to high level. These findings, in part, contradict Bunnell's theory of a gradual shift from intrinsic to extrinsic muscle action in extension of the interphalangeal joints when the metacarpophalangeal joints become more and more flexed. The variable response in extensor digitorum communis demonstrated by electromyography would indicate that some normal subjects, like those with paralysis of the intrinsic muscles, utilize the extensor digitorum communis while others rely more or less exclusively on the intrinsic muscles. Possibly the individual differences are related to the amount of effort employed by the subjects in accordance with the general rule that the more effort that is employed, the more muscles are recruited.

Abduction and Adduction of Digits II-V

NOMENCLATURE

Movements away from the midline of the hand are called *abduction;* movements toward the midline are called *adduction*. The *midline* is a line longitudinally through the center of the forearm and hand and through the middle finger; thus, when the fingers spread apart they are abducted, and when they lie close together they are adducted. The third finger, being in the midline, has radial abduction and ulnar abduction.

RELATION OF ABDUCTION AND ADDUCTION
TO FLEXION AND EXTENSION

Abduction and adduction movements are free when the metacarpophalangeal joints are extended (collateral ligaments are loose); when these joints flex, the fingers automatically adduct, and the range of abduction becomes extremely limited or is absent (collateral ligaments tight). The natural tendency is to abduct the fingers as they extend; it may be said that *extension and abduction belong together,* as do *flexion and adduction.* If the fist is closed and opened in rapid succession, this pattern becomes obvious: the fingers abduct as they extend and adduct as they flex. In slower motions, and with some concentration, it is entirely possible to keep the fingers adducted as they extend. The extension-abduction combination appears to be part of a mass movement which is considerably easier to execute than other combinations.

MUSCLES ACTING IN ABDUCTION OF THE FINGERS

The dorsal interossei, four in number, are responsible for abduction of the second and fourth fingers, and for radial and ulnar abduction of the third finger. The fifth finger has its own abductor, the abductor digiti minimi, located on the ulnar border of the hand and being part of the hypothenar muscle group.

The dorsal interosseous muscles are located between the metacarpal bones, each muscle having a double origin, that is, from the two adjacent bones. The action of the dorsal interosseous muscles as abductors of the fingers may be concluded from their manner of insertion:

First dorsal interosseus—radial side of base of index finger
Second dorsal interosseus—radial side of base of middle finger
Third dorsal interosseus—ulnar side of base of middle finger
Fourth dorsal interosseus—ulnar side of base of ring finger

PALPATION. The muscular portion of the first interosseus is easily observed and palpated in the space between the metacarpal bones of the thumb and the index finger when resistance is applied to abduction of the index finger, by manual resistance or by using a rubber band, as seen in Figure 56. The second, third and fourth dorsal interossei are more difficult to palpate in the narrow spaces between the metacarpal bones, but their insertions at the base of the proximal phalanges may be felt, although some practice is needed to do so. By applying a rubber band around the fingers in various combinations, the action of each of the finger abductors, including the abductor of the fifth finger, may be brought out.

The abductor digiti minimi may be palpated on the ulnar border of the hand.

The extensor digiti minimi, originating above the wrist, inserts at the base of the proximal phalanx in such a manner that it is able

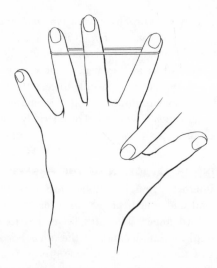

FIG. 56. Palpation of muscular portion of first dorsal interosseus. Rubber band offers resistance to first and fourth dorsal interossei.

both to extend and abduct the little finger. This muscle receives its innervation from the radial nerve. The ability of this muscle to abduct the little finger (in small range) is clearly seen in cases of ulnar nerve paralysis when the hypothenar muscle group is paralyzed. The little finger then tends to maintain a somewhat abducted position, and the subject is unable to adduct it.

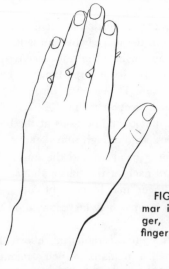

FIG. 57. Testing the palmar interossei of index finger, ring finger and little finger.

MUSCLES ACTING IN ADDUCTION OF THE FINGERS

The palmar interossei are responsible for adduction of the index, ring and little fingers. These muscles, unlike the dorsal interossei, have only a single origin from the metacarpal bone of the digits which they serve. The palmar interossei may be tested by manual resistance to adduction of each finger separately, or by squeezing three small objects between the fingers (Fig. 57). If a piece of paper is slipped between two adjacent fingers and the subject is asked to hold on to it, one palmar and one dorsal interosseous muscle are tested simultaneously.

Some anatomists speak of the deep portion of the flexor pollicis brevis (innervated by the ulnar nerve), or of a division of the adductor pollicis, as the first palmar interosseous muscle. In that case, the index finger is served by the second, the ring finger by the third, and the little finger by the fourth palmar interosseus.

OPPOSITION OF THE LITTLE FINGER

The opponens digiti minimi, aided by the flexor digiti minimi and by the palmaris longus and brevis, is responsible for the motion referred to as opposition of the fifth finger. The movement is not nearly as well developed as that of the thumb with the same name. When both thumb and little finger move toward each other in opposition, "cupping" of the hand results, that is, the hand narrows considerably from side to side (Fig. 58).

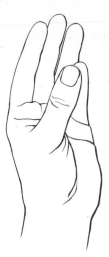

FIG. 58. Opposition of thumb and little finger.

Thumb Movements

The marked mobility which the thumb possesses as compared to the other fingers is made possible, *first*, because the saddle-shaped carpometacarpal joint of the thumb has two degrees of freedom of motion and the capsule is comparatively loose; *second*, because the metacarpal bone of the thumb is not bound to the other metacarpals by ligaments, so that a wide separation between index and thumb can take place; *third*, because the movements which occur at the metacarpophalangeal and interphalangeal joints of the thumb aid substantially to the versatility of thumb movements; and *fourth*, because the many muscles which move the thumb can combine their actions in numerous ways in finely gradated movement combinations.

NOMENCLATURE

There exists a considerable confusion of terms for description of thumb movements, especially for those of the carpometacarpal joint. Movements at this joint have been variously labeled as flexion, extension, abduction, adduction, opposition and reposition, and as taking place either in the plane of the palm or in a plane perpendicular to the palm. To add to the confusion, movements are sometimes defined as related to the entire thumb rather than to movements of separate joints. Clinically, for example, *opposition of the thumb* means the ability to bring the palmar surface of the tip of the thumb in contact with the palmar surfaces of the other digits. Functionally, this is justifiable, but anatomically, each joint has to be dealt with separately.

The *carpometacarpal* joint of the thumb is a saddle joint with two degrees of freedom of motion. If this conception is adhered to, movements at this joint may be defined as *opposition-reposition* and as *abduction-adduction*. The term *flexion-extension* is then reserved for the two distal thumb joints.

The axes of the *carpometacarpal* joint are determined by the shape of the "saddle" of the trapezium; the "rider" is the metacarpal bone. One axis passes longitudinally, the other transversely through the saddle, so that the "rider" may slide from side to side, or tip forward and backward in the "saddle." *Neither of these movements occurs in the plane of the palm.* The custom of defining thumb movements as occurring in the plane of the palm or perpendicular to this plane, therefore, has no anatomical basis.

The *metacarpophalangeal* joint of the thumb, like the corresponding joints of the other digits, has *flexion-extension* and *abduction-adduction*. These movements are oriented to the *plane of the thumb*. They cannot be oriented to the plane of the palm, since flexion and extension of this joint (as well as of the interphalangeal joint) of the thumb can take place in any desired degree of opposition (Fig. 59).

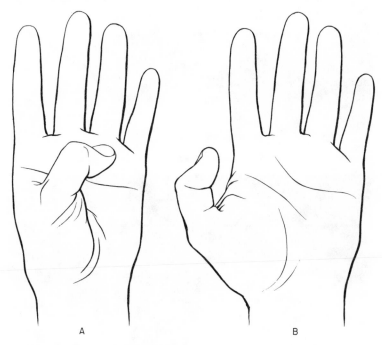

A   B

FIG. 59. Flexion of the thumb refers to interphalangeal and metacarpophalangeal joints and is oriented to the plane of the thumb. It can be performed in all positions between full opposition (A) and full reposition (B). The latter two motions refer to the carpometacarpal joint of the thumb.

MUSCLES ACTING ON THE CARPOMETACARPAL
JOINT OF THE THUMB

All muscles which pass the carpometacarpal joint of the thumb have an influence on its movements. Those muscles which are inserted into the metacarpal bone of the thumb (opponens pollicis,

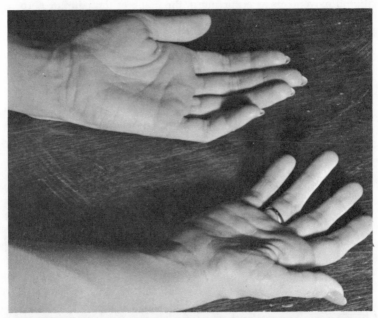

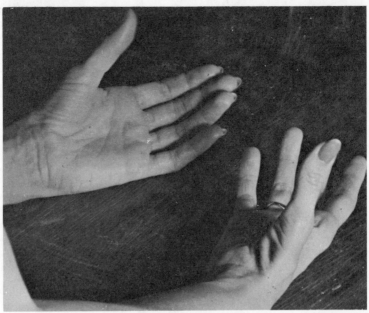

FIG. 60 (see p. 117 for legend).

abductor pollicis longus) are primarily concerned with movement or stabilization of the joint; the muscles which insert into more distal segments act on one or both of the two distal thumb joints as well. To the latter group belong the abductor pollicis brevis, flexor pollicis brevis, adductor pollicis, extensor pollicis longus and brevis, and flexor pollicis longus.

Opposition is performed primarily by the *opponens pollicis* and the *abductor pollicis brevis,* both muscles having approximately the same line of action over the joint. The abductor pollicis brevis is a

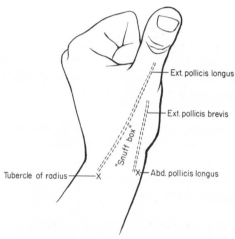

FIG. 61. Anatomical snuff box between tendons of extensor pollicis longus and extensor pollicis brevis.

superficial muscle and it covers the opponens. The two muscles may be palpated in the radial portion of the thenar eminence. The *flexor pollicis brevis* may aid in maintaining opposition, once the joint has been positioned (Fig. 60); the muscle is palpated toward the ulnar side of the thenar eminence.

Reposition is performed mainly by the *extensor pollicis longus* aided by the *extensor pollicis brevis* and *abductor pollicis longus.*

FIG. 60. Partial paralysis, following poliomyelitis, of thenar muscles, particularly opponens pollicis. Upper photograph, Subject is unable to initiate the opposition movement of the thumb. Lower photograph, After thumb has been placed in opposition, subject is capable of maintaining position. It appears as if the flexor pollicis brevis were employed to do so. Note marked atrophy in region of opponens pollicis and abductor pollicis brevis.

The tendon of the *extensor pollicis longus* may be palpated from the tubercle of the radius proximally to its insertion on the base of the distal phalanx. It forms the ulnar boundary of the anatomical "snuff box." The tendon of the *extensor pollicis brevis* is also visible under the skin, forming the radial border of the "snuff box" (Fig. 61). The tendon of the *abductor pollicis longus* lies partially covered by that of the extensor pollicis brevis, but in the wrist region, where the two tendons emerge from their common compartment in the dorsal carpal ligament, the two tendons can usually be separated.

Abduction is performed by the abductor pollicis longus, the extensor pollicis brevis and the abductor pollicis brevis. The movement of *adduction* is executed mainly by the adductor pollicis and part of the flexor pollicis brevis (first palmar interosseus). Under certain circumstances (when the thumb is in a position of complete reposition) the extensor pollicis longus may also adduct.

It should be noted that a rider may slide from side to side in the saddle in various positions of forward and backward tipping of the trunk; similarly, abduction and adduction may be performed in various degrees of opposition and reposition. The muscles activated in abduction-adduction consequently vary in accordance with the amount of opposition present.

MUSCLES ACTING ON THE METACARPOPHALANGEAL JOINT OF THE THUMB

Flexion of the metacarpophalangeal joint of the thumb is performed by the *flexor pollicis brevis* and the *flexor pollicis longus*. Under certain conditions, the abductor pollicis brevis and the adductor pollicis also aid in flexing this joint. These two muscles pass on the flexor side of the joint, inserting into the base of the proximal phalanx of the thumb. They also send expansions to the extensor aponeurosis so that they may act in extension of the interphalangeal joint as well as in flexion of the metacarpophalangeal joint. Note the resemblance with the intrinsic muscles serving the other digits, which also may flex the metacarpophalangeal joint or extend the interphalangeal joints.

Extension of the metacarpophalangeal joint is performed by the extensor pollicis brevis and extensor pollicis longus.

Abduction and *adduction* of the metacarpophalangeal joint of the thumb are performed by the abductor pollicis brevis and the adductor pollicis, respectively, the latter movement being aided by the extensor pollicis longus as its tendon slides toward the ulnar side of the joint.

MUSCLES ACTING ON THE INTERPHALANGEAL JOINT OF THE THUMB

The *flexor pollicis longus* flexes the interphalangeal joint, the *extensor pollicis longus* extends it. Those thenar muscles which send expansions into the dorsal aponeurosis (abductor pollicis brevis, flexor pollicis brevis and adductor pollicis) also aid in extension. These latter muscles may, unaided by the extensor pollicis longus, extend the interphalangeal joint. Such extension has been observed in patients with radial nerve injuries, when extensor pollicis longus and brevis are paralyzed. Strong and Perry (1966) investigated this observation by blocking the nerve to extrinsic muscles of the thumb in 11 subjects and noting the subsequent performance. They examined electromyographically the extensor pollicis longus, abductor pollicis brevis, flexor pollicis brevis and adductor pollicis. Their results showed the abductor pollicis brevis to be the prime extensor when the extensors pollicis longus and brevis were inactive. They observed individual variations in the amount of interphalangeal joint extension and they noted that this extension was accompanied by abduction and medial rotation of the thumb.

COORDINATED MOVEMENTS OF THE THREE THUMB JOINTS

When flexion and extension of the interphalangeal joint of the thumb are carried out without attention being paid to the manner of execution of the motion, the metacarpophalangeal and carpometacarpal joints become involved as well. The former moves in the same direction as, the latter in the opposite direction to, that of the interphalangeal joint. At the onset of the observations, the hand should be relaxed so that the digits assume their natural positions. The carpometacarpal joint will then be in a midposition between opposition and reposition. The interphalangeal and metacarpophalangeal joints will be slightly flexed. If in this position the interphalangeal joint is voluntarily and somewhat forcibly extended, the metacarpophalangeal joint will also extend. This is understandable since the extensor pollicis longus passes on the extensor side of that joint. The carpometacarpal joint will move in the direction of opposition by the action of the thenar muscles, including the opponens pollicis. (The contraction of these muscles may be ascertained by inspection and palpation.) Conversely, flexion of the interphalangeal joint is accompanied by a reposition movement, effected by the extensor pollicis longus, extensor pollicis brevis and abductor pollicis longus; the tensing of the tendons of these muscles should be observed.

Interestingly enough, the functional relationship of the various muscles observed clinically in flexion and extension of the interphalangeal joint of the thumb is reflected by electromyographic studies by Weathersby and associates (1963). In flexion of the interphalangeal joint (performed slowly and without resistance), these investigators recorded activity in the extensor pollicis longus, extensor pollicis brevis and abductor pollicis longus, while the opponens pollicis was silent electromyographically. In extension of the interphalangeal joint of the thumb, the opponens pollicis became active while the abductor pollicis longus and the extensor pollicis brevis were inactive.

The functional advantage of this arrangement is easily recognized. The movements of opposition and reposition performed in conjunction with extension and flexion of the interphalangeal joint, respectively, enable the extensor pollicis longus and the flexor pollicis longus to utilize a favorable portion of the length-tension diagram. A mechanism governing the closing and opening of the fist and serving the same purpose has previously been discussed (see pp. 96 and 104).

The Cleveland research group (Long and associates) is presently engaged in extensive electromyographic studies of the muscles moving the thumb. These studies are expected to further elucidate the functional associations of the extrinsic and intrinsic muscles of the thumb (personal communication to author).

SYNERGIC ACTION OF WRIST MUSCLES IN MOVEMENTS OF THUMB AND LITTLE FINGER

Synergic actions of the wrist muscles should be noted in the following movements:

1. When the little finger is abducted (by abductor digiti minimi), the flexor carpi ulnaris contracts to furnish counter-traction on the pisiform bone (Fig. 62). To prevent the flexor carpi ulnaris from

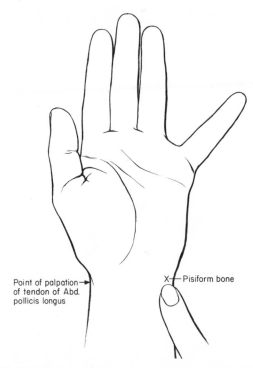

Point of palpation→ of tendon of Abd. pollicis longus

X—Pisiform bone

FIG. 62. Palpation of flexor carpi ulnaris proximal to pisiform bone in abduction of little finger. Abductor pollicis longus contracts synergically.

ulnar-abducting the wrist, the abductor pollicis longus contracts. Its tendon may be palpated as indicated in the illustration.

2. When the thumb is abducted to the position seen in Figure 63, the tensed tendon of the extensor carpi ulnaris is palpated on the opposite side of the wrist. This muscle springs into action to prevent radial-abduction of the wrist by the abductor pollicis longus. The points of palpation of the tendons of both muscles are indicated. The tendon of the abductor pollicis longus lies close to, and is partially covered by, the tendon of the extensor pollicis brevis.

3. When the entire thumb is brought in a palmar direction by the thenar muscles, the palmaris longus aids the movement by tensing the fascia of the palm. To prevent the palmaris longus from flexing the wrist, the extensor carpi radialis brevis contracts (compare p. 91).

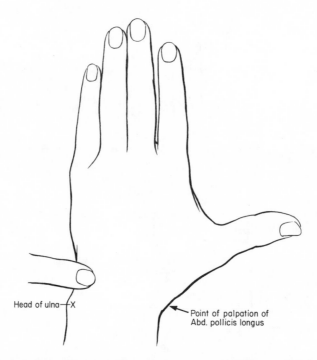

Head of ulna—X

Point of palpation of
Abd. pollicis longus

FIG. 63. Palpation of extensor carpi ulnaris distal to the head of the ulna in abduction of the thumb. Abductor pollicis longus may be palpated as indicated by the arrow.

Peripheral Nerve Injuries Affecting Wrist and Hand

In *radial nerve paralysis* the extensors of the wrist and the long extensors of the digits are paralyzed. A wrist drop develops causing a hand position much like the one seen in Figure 42B. The wrist cannot be actively extended nor can it be stabilized for effective grasp. In the drop-wrist position the digits are partially extended, but such extension is due to tendon action, not to active contraction. The grasp becomes awkward and weak (Fig. 48), but if the wrist is supported in extension by means of a splint, the strength of the grip is good because the flexor muscles are intact.

In *ulnar nerve paralysis*, the habitual position of the hand is a characteristic one (Fig. 64). The fourth and the fifth digits are the ones mostly affected since the flexor digitorum profundus, the lum-

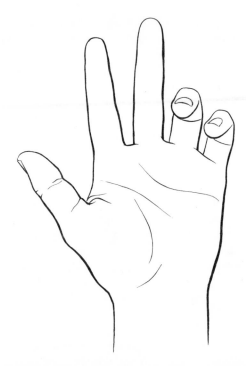

FIG. 64. Characteristic hand posture in ulnar nerve paralysis. The fourth and the fifth fingers cannot be extended, since the long extensors of these digits, in the absence of the intrinsic muscles, cause hyperextension of the metacarpophalangeal joints but are incapable of extending the interphalangeal joints.

bricals and the interossei belonging to these fingers are paralyzed and the hypothenar group is also out of function. The extensor digitorum communis tends to keep the metacarpophalangeal joints of digits IV and V hyperextended. If the examiner holds the metacarpophalangeal joints in a flexed position, however, the subject is capable of extending the interphalangeal joints by using the extensor digitorum communis. Although the abductor of the little finger is paralyzed, this finger is maintained somewhat abducted (by the extensor digiti minimi proprius), but it cannot be adducted because the action of the palmar interosseus cannot be taken over by any other muscle. Abduction and adduction movements of all digits served by the interosseous muscles are affected. Occasionally, however, there is some median nerve supply to the more radially located interossei, in which case some movements may be preserved.

A *median nerve paralysis* causes most of the flexors of the digits to lose action and therefore seriously affects the grasp. The digits on the radial side, having medial nerve supply only, are affected to a greater extent than those on the ulnar side. Flexion and opposition of the thumb are lost, the thenar muscles atrophy, and the entire thumb is pulled in a dorsal direction by the extensor muscles so that it remains in the plane of the palm or is taken even further back toward the dorsum of the hand. The adductor is the only useful thenar muscle, and with the first dorsal interosseous muscle may enable the subject to hold a small object between the thumb and the index finger. Since the flexor digitorum superficialis and profundus, and also the lumbricals of the index and middle fingers, have median nerve supply, these two fingers lose their ability to flex. The index finger tends to remain in an extended position while the middle finger, when the two ulnar fingers flex, may be drawn into some flexion. However, if the subject extends the wrist as far as possible, both index and middle finger may flex by tendon action, but this is not an active grasp.

Types of Prehension Patterns

The hand may be used in a multitude of postures and movements which in most cases involve both the thumb and the other digits. Schlesinger (1919), in investigating designs for terminal devices for artificial arms, studied the versatility of the human hand in grasping and holding objects of various sizes and shapes. He distinguished between twelve different types of prehension, of which the following seven are cited:

Hook grasp. Digits II to V are used as a hook, as in carrying a brief case. The thumb is not necessarily active.

Cylindrical grasp. The entire palmar surface of the hand grasps around a cylindrical object, such as a glass jar. The thumb closes in over the object.

Fist grasp. The fist closes over a comparatively narrow object and the grip is secured by the thumb over the other digits, as in grasping a golf club.

Spherical grasp. The grasp is adjusted to a spherical object, such as a ball or an apple.

Tip prehension. The tip of the thumb is used against the tip of one or the other digits to pick up a small object, such as a bead or a pin.

Palmar prehension. The thumb opposes one or more of the other digits; contact is made by the palmar surfaces of the distal phalanges of the digits. This grip is used to pick up and hold small objects, such as an eraser or a pen. Larger objects may also be held in this manner by widening the grip.

Lateral prehension. A thin object, such as a card, is grasped between the thumb and the lateral side of the index finger.

Schlesinger also points out that some of these prehension types may be compared to simple tools, such as a hook (hook grasp), pincers (tip prehension), and pliers (palmar prehension).

Keller, Taylor and Zahm, cited by Taylor and Schwartz (1955), investigated the frequency of three types of common prehension patterns in picking up objects and holding them for use. Their findings were as follows:

	Palmar	*Tip*	*Lateral*
Pick up	50%	17%	33%
Hold for use	88%	2%	10%

This study showed that palmar prehension is by far the most commonly used type for both picking up and holding small objects. An adaptation of this grasp was subsequently used in the design of terminal devices for artificial arms.

Palmar and tip prehension require that thumb and fingers be opposed to each other, and their frequency in daily activities points to the importance of opposition of the thumb in the human hand.

Patients who have lost their ability to oppose the thumb but who are capable of adducting it, however, may use lateral prehension for grasping and holding small objects. Lateral prehension makes use of pressure of the thumb against the radial side of the index finger, which is held semiflexed. It is the prehension pattern of choice for patients with upper motor neuron lesions, in whom contact on the palmar surface of the fingers causes spasticity of the finger flexors, which is frequently the case. Such patients may be able to release an object held with lateral prehension, while an object which touches the palm of the hand may be very difficult to release.

Strength of Grip

The compressive force in grip is markedly influenced by the position of the wrist. Measurements on normal male subjects at the University of California at Berkeley, quoted by Taylor and Schwarz

(1955) indicate that maximum grip strength is obtained at an arm-hand angle of 140 to 150 degrees, that is, with the wrist in 30 to 40 degrees of extension. At this angle the finger flexors appear to be at their optimum length for producing tension. Grip strength declines rapidly when the wrist is flexed and also when it is in extreme extension. Maximum isometric grip force in three male subjects varied from 100 to 120 pounds.

CHAPTER 5

Shoulder Region

BONES

The osseous parts participating in movements of the upper extremity in relation to the trunk are:

Sternum (breast bone)	(Gr. *sternon,* chest)
Costae (ribs)	(L. *costa,* rib)
Clavicle (collar bone)	(L. *clavicula,* dimin. of *clavus,* key)
Scapula (shoulder blade)	(L. *scapula,* shoulder blade)
Humerus (bone of upper arm)	(L. *humerus,* shoulder)

PALPATION

STERNUM. The sternum may be palpated anteriorly on the thorax from the *xiphoid process* at its lower end to the *manubrium sterni* at its upper end (Gr. *xiphos,* sword, and *eidos,* appearance; L. *manubrium,* handle).

CLAVICLE. The sternal portion of the clavicle is prominent where it articulates with the manubrium sterni (sternoclavicular joint). From this point the clavicle may be followed laterally to its acromial end. The curved shape of this bone should be noted—it is convex forward medially and concave forward laterally. The acromial end, like the sternal end, is enlarged and may be palpated as a protuberance.

SCAPULA. At the tip of the shoulder, the broad *acromion process* which extends like a shelf over the shoulder joint is palpated (Gr. *acron,* tip, and *omos,* shoulder). Anteriorly, its free edge may be felt. Its junction with the clavicle (acromioclavicular joint) lies somewhat protected, being covered by the acromioclavicular ligament; hence, it is difficult to palpate with accuracy. In most individuals, two bony enlargements may be felt in this region, one on the acromion, the other on the clavicle, and in the area between these two prominences is the joint.

By following the acromion process posteriorly the *spine of the scapula* is palpated; it is continuous with the acromion process. The spine of the scapula may be followed transversely across the scapula to the medial (vertebral) border of the scapula where it flattens out to form a smooth triangular-shaped area. The *supraspinous fossa* of the scapula, above the spine, and *infraspinous fossa*, below the spine, should be identified, but since both are filled with muscles their depths cannot be appreciated. This applies particularly to the supraspinous fossa which is not accessible to palpation in its deeper parts. The *medial* (vertebral) *border* of the scapula and its *lateral* (axillary) *border* are easily palpable if the scapular muscles are relaxed. The *inferior angle* of the scapula is the lowest part of the scapula where the medial and lateral borders join. The *superior angle* of the scapula is well covered by muscles and therefore more difficult to palpate. Anteriorly, below the clavicle, where the roundness of the shoulder begins, the *coracoid process* is palpated (Gr. *korax*, raven, curved door handle, and *eidos*, appearance).

The *glenoid cavity* of the scapula (Gr. *glene*, a socket), which receives the head of the humerus, cannot be palpated. This also applies to the *supraglenoid tubercle* which serves as origin for the long head of the biceps, and to the *infraglenoid tubercle* where the long head of the triceps originates.

HUMERUS.   The name *anatomical neck* is applied to a narrow area distal to the articular surface of the humeral head. Fractures in this region tend to occur at the *surgical neck,* below the tubercles. If the humerus is internally rotated while the arm is at the side of the body, the *greater tubercle* of the humerus may be palpated just distal to the acromion process. Once this tubercle has been identified, the palpating fingers may follow its changing position as the shoulder is rotated externally. In full external rotation this tubercle is no longer palpable because it disappears under the heavy portion of the deltoid muscle. The greater tubercle has three facets, serving as insertion for muscles, but these facets cannot be distinguished by palpation. The *lesser tubercle* is best felt when the shoulder is externally rotated and may be followed during internal rotation. The proximal portion of the humerus may also be approached from the axilla but palpation must be done gently because of the many nerves and vessels in this area.

On the proximal portion of the shaft of the humerus the *crest of the greater tubercle* and the *crest of the lesser tubercle* should be noted. Between the two crests is the *intertubercular* (bicipital) *groove.* These structures should be studied on the skeleton as they are difficult to palpate through the muscles. Note the changing position of the intertubercular groove during humeral rotation; in complete external rotation the groove is in line with the acromion process.

JOINTS

The bones of the shoulder region are joined together at three articulations: the clavicle articulates with the manubrium sterni at the *sternoclavicular joint;* the clavicle and the scapula join at the *acromioclavicular joint;* and the humerus articulates with the scapula at the *glenohumeral joint.* During movements of the upper extremity the scapula also slides freely on the thorax, but this scapulo-thoracic relationship can hardly be classified as a joint.

DEFINITION OF SHOULDER GIRDLE MOVEMENTS

Functionally, the sternoclavicular and the acromioclavicular joints must be considered together since both joints contribute to movements of the shoulder girdle. It is customary to speak of the following movements:

Elevation—The shoulder moves in direction toward the ear.

Depression—The reverse movement of elevation. In the upright position, gravity lowers the shoulder girdle as the elevating muscles cease to contract. The term *depression* is mainly applicable when a downward movement is resisted.

Retraction—The shoulder girdle moves in a backward direction, so that the medial border of the scapula approaches the vertebral column. This movement is sometimes referred to as adduction of the scapula.

Protraction—The reverse movement of retraction. This movement is sometimes referred to as abduction of the scapula.

A circling movement may be performed by moving the shoulder girdle upward-forward-downward-backward (involving a combination of elevation, protraction, depression and retraction) or in the opposite direction. During these movements the sternoclavicular joint is the pivot point and the tip of the shoulder moves in a circular path. The scapula, because it articulates with the clavicle at the acromioclavicular joints, adjusts its position and stays close to the thorax.

Upward rotation, usually referred to as upward rotation of the scapula, is the movement which causes the glenoid cavity of the scapula to face forward and upward. The inferior angle of the scapula moves laterally away from the vertebral column, and the entire scapula slides forward on the thorax.

Downward rotation is the reverse of upward rotation. Complete range in downward rotation obtains if the hand is placed in the small of the back, as seen in Figure 67.

STERNOCLAVICULAR JOINT

This is the only joint which connects the upper extremity directly with the thorax. The shoulder girdle, together with the entire upper extremity, is suspended from the skull and the cervical spine by muscles and fascia. The position of this hanging structure is determined partly by the action of gravity and partly by the clavicle, which restricts shoulder girdle movements in all directions, particularly in a forward direction. Cases of absence of the clavicle have been reported in medical literature—these individuals were able to move their shoulders so far forward that the tips of the shoulders almost met in front of the body. If fractures of the clavicle heal with overriding fragments, the posture of the shoulder is permanently altered.

TYPE OF JOINT. The enlarged sternal end of the clavicle and the articular notch of the sternum are separated by an articular disk. Motions thus take place both between the clavicle and the disk and between the disk and the sternum. Many ligaments protect the joint. This double joint has three degrees of freedom of motion.

AXES OF MOTION AND MOVEMENTS. The axis for *elevation and depression* of the shoulder girdle is an oblique one which pierces the sternal end of the clavicle and takes a backward-downward course. Movement about this axis takes place between the sternal end of the clavicle and the articular disk. Owing to the obliquity of this axis, shoulder girdle elevation occurs in an upward-backward, and depression in a forward-downward, direction.

The joint between the articular cartilage and the sternum is involved mainly in *retraction-protraction* of the shoulder girdle. These motions take place about a nearly vertical axis which pierces the manubrium sterni close to the joint.

TRANSVERSE ROTATION OF THE CLAVICLE. According to Inman and associates (1944), about 40 degrees of rotation of the clavicle around its long axis is permitted. This rotation contributes considerably to the total mobility of the shoulder complex.

ACROMIOCLAVICULAR JOINT

TYPE OF JOINT. The acromioclavicular joint is a single arthrodial joint involving the medial margin of the acromion and the acromial end of the clavicle. Individual variations in the shape of the joint surfaces are common. Usually the clavicle overrides the acromion somewhat, in which case the prominence at the acromial end of the clavicle appears quite large.

MOVEMENTS PERMITTED. The joint effect of acromioclavicular and sternoclavicular motions is to permit scapular rotation so that the glenoid cavity may face forward and upward, or downward, as the need may be, while its costal surface remains close to the thorax. Excess acromioclavicular motion is prevented by ligaments.

SHOULDER JOINT (Glenohumeral Joint)

TYPE OF JOINT. The glenohumeral joint is a ball-and-socket joint (also called spheroidal or universal joint) possessing three degrees of freedom of motion. The hemispherical-shaped head of the humerus articulates with the shallow glenoid cavity which is enlarged by a ring of cartilage around its periphery, serving to deepen the joint cavity. The joint capsule is loose to permit wide range of motion. Protection of the joint is provided by the acromion and coracoid processes, and coracoacromial, coracohumeral and other ligaments. Muscular tension is necessary to keep the head of the humerus in proper relation to the glenoid cavity. When the protecting muscles are paralyzed, the weight of the hanging arm tends to separate the head of the humerus from the glenoid cavity, resulting in a subluxation of the joint. It is then possible to palpate the head of the humerus underneath, and below, the acromion process. This clinical observation gives support to the contention that the capsular ligaments are not sufficiently strong or tense to prevent a glenohumeral separation and that muscles play an important role in maintaining the integrity of the glenohumeral joint.

AXES OF MOTION. Conventionally, the movements of the gleno-humeral joint are described as occurring about three axes perpendicular to each other, all of which pass through the center of the head of the humerus. But movements in other directions about any number of oblique axes passing through the head of the humerus may also take place, and the choice of describing movements about three axes is merely one of convenience.

It is customary to use the erect standing position for defining shoulder motions, in which two of the chosen axes are horizontal and one is vertical. The clinical definitions given in the next paragraphs include both scapular and glenohumeral motions so that the entire range of motion may be measured by the arm-trunk angle. To simplify definitions, it is here assumed that the arm moves in relation to the trunk, but it is understood that the trunk may also move in relation to the arm, or both segments may move simultaneously, as in swimming, in climbing a rope and in other activities.

DEFINITIONS OF SHOULDER MOVEMENTS

Flexion of the shoulder takes place in the sagittal plane about a transverse axis through the head of the humerus. The arm is elevated forward and overhead.

Extension of the shoulder is the reverse of flexion. When the arm passes behind the body the movement is known as *hyperextension.*

Abduction of the shoulder is a movement in the frontal plane about a horizontal axis directed dorsoventrally. The arm moves laterally and overhead, the final position being identical with complete flexion.

Adduction of the shoulder is the reverse of abduction. When performed strictly in the frontal plane and the arm is lowered to the side, adduction is arrested by contact with the body. With the arm slightly in front or in back of the body, the movement range increases but then is no longer pure adduction.

The term *horizontal abduction* is often used to indicate a movement in the horizontal plane, starting with 90 degrees flexion and moving laterally to 90 degrees abduction. *Horizontal adduction* is the reverse movement.

External (lateral) *rotation of the shoulder* takes place about an axis longitudinally through the head and the shaft of the humerus. If the arm is hanging at the side of the body, external rotation causes the medial epicondyle to be close to the body and the lateral epicondyle to be away from the body. When the elbow is extended, supination of the forearm and external rotation of the shoulder tend to occur together. External rotation may be isolated from supination by holding the elbow flexed at 90 degrees.

Internal (medial) *rotation of the shoulder* is the reverse of external rotation. Functionally, internal rotation works together with pronation. When it is desirable to isolate internal rotation, the elbow should be flexed to 90 degrees. Complete range of internal rotation is achieved when the hand is placed in the small of the back.

SCAPULOTHORACIC AND SCAPULOHUMERAL
COMPONENTS OF ABDUCTION

As previously mentioned, clinical measurements of abduction of the shoulder refer to the arm-trunk angle, since exact determination of the *scapulohumeral angle* (angle between the spine of the scapula and the long axis of the humerus) is more difficult to obtain. Braune and Fischer (1887) used x-ray photographs to determine the relationship between scapular and glenohumeral motion during abduction. The following data, from Braune and Fischer, quoted by Lantz and Wachsmuth (1935, p. 94) show that motions of both scapula and humerus take place throughout abduction and that glenohumeral contribution exceeds that of scapular contribution:

Arm-trunk Angle (degrees)	Scapular Contribution (degrees)	Glenohumeral Contribution (degrees)
45	17	28
90	36	54
135	57	78
155	60	95

Inman and associates (1944) substantiated the findings that both segments participate throughout the motion. It was found that the early phase of abduction was irregular, but "once 30 degrees of abduction . . . has been reached . . . a ratio of two of humeral to one of scapula obtains; thus between 30 and 170 degrees of elevation (abduction), for every 15 degrees of motion, 10 degrees occurs at glenohumeral joint, and 5 degrees by rotation of the scapula on the thorax."

More recently other investigators (Freedman and Munro, 1966; Doody, Freedman and Waterland, 1970) studied the relative contributions of scapular and glenohumeral movements to scapular plane abduction and they found only slight differences from earlier studies. Movements of upward rotation of the scapula and humeral elevation were simultaneous and the glenohumeral component was almost twice that of scapular rotation. This synchronous movement of scapula and humerus varied for different individuals and some subjects showed a reversal of scapular rotation during the first 30 to 60 degrees. Doody, Freedman and Waterland (1970) used a direct goniometric method of measurement in place of x-ray studies and they investigated, also, the influence of increased resistance on the relationship between scapular and glenohumeral movements. With stress or resistance, the major contribution of scapular rotation occurred in the earlier phase of abduction (from 60 to 90 degrees) and total scapular rotation decreased slightly.

MUSCLES OF THE SHOULDER REGION

The muscles of the shoulder region give fixation to, and produce movements of, the shoulder girdle and control scapulohumeral relationships. All three joints previously discussed, to a variable extent, participate in such movements. The resulting mobility of the shoulder is largely responsible for the ability of using the hand in all desired positions—in front of the body, overhead, behind the body, etc. The muscles of the shoulder girdle also participate significantly in skilled movements of the upper extremity, such as writing, and are essential in activities requiring pulling, pushing and throwing, to mention only a few of the important activities of the upper extremity.

The shoulder region muscles are divided in three groups for study:
- Group I.   Muscles connecting the shoulder girdle with the trunk, the neck and the skull.
- Group II.   Muscles connecting the scapula and the humerus.
- Group III. Muscles connecting the trunk and the humerus, having little or no attachment to the scapula.

Group I.   Muscles from Trunk to Shoulder Girdle

SERRATUS ANTERIOR
Serratus anterior (L. *serra,* saw) is one of the most important muscles of the shoulder girdle. Without it, the arm cannot be raised overhead. *Origin:* By nine muscular slips from the anterolateral as-

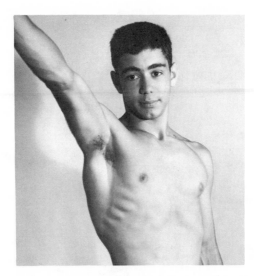

FIG. 65. Showing lower digitations of serratus anterior near their origins on the ribs. The upper portion of the muscle is covered by the pectoralis major.

pect of the thorax, from the first to the ninth ribs—hence its name, the saw muscle. The lowest four or five slips interdigitate with the external oblique abdominal muscle. Lying close to the thorax, the muscle passes underneath the scapula to be *inserted* along the medial border of the scapula. The lowest five digitations converge on the inferior angle of the scapula, attaching to its costal surface. This is the strongest portion of the muscle. *Innervation:* Long thoracic nerve.

Inspection and palpation: On well-developed individuals the lower digitations may be seen and palpated near their origin on the ribs when the arm is overhead (Fig. 65). The middle and upper portions of the muscle are largely covered by the pectoral muscles but may be palpated in the axilla close to the ribs, posterior to the pectoralis major. For palpation of the muscle in the axilla, the subject first elevates the arm to a horizontal position halfway between flexion and abduction, then reaches forward so that the scapula slides forward on the thorax.

TRAPEZIUS

The trapezius is a superficial muscle of the neck and upper back and is accessible for observation and palpation in its entirety. Be-

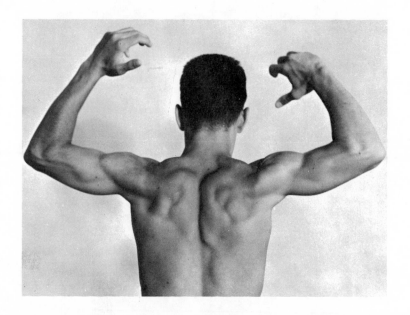

FIG. 66. Showing all portions of the trapezius in contraction. For strong action of this muscle, subject inclines trunk forward. Note also the contraction of posterior deltoid, infraspinatus and teres minor.

cause of its shape, it has been called the "shawl" muscle. The old anatomists named it "musculus cucullaris" (shaped like a monk's hood). The name presently used refers to a geometrical figure. *Origin:* Occipital bone, ligamentum nuchae and spinous processes from C7 to T12. From this widespread origin the muscle fibers converge to be *inserted* into the acromial end of the clavicle, into the acromion, and into the spine of the scapula. The fibers of the upper portion course downward and laterally, those of the middle portion more horizontally, and those of the lower portion obliquely upward. *Innervation:* Spinal accessory nerve.

Inspection and palpation: For observation of the entire muscle in action bilaterally, the subject abducts the shoulders and retracts the shoulder girdles, as seen in Figure 66. This position requires the action of all parts of the trapezius: retraction of the shoulder girdle by the entire muscle, and upward rotation of the scapula by the upper and lower portions of the muscle. If the trunk simultaneously is inclined forward or the subject lies prone, the muscle has to act against the force of gravity to hold the shoulders back, and the intensity of the contraction increases. The upper portion of the trapezius should also be observed and palpated as it performs its functions of shoulder elevation, and the lower portion, also, as it carries out its function of shoulder depression.

RHOMBOIDEUS MAJOR AND MINOR

The rhomboids (Gr. *rhombos,* a lozenge-shaped figure), which connect the scapula with the vertebral column, lie underneath the trapezius. The upper portion is known as the *rhomboideus minor,* the lower (larger) portion as *rhomboideus major. Origin:* Ligamentum nuchae and the spinous processes of the lowest two cervical and the upper four thoracic vertebrae. *Insertion:* Medial border of scapula. The oblique direction of the muscles indicates that they serve to elevate as well as retract the scapula. The rhomboideus major also has the important function of downward rotation of the scapula since it attaches to the inferior angle of the scapula. The rhomboids are made up of parallel fibers, the direction of which is almost perpendicular to those of the lower trapezius. *Innervation:* Dorsal scapular nerve ("the nerve to the rhomboids").

Inspection and palpation: Since this muscle is covered by the trapezius, it is best palpated when the trapezius is relaxed. The subject's hand is placed in the small of the back. The investigator places the palpating fingers underneath the medial border of the scapula, which can be done without causing discomfort to the subject provided that the muscles in this region are relaxed (Fig. 67A). If now the subject raises his hand just off the small of the back, the rhomboideus major contracts vigorously as a downward rotator of the scapula and pushes the palpating fingers out from underneath the medial border of the scapula (Fig. 67B). If the lower trapezius is not too bulky, the direction of the contracting fibers of the rhomboids may be seen under the skin. In the case of trapezius paralysis, the course of the rhomboids is even better observable (Fig. 68).

PECTORALIS MINOR

The pectoralis minor (L. *pectus,* breast bone, chest) is located anteriorly on the upper chest, being entirely covered by the pectoralis major. *Origin:* By four tendomuscular slips from the second to the fifth ribs. These muscular slips converge to be inserted into the coracoid process of the scapula. This gives the muscle a triangular

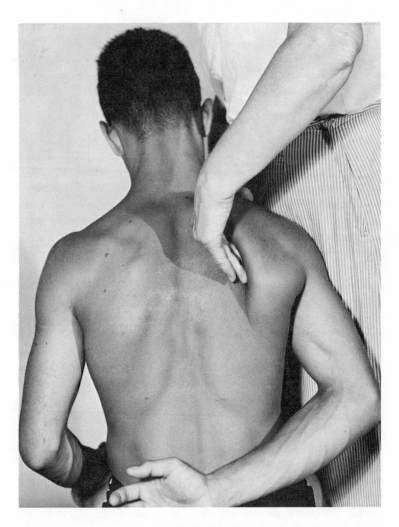

A

FIG. 67A. Palpation of rhomboids. When trapezius and rhomboids are relaxed, examiner's finger may be placed under medial border of scapula.

shape. *Innervation:* Anterior thoracic nerve.

Inspection and palpation: The forearm is placed in the small of the back. In this position the pectoralis major is relaxed, a prereq-

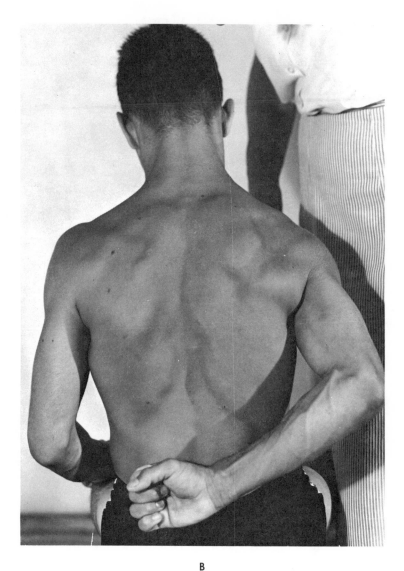

B

FIG. 67B. Palpation of rhomboids. As subject raises hand off the back, examiner's fingers are pushed out from underneath the scapula by the contraction of the rhomboideus major. Note also the contraction of teres major.

uisite for palpation of the pectoralis minor. The examiner places one finger just below the coracoid process of the scapula, as seen in

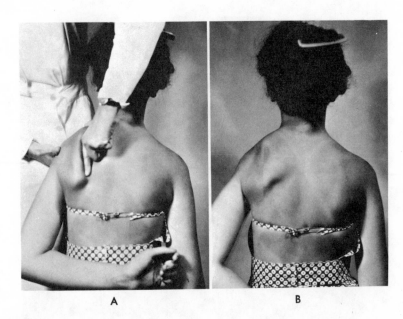

FIG. 68. Testing the rhomboids in subject with trapezius paralysis. When subject raises hand off back, the lower border of the rhomboideus major is well visible. Reproduced by permission of J. Bone Joint Surg. (Brunnstrom, 1941)

Figure 69, pressing down gently so as to let the finger sink in as far as possible.

In this position the finger lies across the tendon of the pectoralis minor, which muscle is relaxed as long as the forearm rests in the small of the back. When the subject raises the forearm off the back, the pectoralis minor contracts and its tendon becomes tense under the palpating fingers.

LEVATOR SCAPULAE

The levator scapulae, as its name indicates, is an elevator of the scapula, an action which it shares with the upper portion of the trapezius and with the rhomboids. *Origin:* Transverse processes of the upper four cervical vertebrae. *Insertion:* Medial border of the scapula, above the spine, near the superior angle. *Innervation:* Dorsal scapular nerve.

Inspection and palpation: The levator is covered by the upper trapezius and in its upper portion also by the sternocleidomastoid

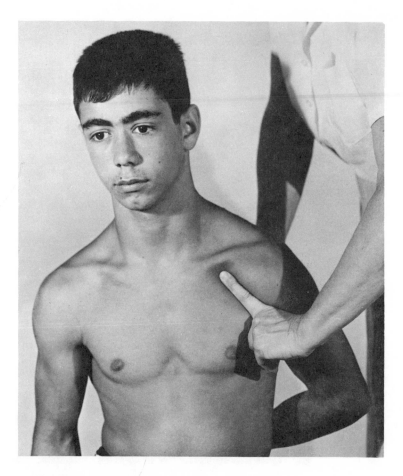

FIG. 69. Palpation of pectoralis minor. With the subject's hand resting in the lumbar region of the back, both pectoralis major and pectoralis minor are relaxed. The tendon of pectoralis minor is palpated below the coracoid process when the subject raises the hand off the back.

muscle. Posteriorly, its border extends to the rhomboideus minor and the splenius muscle of the neck. Ordinarily, in elevation of the shoulder girdle, the upper trapezius and the levator contract together. To bring out levator action with a minimum of trapezius participation, the subject places his forearm in the small of the back, then shrugs the shoulder. The levator may then be palpated in the neck region, anterior to the trapezius but posterior to the sternocleidomastoid muscle (Fig. 70). In the illustration the latter muscle is being pushed

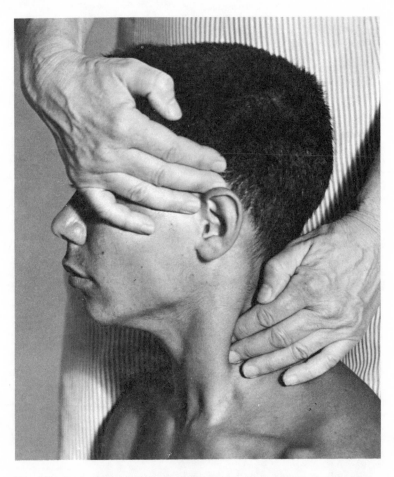

FIG. 70. For palpation of the levator scapulae, the posterior border of the sternocleidomastoid muscle is first identified. The examiner's fingers are then moved a short distance in a posterior direction and the levator palpated as the subject shrugs the shoulder (see text).

forward by the examiner. The palpating fingers are then moved in a posterior direction across the posterior triangle of the neck until they are located at, or beneath, the anterior margin of the upper trapezius. In this region the levator may be identified when the patient shrugs the shoulder. For best result, the patient's hand should be resting in the lumbar region of the back which secures a downward-rotated position of the scapula, favorable for levator action.

It will be recalled that the line of action of the upper trapezius is such as to produce *elevation and upward rotation of the scapula* while the levator, at least in a certain range, has a *downward-rotary* action on the scapula (compare p. 151). Therefore, the latter muscle will more likely be utilized as an elevator when elevation is carried out with the scapula in a downward-rotated position, as in shrugging the shoulder when the hand is behind the body. A comparatively isolated action of the levator may be obtained if the shrug is made briefly and quickly and in short range. If much effort is exerted in raising the shoulder and if the elevated position is maintained, the trapezius will contract in spite of above precautions.

Inspection and palpation of the sternocleidomastoid muscle will be discussed on page 258.

SUBCLAVIUS

This small muscle, as its name indicates, is located underneath the clavicle, and it connects the clavicle to the first rib. From its *origin* on the first rib the fibers course laterally to be *inserted* into the lower surface of the clavicle. The muscle is difficult to palpate.

The muscles of Group I course from the skull, the neck and the rib cage to the shoulder girdle. Most of these muscles insert into the scapula and are thus concerned not only with stabilization, but also with movements of this bone. The subclavius muscle, having a very short range of contraction, is concerned mainly with stabilization.

Discussion of Function of Muscles of Group I

SUPPORT OF THE UPPER EXTREMITY

It has been pointed out previously that the shoulder girdle is suspended from the skull and neck by means of muscles and fascia, and that the only joint connecting the upper extremity with the trunk is the sternoclavicular joint. Several muscles are involved in this suspension and the same muscles also act in elevation of the shoulder girdle.

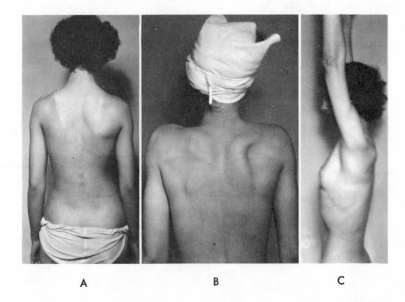

A   B   C

FIG. 71. Left trapezius paralysis of long duration due to injury to spinal accessory nerve. A, In the relaxed standing position, the scapula has a downward-rotated position. The superior angle of the scapula is seen as a protuberance under the skin. The distal portion of the clavicle is visible. B, In spite of the loss of the upper trapezius, the shoulder girdle can be elevated quite well (by the levator scapulae and the rhomboids). Note neck contour. C, The serratus anterior without the aid of the trapezius is capable of rotating the scapula upward full range so that the arms may be elevated above the head. This patient experienced no difficulty in doing so.

TRAPEZIUS. Those portions of the trapezius, which attach to the acromial end of the clavicle and to the acromion process, normally support the shoulder girdle and prevent sagging of the shoulder. When the trapezius is paralyzed, this support is missing and the shoulder slopes down more than it would normally (Brunnstrom, 1941). The weight of the arm tends to draw the tip of the shoulder down, causing the scapula to rotate downward beyond its normal hanging position (Fig. 71A). The leverage action of the weight of the arm on the clavicle may cause a subluxation of the sternoclavicular joint (Fig. 72).

In spite of paralysis of the trapezius, the shoulder girdle can be elevated without difficulty (Fig. 71B). The levator scapulae and the rhomboids are capable of doing so without the aid of the upper trapezius.

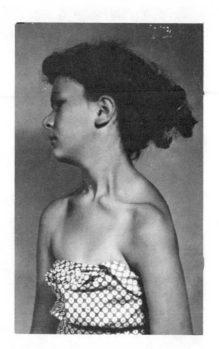

FIG. 72. Paralysis of trapezius. Note subluxation of sternoclavicular joint and sharp outline of posterior border of clavicle, also skin fold in anterior axillary region, characteristic of trapezius paralysis. Reproduced by permission of J. Bone Joint Surg. (Brunnstrom, 1941)

DEPRESSION OF THE SHOULDER GIRDLE

In the upright position, when the elevators of the shoulder girdle release their tension the shoulder is lowered by the weight of the limb. Some additional lowering may be brought about by deliberately depressing the shoulder and, when this is done, a considerable tension is experienced in muscles of the trunk, both in front and in back. The *lower portion of the trapezius* then springs into action and simultaneously the *latissimus dorsi* and the *lower portion of the pectoralis major* are felt contracting. These two latter muscles apply their action not to the scapula but to the humerus.

Such action of depression is utilized in push-ups on parallel bars, in crutch walking, and in getting up from the sitting position when the arms aid the motion by pushing down on the chair.

PROTRACTION OF THE SHOULDER GIRDLE

This movement is effected mainly by the *serratus anterior* which pulls the scapula forward on the rib cage, and also by the *pectoralis major* exerting its pull on the humerus. In protraction of the shoulder

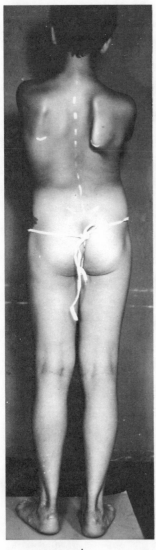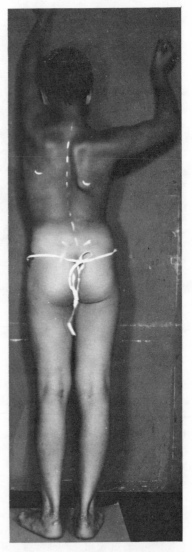

A   B

FIG. 73. Isolated paralysis of serratus anterior. A, Forward reach is poor. The scapula fails to slide forward on the rib cage and there is a typical winging of its medial border. B, In retraction of the shoulder girdle, the medial border of the scapula does not stay close to the rib cage. The right arm cannot be raised overhead since the trapezius does not provide sufficient upward rotation of the scapula. Reproduced by permission of J. Bone Joint Surg. (Brunnstrom, 1941)

girdle with the arms at the side of the body, the action of the two muscles can hardly be isolated. The two muscles also act simultaneously in reaching forward with the arm elevated to a horizontal position. If the reaching is done obliquely outward, however, the pectoralis ceases to contract and the serratus assumes the responsibility alone. When the serratus is paralyzed and forward reaching is attempted (Fig. 73A), a typical "winging" of the medial border of the scapula is seen and the scapula fails to slide forward on the rib cage (Brunnstrom, 1941).

RETRACTION OF THE SHOULDER GIRDLE

Retraction of the shoulder girdle is carried out by the combined action of the *trapezius* and the *rhomboids*. The upward rotary action of the trapezius is counteracted by the downward rotary action of the rhomboids, and by the weight of the arm applied to the tip of the shoulder. The tendency of the upper trapezius and the rhomboids to elevate the shoulder girdle is checked by the depressor action of the lower trapezius and by the weight of the arm. The result is that the scapula moves backward on the rib cage, with the medial border remaining approximately parallel to the vertebral column. Normally, the serratus anterior also plays a part in this motion by keeping the medial border of the scapula close to the rib cage. That this is so may be deducted from observing the effect of serratus paralysis on retraction of the shoulder girdle (Fig. 73B).

When the arms are elevated to a horizontal position (i.e., the scapula is rotated partially upward) and the trunk is inclined forward, retraction of the shoulder girdle requires strong action by the trapezius (Fig. 66). A subject with trapezius paralysis is unable in this position to hold the scapula back (Fig. 74).

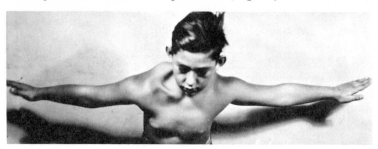

FIG. 74. Paralysis of the right trapezius. Subject is unable to retract the shoulder girdle when the trunk is inclined forward. Reproduced by permission of J. Bone Joint Surg. (Brunnstrom, 1941)

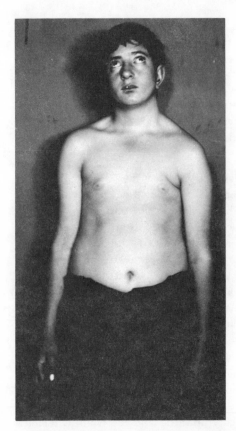

FIG. 75. Partial paralysis of left trapezius. Note fold in skin anterior to axilla.

The effect of loss of the trapezius as a retractor of the shoulder girdle is also seen in erect standing with the arms hanging at the sides. The shoulder girdle then tends to slide somewhat forward, causing a fold in the skin near the axilla (Fig. 75). Such a fold is particularly noticeable on obese individuals.

UPWARD ROTATION OF THE SCAPULA

In the erect position with the arms at the sides, the medial border of the scapula is more or less parallel to the vertebral column. When the arm is raised overhead, the scapula rotates upward while simultaneously sliding forward on the rib cage, so that its medial border assumes an oblique position and its inferior angle comes to lie approximately in the axillary line. The serratus anterior and the trapezius work together to bring about this movement. These muscles also act together to give fixation to the scapula in any partially upward rotated position that the occasion may demand.

The serratus and trapezius both have definite functions to fulfill but, as far as upward rotation of the scapula is concerned, the serratus appears to be the more important of the two. When the serratus is paralyzed, the subject is unable to raise the arm overhead, as the trapezius cannot bring about enough upward rotation for complete abduction (Fig. 73B). On the other hand, when the trapezius is paralyzed and the serratus intact, the arms can be raised overhead without difficulty (Fig. 71C).

If both trapezius and serratus are paralyzed, the scapula has lost its most important stabilizing muscles and its position will be determined mainly by the weight of the arm acting at the tip of the shoulder. When such a subject stands with the arms relaxed at the

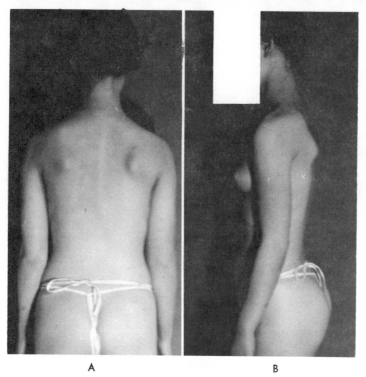

A   B

FIG. 76. Bilateral paralysis of trapezius and serratus anterior. The scapulae assume downward-rotated positions (A) and also tip forward so that the inferior angles protrude backward (B).

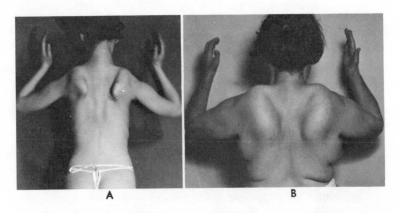

A   B

FIG. 77. Bilateral paralysis of trapezius and serratus. Maximum elevation of the arms of which these subjects are capable is demonstrated. Note
downward rotated position of scapulae. Illustration A is reproduced by permission of J. Bone Joint Surg. (Brunnstrom, 1941)

sides, the scapula assumes a downward rotated position and also
tips forward so that its inferior angle protrudes backward (Fig. 76).
The effect of bilateral paralysis of the trapezius and the serratus
on abduction of the shoulders is seen in Figure 77. When flexion or
abduction of the shoulders is attempted, satisfactory *glenohumeral*
motion takes place, but the scapula rotates *downward* instead of
upward. The result, in terms of arm elevation, is extremely poor. The
deltoid in this instance becomes a downward rotator of the scapula as
it exerts traction on the acromial process in a distal direction. Such
action of the deltoid, of course, never occurs under normal conditions owing to synergic action of the upward rotators of the scapula.

DOWNWARD ROTATION OF THE SCAPULA

When resistance to the downward movement of the arm is encountered (as in swimming the crawl, pulling down a window, using
an overhead pulley to lift a weight, or in chinning oneself), the
downward rotators of the scapula (together with the shoulder adductors and extensors) come into action. Manual resistance may
also be applied to bring out action of the downward rotators. Ideally,
such resistance should be applied to the scapula, but if this proves
difficult, shoulder adduction may be resisted.

The most important muscle for downward rotation of the scapula
is the *rhomboideus major*. This muscle, because of its attachment

to the lower portion of the medial margin of the scapula, maintains a downward rotary action throughout the range of motion. The *rhomboideus minor* downward rotates in the early range (from the fully upward rotated position) but its rotary effect decreases as the movement progresses: when the medial border of the scapula is vertical, the rotary effect becomes *nil;* beyond this point, the rhomboideus minor retracts and elevates the scapula without rotation. The *levator scapulae,* like the minor rhomboid, has a downward rotary action in the early range, then loses it to become an elevator of the scapula exclusively.

In the last range of motion, downward rotation proceeds beyond the vertical position of the medial border of the scapula. In this range the scapula also tips forward by the combined actions of the rhomboideus major in back and the *pectoralis minor* in front, the latter exerting downward traction on the coracoid process.

It should also be recalled that the *latissimus dorsi,* to a greater or lesser extent, attaches to the inferior angle of the scapula; sometimes this angle is held in place by a pocket formed by the fascia around the latissimus. Thus the latissimus may act on the scapula in the sense of downward rotation as it contracts in adduction and extension of the shoulder.

Group II. Muscles from Shoulder Girdle to Humerus

DELTOID

The deltoid (Gr. *delta,* the letter △ and *eidos,* resemblance) is a superficial muscle of the shoulder consisting of three parts: *anterior, middle,* and *posterior.* The muscle fits over the glenohumeral joint like the upper portion of a sleeve, covering the joint on all sides except in the axillary region. *Origin:* The acromial end of the clavicle, the acromion process and the spine of the scapula. From this widespread origin the three portions of the muscle converge to be *inserted* into the deltoid tuberosity, a rather rough area about halfway down the shaft of the humerus. *Innervation:* Axillary nerve.

Inspection and palpation: The muscle is covered by skin only and may therefore be observed and palpated in its entirety. The characteristic roundness of the normal shoulder is due to the deltoid muscle. All parts of the deltoid are easily identified in Figures 36 and 37.

The *anterior deltoid* may be observed and palpated when the arm is held in a horizontal position (Fig. 78). Note that its inferior border lies close to the upper portion of the pectoralis major. The anterior deltoid contracts strongly when horizontal adduction is resisted.

The *middle deltoid* has the best anatomical position for abduction and is seen contracting whenever this movement is carried out or the abducted position is maintained.

The *posterior deltoid* contracts strongly when the shoulder is hyperextended against resistance, or resistance is given to horizontal abduction. The inferior border of the posterior portion of the deltoid has a close relation to the long head of the triceps and to the teres muscles (Figs. 38, 83). Isolated action of the posterior deltoid may be seen in Figure 79. The patient (post-poliomyelitis) had extensive paralysis of the shoulder muscles, including the middle and anterior portions of the deltoid, while the posterior portion was more or less preserved.

The three portions of the deltoid should be observed in action while horizontal abduction and adduction are performed and in pulling and pushing activities. It will then be seen that the anterior

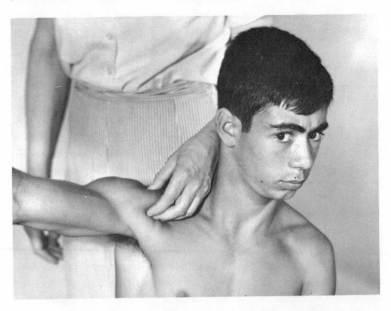

FIG. 78. The examiner grasps around the anterior portion of the deltoid, separating it from the middle deltoid and from the pectoralis major.

Clinical Kinesiology

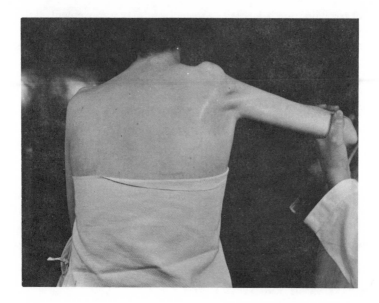

FIG. 79. Isolated action of posterior deltoid in post-poliomyelitis patient. Examiner holds arm abducted while patient pushes back against resistance.

and posterior portions often act antagonistically—the anterior portion exerting traction forward, the posterior portion backward—on the arm.

SUPRASPINATUS

As its name indicates, this muscle is located above the spine of the scapula. It is hidden by the trapezius and the deltoid, the trapezius covering its muscular portion, the deltoid its insertion. *Origin:* Supraspinous fossa of the scapula, which it completely fills. The muscle fibers converge toward the tip of the shoulder to form a short tendon which passes underneath the acromion and which adheres to the capsule of the shoulder joint. *Insertion:* The uppermost facet of the greater tubercle of the humerus. *Innervation:* Suprascapular nerve.

Palpation: The deepest portion of the supraspinatus lies too deep in the supraspinous fossa to be palpated, but its more superficial fibers may be felt through the trapezius. The spine of the scapula is first identified, and the palpating fingers are placed above the spine (they should be moved to various positions so that the best spot for palpation is located). A quick abduction movement in short range is carried out and a momentary contraction of the muscle is felt. In wider range of abduction the supraspinatus is more difficult to palpate because the trapezius becomes increasingly tense and it is then not easy to distinguish one muscle from the other.

It is suggested that palpation of the supraspinatus also be done with the subject prone and the arm hanging over the edge of the table. In this position, the scapula has moved forward on the rib cage by the weight of the arm and is already partially upward rotated. When abduction is carried out in this position, a contraction of the supraspinatus muscle may be felt with little or no interference by the trapezius. The supraspinatus may also be palpated when the subject lifts a heavy briefcase or the like, preferably with the trunk inclined forward. As the weight of the object exerts its downward traction, the supraspinatus becomes tense, apparently for the purpose of preventing excessive separation of the glenohumeral joint.

INFRASPINATUS AND TERES MINOR

These two muscles, although supplied by two different nerves, are described together because they are closely related in location and action. *Origin:* Infraspinous fossa and lateral border of the scapula. The infraspinatus lies closest to the spine of the scapula and occupies most of the infraspinous fossa. The teres minor (L. *teretis,* round and long) takes its origin mainly from the lateral border of the scapula. *Insertion:* The greater tubercle of the humerus, the infraspinatus into its middle facet, the teres minor into its lower (posterior) facet. The tendons of both muscles are adherent to the capsule. *Innervation:* Infraspinatus by the suprascapular, teres minor by the axillary nerve.

Inspection and palpation: The largest parts of the infraspinatus and the teres minor are superficial and may be palpated; some portions are covered by the trapezius and the posterior deltoid. In order to have as large parts of the muscles as possible available for palpation, the arm must be away from the body and the posterior deltoid must be relaxed. This is accomplished if the subject lies prone or stands with the trunk inclined forward and if the arm hangs vertically (Fig. 80). The margin of the posterior deltoid is first identified. The palpating fingers are placed below the deltoid on the scapula, near its lateral margin. While the subject maintains the arm in a vertical position, he externally rotates the shoulder by turning the

Clinical Kinesiology

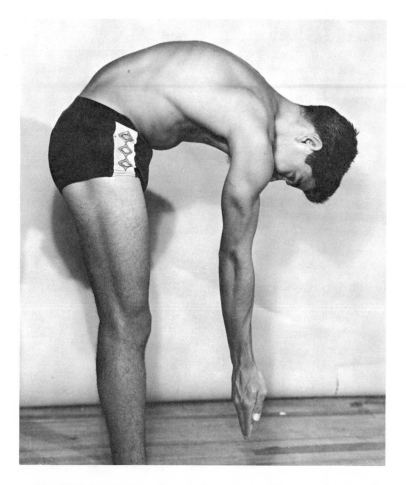

FIG. 80. Infraspinatus and teres minor may be felt contracting near the lateral border of the scapula when the shoulder is externally rotated. Vertical position of arm allows activation of these two muscles in a rather isolated fashion.

palm forward. The two muscles then rise under the palpating fingers, the teres minor being felt next to the infraspinatus, but further away from the spine of the scapula than the infraspinatus. External rotation in this position requires only a mild contraction of these muscles, and consequently they do not show beneath the skin in the illustration. A more vigorous contraction is seen in Figure 66, where a large number of other muscles are also activated.

SUBSCAPULARIS

The subscapularis is located underneath the scapula, close to the rib cage, but it is not attached to the rib cage. The smooth connective-tissue covering of the subscapularis provides a sliding surface

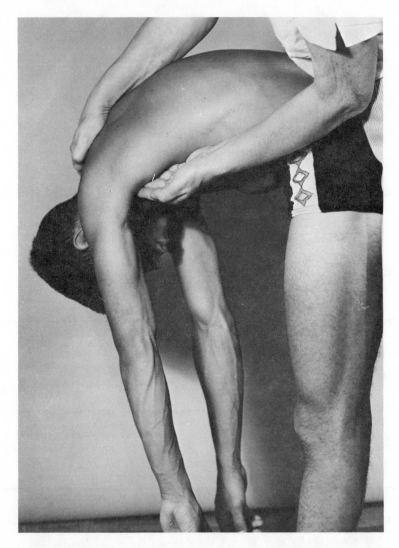

FIG. 81. Subscapularis is palpated in internal rotation of the shoulder. The palpating fingers are placed in the axilla and are moved in direction toward the costal surface of the scapula.

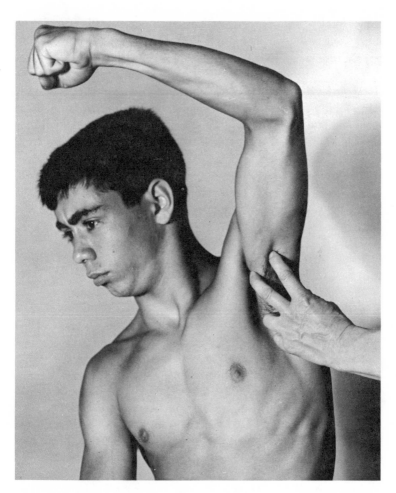

FIG. 82. Identification of coracobrachialis. This muscle emerges from underneath the inferior border of the pectoralis major, where it lies close to the tendon of the short head of the biceps.

for the scapula on the rib cage. *Origin:* Costal surface of scapula. Fiber bundles converge toward the axilla to form a broad tendon which passes over the anterior aspect of the capsule of the gleno-humeral joint. *Insertion:* The lesser tubercle of the humerus and the shaft below the tubercle. *Innervation:* Subscapular nerves.

Palpation: With the subject in the erect standing position the mus-cle cannot very well be reached for palpation, but if the trunk is inclined forward so that the scapula slides forward on the rib cage by the weight of the hanging arm, a portion of this muscle may be palpated. The fingers are placed in the axilla anterior to the latissimus dorsi, and with gentle pressure are moved in the direction of the costal surface of the scapula. With the arm hanging vertically, the subject internally rotates the shoulder by turning the palm backward and laterally (Fig. 81). The firm round belly of the subscapularis can then be felt rising under the palpating fingers. If a person wishes to feel the muscle on himself, the thumb is used for palpation. As far as can be ascertained by palpation, the size of the muscle varies considerably from person to person. According to Fick (1911, p. 82) the subscapularis has a cross section approximately equal to that of the middle deltoid, which indicates that it is a muscle of considerable size.

"CUFF MUSCLES"

The shoulder joint permits a larger range of motion than any other joint in the body. Such wide range is made possible by the shallowness of the glenoid cavity and the relative looseness of the joint capsule. The acromion, the coracoid process and various strong ligaments, such as the coraco-acromial, coracohumeral and glenohumeral ligaments, provide protection for the joint. Those muscles whose tendons are blended with the capsule, namely, the *supraspinatus,* the *infraspinatus* and the *teres minor,* protect the joint by reinforcing the capsule. The tendon of the *subscapularis,* although separated from the capsule, guards the joint anteriorly. These four muscles are known as the "cuff muscles." Note that they insert close to the joint, into the greater and lesser tubercles of the humerus. In a wider sense, all muscles around the shoulder joint aid in protecting it, but those located closest to the joint are particularly important.

TERES MAJOR

The teres major is located at the axillary border of the scapula near the teres minor. It is round like the minor, but larger. *Origin:* Inferior angle of scapula. The muscle fibers course upward and laterally to be *inserted* with a strong broad tendon into the crest of the lesser tubercle of the humerus. *Innervation:* Subscapular nerves

Inspection and palpation: The muscular portion of the teres major is well accessible to palpation, but its tendon of insertion is not. There are many ways of demonstrating and palpating the teres major. It acts in most pulling activities when the shoulder is extended or adducted against resistance. If the examiner gives manual resistance to adduction, as seen in Figure 38, the muscle may be palpated lateral to the inferior angle of the scapula. In this illustration, resistance is given simultaneously to extension of the elbow and adduction of the shoulder so that the triceps as well as the teres major contracts. The teres major is also seen in Figure 83.

CORACOBRACHIALIS

Origin: Coracoid process of scapula. *Insertion:* Medial surface of humerus, about halfway down the shaft of the humerus. *Innervation:* Musculocutaneous nerve.

Inspection and palpation: Part of this rather thin muscle is covered by the deltoid and the pectoralis major. The coracobrachialis may be palpated in the distal portion of the axillary region if the arm is elevated above the horizontal, as seen in Figure 82. It emerges from underneath the inferior border of the pectoralis major where it lies medial to, and parallel with, the tendon of the short head of the biceps. The biceps is first identified by supination of the forearm; the palpating fingers then follow the short head of the biceps proximally until the muscle tapers off, and this is the height best suited for palpation of the coracobrachialis. In the illustration the subject is bringing his arm in a direction toward the head.

BICEPS AND TRICEPS

These two muscles do not belong to the scapulohumeral group, since they do not insert into the humerus; however, the two heads of the biceps and the long head of the triceps cross the shoulder joint and therefore act on it. It should be recalled that the heads of the biceps originate from the supraglenoid tubercle and from the coracoid process, respectively, and that the triceps originates from the infraglenoid tubercle.

Group III. Muscles from Trunk to Humerus

These muscles take their origin on the trunk and insert into the humerus, having little or no attachment to the scapula. They act primarily on the humerus, but indirectly also affect the position of the shoulder girdle. There are only two muscles in this group, the *latissimus dorsi* and the *pectoralis major,* both acting in adduction and internal rotation of the shoulder.

LATISSIMUS DORSI

The name is derived from the Latin *latus,* meaning broad, *latissimus* being the superlative of *latus.* This muscle is the broadest

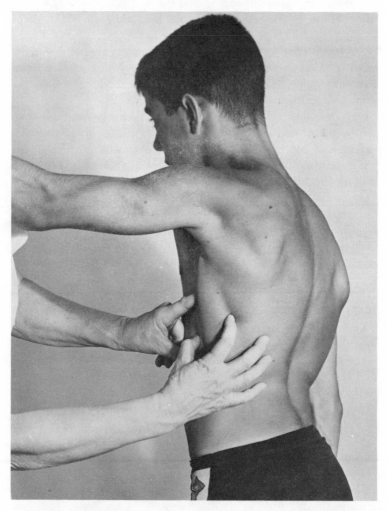

FIG. 83. Palpation of the lower portion of the latissimus dorsi. The subject presses downward on the examiner's shoulder. The teres major may also be seen contracting strongly.

muscle of the back and the lateral thoracic region. It lies superficially, except a small part which is covered by the lower trapezius. *Origin:* Spinous processes of the thoracic vertebrae from T6 downward; dorsolumbar fascia; crest of ilium (posterior portion), and the lowest ribs, here interdigitating with the external oblique abdominal muscle. The fibers converge toward the axilla, some fibers passing over or near the inferior angle of the scapula, often adhering to it. The tendon of *insertion* courses in the axilla and attaches to the crest of the lesser tubercle of the humerus, proximal to that of the teres major. *Innervation:* Thoracodorsal nerve.

Inspection and palpation: The largest part of this muscle is thin and sheetlike, which makes it difficult to distinguish from the fascia and from the deeper muscles of the back. Laterally, in the axillary line and where the fibers converge, the muscle has considerable bulk and here it is easy to observe and palpate (Fig. 83). The latissimus and the teres major contract when adduction or extension of the shoulder is resisted as seen in the illustration, where the subject is pressing down on the examiner's shoulder. The latissimus forms the posterior fold of the axilla. Its relation to the teres major and the long head of the triceps in this region should be noted.

PECTORALIS MAJOR

Its name (L. *pectus,* breast bone, chest) indicates that it is a large muscle of the chest. It has an extensive origin but does not cover nearly as large an area as the latissimus dorsi. *Origin:* Clavicle (sternal half), sternum and costal cartilages of the second to seventh ribs, and the aponeurosis over the abdominal muscles. The muscle is usually described as consisting of three parts: the clavicular, sternocostal and abdominal. From the standpoint of action, it suffices to think of it as having an *upper portion* (clavicular) and a *lower portion* (sternocostal and abdominal). Because of its wide origin and the convergence of its fibers toward the axilla, the muscle takes the shape of a fan. *Insertion:* Crest of the greater tuberosity of the humerus, on an area several inches long. Before reaching its insertion, the tendon bridges the intertubercular (bicipital) groove. The manner in which the muscle fibers approach their insertion should be noted—the tendon of insertion appears to be twisted around itself, so that the uppermost fibers insert lowest on the crest and the lower fibers more proximally. *Innervation:* Medial and lateral anterior thoracic nerves.

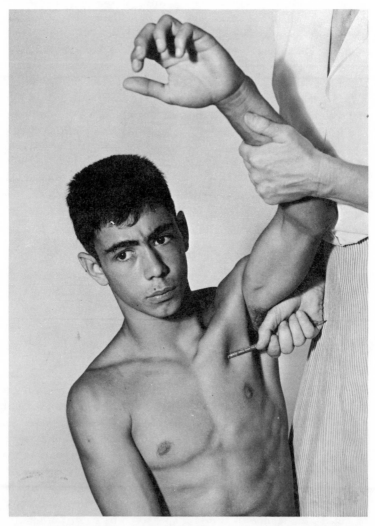

FIG. 84. The upper portion of the pectoralis major is seen contracting as the subject is pulling his arm in direction toward his head against resistance. A pencil has been placed across the lower portion of pectoralis major to show that it is relaxed.

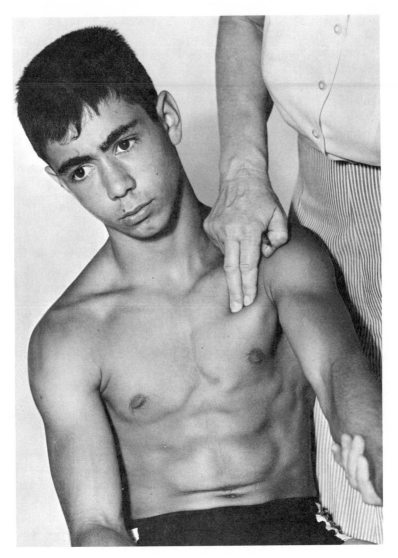

FIG. 85. The lower portion of the pectoralis major contracts as the subject adducts the arm against resistance. The examiner's fingers are separating the lower portion from the upper.

Inspection and palpation: The muscle is easily observed and palpated since it is superficial and of considerable bulk. It is best palpated where the fibers converge toward the axilla. The entire muscle contracts when horizontal adduction is resisted, as in pressing the palms together in front of the body.

The *upper portion* acts separately if the arm is brought obliquely upward toward the head against resistance, as seen in Figure 84. A pencil has been placed across the lower portion of the muscle to show that it is not contracting. The *lower portion* contracts separately when the arm is adducted in a lower position (Fig. 85). The examiner's fingers are placed across the upper portion to show that it is relatively relaxed. The external oblique abdominal muscle is also seen contracting (note its interdigitations with the serratus anterior).

Discussion of Function of Muscles of Groups II and III

Muscles of Group II (connecting the scapula and humerus) are concerned with movements of the shoulder joint and may be thought of as primarily moving the humerus in relation to the scapula, although the reverse may also take place (Fig. 77).* In moving the humerus the muscles of Group II work synergically with muscles of Group I which stabilize or move the scapula in relation to the thorax. Observation of the relative length of lever arms of scapular and humeral muscles shows those of the deltoid and supraspinatus to be small while those of the caudal portion of the serratus anterior and the cranial part of the trapezius are considerably longer. This suggests that scapular muscles are organized for force and that the deltoid and supraspinatus are organized for movement of greater range (Doody, Freedman and Waterland, 1970). The effect of length-tension relationships of these muscles is apparent also. Simultaneous movements of the scapula and humerus enable the muscles of Group II to move the shoulder joint through a large range while maintaining relative lengths since they are continuously being elongated by the scapular movement. By means of this arrangement, the muscles maintain their strength through a large range. The effectiveness of the scapulohumeral muscles, therefore, depends a great deal upon the scapulothoracic muscles. Without these muscles, arm movements are severely affected.

Muscles of Group III (from the trunk to humerus) act mainly on the humerus, having a firm fixation on the trunk. Under certain circumstances, they may move the trunk in relation to the humerus.

*Cross sections and work capacities of muscles passing the glenohumeral joint are given in Table VII in the Appendix.

ABDUCTION OF THE SHOULDER

The *deltoid* and the *supraspinatus* are the most important muscles acting in abduction of the shoulder. When the shoulder is fully externally rotated, the *long head of the biceps* may also aid in abduction. The shoulder abductors also aid in the suspension of the humerus, preventing glenohumeral separation by the weight of the upper extremity and of objects carried in the hand. Electromyographic studies indicate that the supraspinatus in particular increases its activity when a heavy object is carried in the hand (Basmajian, 1967).

The effectiveness of the deltoid and the supraspinatus in abduction and flexion of the shoulder depends largely upon synergic action of the serratus anterior and the trapezius. Without the action of at least one of the latter muscles a contraction of the deltoid and supraspinatus would cause the scapula to rotate downward, and these muscles would become so shortened that their ability to produce tension would diminish markedly, or even become exhausted. Fortunately, under normal conditions this does not occur because of the strong linkage with their scapulothoracic synergists. The devastating effect of paralysis of the shoulder blade fixators is illustrated in Figure 77.

DELTOID PARALYSIS (supraspinatus intact). During World War II, the author observed three patients with gunshot injuries to the

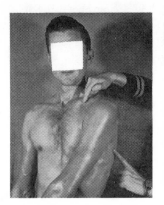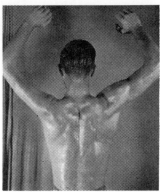

FIG. 86. Deltoid and teres minor paralysis due to gunshot injury to axillary nerve. Note flaccidity of left deltoid. Subject was able to abduct arm full range. (Brunnstrom, 1941)

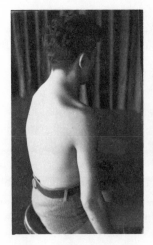
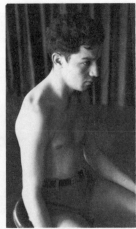

FIG. 87. The emptiness in the supraspinous region is well observable in this boy who had involvement of the trapezius and the supraspinatus following an attack of poliomyelitis. The subject experienced no difficulty in raising arm over head.

axillary nerve, with resulting paralysis of the deltoid and the teres minor. All three men were capable of abducting the shoulder full range. One of these cases is illustrated in Figure 86. Note the normal contour on the right side and the flaccidity of the deltoid on the left side.

SUPRASPINATUS PARALYSIS (deltoid intact). When the supraspinatus is paralyzed and atrophied, the region above the spine of the scapula becomes flat or even hollow (Fig. 87). In the case illustrated (post-poliomyelitis), the trapezius was also partially affected which accounts for the marked emptiness in the supraspinous region. The serratus functioned satisfactorily and the subject experienced no difficulty in raising the arm overhead.

Van Linge and Mulder (1963) observed the effect of a temporary and complete paralysis of the supraspinatus following suprascapular nerve block by local anesthesia. All subjects (10 healthy males) experienced no difficulty in raising the arm overhead, but a decrease in strength and endurance resulted. The authors conclude that loss of abduction as seen in patients with rupture of the supraspinatus tendon is due to pain, possibly impingement of the tendon between the humeral head and the acromion, not primarily to absence of supraspinatus function.

Clinical Kinesiology

The cases discussed in the previous paragraphs demonstrate that either of the two abductors can perform well without the other, although strength in abduction is reduced; but if both deltoid and supraspinatus are out of function, shoulder abduction is seriously affected. No true abduction is then possible unless the shoulder is fully externally rotated. In the externally rotated position, the long head of the biceps, coursing in the intertubercular groove, has a good line of action (but poor leverage) for abduction. That this muscle is capable of abduction was demonstrated by a patient whose deltoid and supraspinatus were paralyzed (Brunnstrom, 1946). Abduction was performed in external rotation but was lost in the internally rotated position.

FLEXION OF THE SHOULDER

When the shoulder is flexed (that is, the arm is raised forward in the sagittal plane), the *anterior and middle deltoid,* the *supraspinatus,* the *clavicular portion of the pectoralis major,* the *coracobrachialis* and the *biceps brachii* (both heads) have a favorable line of action. The first two muscles are the most important flexors, capable of carrying out a full range of flexion. The other muscles act mainly in the first 90 degrees of flexion and their actions decline or cease altogether in flexion beyond 90 degrees.

THE ROLE OF THE INFRASPINATUS, TERES MINOR AND SUBSCAPULARIS IN FLEXION AND ABDUCTION OF THE SHOULDER

So far, those muscles which are primarily responsible for abduction and flexion of the shoulder have been discussed. Electromyograms of the shoulder muscles in these two movements reveal that the infraspinatus, teres minor and subscapularis act continuously during flexion and abduction (Inman and associates, 1944). Their function as a group is to *depress the humerus* to prevent the traction of the deltoid from causing the head of the humerus to jam against the acromion process. The infraspinatus and teres minor also produce the necessary *external rotation* for complete elevation of the arm.

ADDUCTION AND EXTENSION OF THE SHOULDER

The main muscles involved in these movements are the *latissimus dorsi, teres major,* lower portion of the *pectoralis major,* the *posterior deltoid,* and the *long head of the triceps.*

When the arm is brought down to the side of the body from the overhead position, it may be lowered laterally (adducted) or forward (extended), and these movements require essentially the same muscles, although in variable proportions. In the erect position, resistance must be applied to the movements to bring out the action of the adductors-extensors.

The latissimus and pectoralis major have a firm origin on the trunk while the teres major requires simultaneous action of the scapula-fixators, mainly the rhomboideus major. The rhomboids and the teres major in their synergic actions are comparable to the combination of the serratus anterior and the deltoid. In each case, rela-

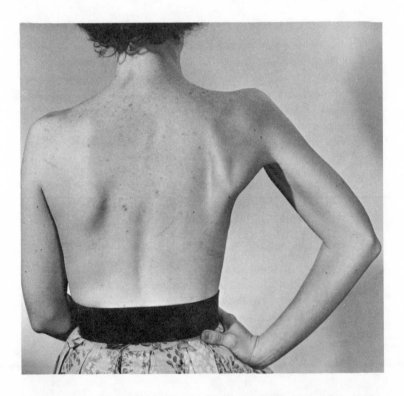

FIG. 88. Contraction of the teres major without synergic action of the rhomboids results in upward rotation and forward sliding of the scapula on the rib cage. Movement performed by a normal individual capable of breaking up the strong linkage between the teres major and rhomboids.

tive elongation of the scapulohumeral muscles, with maintenance of their strength, is achieved. Without the rhomboids, the teres major would rotate the scapula upward and lose its effectiveness on the humerus, which is indeed the case when the rhomboids are paralyzed. In such a case, resistance to adduction of the shoulder causes the inferior angle of the scapula to slide forward owing to the action of the teres major. A similar position of the scapula is seen in a normal individual in Figure 88, but to break up the strong linkage between the rhomboids and the teres major requires a coordination of which few individuals are capable.

The latissimus and the teres major adduct and extend the shoulder, drawing the arm backward; the pectoralis major, mainly its lower portion, draws the arm forward as it adducts. The coracobrachialis appears to be active during the first half of the movement of extension—from overhead position to the horizontal position of the arm—but its activity is difficult to assess by palpation.

When the movement of extension continues into *hyperextension,* the activity of the pectoralis declines and the *posterior deltoid* springs into action. If the posterior deltoid is paralyzed, hyperextension is of very limited range (Brunnstrom, 1946).

EXTERNAL ROTATION OF THE SHOULDER

The *infraspinatus, teres minor,* and *posterior deltoid* are responsible for external rotation. The first two muscles contract in a fairly isolated fashion when the arm hangs vertically, and external rotation is performed without much effort (Fig. 80). The posterior deltoid, if acting alone in external rotation, would simultaneously hyperextend the shoulder. In resisted external rotation all three muscles act in variable proportions, depending upon the position of the joint.

FUNCTIONAL ASSOCIATION: EXTERNAL ROTATION AND SUPINATION. The external rotators of the shoulder and the supinators of the forearm are strongly linked. When the elbow is extended, these two muscle groups serve the same purpose, namely, to cause the palm to face upward, or forward, and they tend to be innervated together. This is well demonstrated if the forearm is supinated while the arm is hanging at the side of the body in which case external rotation of the shoulder occurs invariably with supination. It requires good concentration, indeed, to perform an isolated supination of the forearm whenever the elbow is extended.

INTERNAL ROTATION OF THE SHOULDER

There are five muscles for internal rotation: the *subscapularis, teres major, latissimus dorsi, pectoralis major* and *anterior deltoid.* Of these, the subscapularis is the only one which comes close to being a pure internal rotator.

If, in the forward-bent position with the arm hanging relaxed, an internal rotation of the shoulder is carried out, the subscapularis is likely to perform the movement alone, with little or no assistance from the other four muscles. This can be ascertained by palpation (Fig. 81). Note that comparatively little effort should be used if the subscapularis is to act alone.

The pectoralis major combines internal rotation with adduction of the shoulder so that its action carries the arm in front of the body, the anterior deltoid flexes the shoulder as it internally rotates, the latissimus and teres major combine internal rotation with adduction and extension.

FUNCTIONAL ASSOCIATION: INTERNAL ROTATION AND PRONATION. Internal rotation and pronation are closely linked and tend to occur simultaneously for the purpose of turning the palm downward or backward. Isolated pronation seldom takes place.

Internal rotators and pronators often combine with other muscle groups in typical fashions. For example, in throwing a ball or in serving a ball in tennis, protraction of the shoulder girdle, internal rotation and adduction of the shoulder, extension of the elbow, pronation of the forearm, and trunk rotation combine. Preceding the throw, there is retraction of the shoulder girdle, external rotation and abduction of the shoulder, flexion of the elbow, supination of the forearm, and trunk rotation to the side of the raised arm. It is seen that, in preparing for the throw, exactly the reverse movement combination is used as needed for the throw itself. The muscles responsible for the throw are first elongated, which contributes materially to the effectiveness of the throw. If the movement analysis is carried to the hips and the lower extremities, it will be seen that the entire body contributes to an effective throw and that all muscles needed for the throw are first elongated.

LATISSIMUS DORSI AS AN ELEVATOR OF THE PELVIS

The latissimus dorsi originates, in part, from the crest of the ilium. When the arms are stabilized as in pushing down on crutch handles, this muscle may aid in lifting the pelvis so that the foot clears the ground in walking. This function is of particular importance to the paraplegic patient, whose lower extremity muscles, including the hip-hikers, are paralyzed owing to an injury of the spinal cord. It should be recalled that the latissimus dorsi is innervated by the thoracodorsal nerve, derived from C6, C7, and C8, and therefore not involved in injuries to the spinal cord below C8.

WORK CAPACITY OF SHOULDER MUSCLES

The maximal work capacity of the shoulder muscles and the contribution of these muscles to the various shoulder movements, as determined by R. Fick, are seen in Table VII, Appendix. Since several important muscles are omitted (deltoid, latissimus, pectoralis major) and the investigation concerned glenohumeral motion without regard to scapular motion, only limited practical application in terms of *work* can be derived from the table. However, a glance at the cross sections of the various muscles is of interest. Note, for example, the large cross section of the subscapularis. This muscle's large work capacity in internal rotation of the shoulder as compared to its very small work capacity for other motions clearly indicates that its main function is internal rotation. It is obviously the most powerful of the internal rotators.

SYNERGISM AND ANTAGONISM OF SHOULDER MUSCLES

Previous discussions in this section indicate that muscles and muscle groups of the shoulder region (as elsewhere) can combine their actions in many different ways. In other words, two muscles acting on the scapula (or the shoulder joint) in opposite directions are antagonistic for a particular movement only—they may act as synergists in other combinations. For example:

The *trapezius and serratus anterior* act as synergists in upward rotation of the scapula, but as antagonists in retraction and protraction of the shoulder girdle.

The *trapezius and rhomboids* act as synergists in retraction of the shoulder girdle, but as antagonists in upward and downward rotation of the shoulder blade.

The upper and lower portions of the trapezius act synergically in upward rotation of the scapula, but antagonistically in elevation and depression of the shoulder girdle.

The anterior and posterior portions of the deltoid act synergically in abduction of the arm in the frontal plane, the flexor component of the anterior deltoid being balanced by the extensor component of the posterior deltoid. The two portions of the muscle act antagonistically in flexion and extension, as in swinging the arm forward and backward in the sagittal plane.

The *subscapularis and the infraspinatus* act together to depress the head of the humerus in shoulder abduction, but they are antagonistic as far as internal and external rotation of the shoulder is concerned.

CHAPTER 6

Knee Region

BONES

PALPABLE STRUCTURES

The distal enlargements of the femur, the *condyles,* are best palpated when the knee is flexed and best approached from the medial and lateral sides. The most prominent parts of the condyles are the *epicondyles* (Gr. *epi,* upon, and *kondylos,* condyle) which serve as landmarks for the knee region.

If the index finger is placed on the lateral epicondyle of the femur, the middle finger will find the *head of the fibula* in a distal direction as seen in Figure 89. The *fibular collateral ligament* of the knee joint extends between these two points. If now the thumb of the other hand is placed on the prominent part of the *lateral condyle of the tibia,* it will be seen that these three bony prominences form an equilateral triangle (Fig. 89).

On the medial side of the knee, below the medial epicondyle, is an impression which indicates the line of the knee joint. This is the point where the edge of the *medial meniscus* is palpated. It may not be easy to distinguish the meniscus with certainty, but in injuries to the meniscus, this spot is extremely sensitive to pressure. The *tibial collateral ligament* spans the joint in this region, extending from the medial epicondyle of the femur to an area on the shaft of the tibia, below the medial condyle of the tibia. Proximal to the medial epicondyle and rather close to it, the *adductor tubercle* of the femur may be recognized, although this tubercle is imbedded in soft tissue.

Anteriorly on the tibia and below the tibial condyles is a large rough area, the *tuberosity of the tibia,* the upper part of which serves as insertion for the quadriceps muscle by means of the patellar ten-

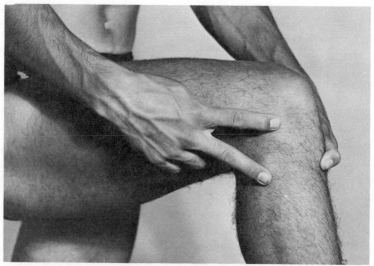

FIG. 89. Subject's index finger is on the lateral epicondyle of the femur; middle finger on the head of the fibula; and left thumb on the protuberance of the lateral condyle of the tibia.

don. Distal to the tibial tuberosity, the sharp *anterior margin of the tibia* is felt. If the knee is extended and the quadriceps muscle is relaxed (best achieved in the supine position), the *patella* (knee cap) may be passively moved, a movement which can be performed freely from side to side and, less freely, in proximal and distal directions. But when the quadriceps muscle is tensed, the patella cannot be passively moved. The *patellar tendon* may be palpated from the inferior margin of the patella to the tuberosity of the tibia, both when the quadriceps muscle is relaxed and when it is tensed. The triangular shape of the patella, its apex being directed downward, is easily palpable.

NONPALPABLE STRUCTURES

Note the following nonpalpable structures: *articular surfaces and patellar surfaces of the condyles of the femur; intercondyloid fossa; lateral and medial supracondylar lines,* extending proximally from the condyles and enclosing an area which forms the floor of the *popliteal fossa* (L. *poples,* back of knee) ; *articular surfaces of the condyles of the tibia* ("tibial plateau"), separated by the *intercondylar eminence; lateral meniscus,* nearly circular in form (Gr. *menis-*

kos, crescent) ; *medial meniscus* ("semilunar cartilage") ; *anterior and posterior cruciate ligaments;* and *transverse ligament,* connecting the menisci anteriorly.

KNEE JOINT (ARTICULATIO GENU)

ORIENTATION

The distal enlarged end of the femur articulates with the proximal enlarged end of the tibia. The fibula takes no part in the formation of this joint. Two cartilages, the medial and lateral menisci, are interposed between the joint surfaces of the two bones.

An anterior or posterior view of the femur and the tibia reveals an angle, open laterally, between the shafts of the two bones. The size of this angle varies in different individuals; about 170 degrees is regarded as normal (Fig. 111).

When an individual stands with the feet close together, both shafts have a lateral slant, the femur slanting more than the tibia. In this position, the joint surfaces stand horizontally. But if the feet are slightly apart, which is more comfortable than holding them together, the shaft of the tibia stands vertically so that the weight from above passes perpendicularly through its shaft. The tibial plateau then has a slight slant. The further the feet are apart, the more slanting the joint surface.

In general, the movements of the knee joint are dictated by the shape of the articular surfaces and the interposed cartilages. The collateral ligaments prevent lateral motions when the knee is extended; the cruciate ligaments are important for stabilization in the flexed position—they particularly guard against undue sliding motions in an anteroposterior direction. In this task they are supported by the popliteus muscle (see pp. 188 and 195).

TYPE OF JOINT

The knee permits mainly flexion and extension, movements characteristic of hinge joints. However, the knee is not a hinge joint, *first,* because it does not have a fixed axis of motion for flexion and extension; *second,* because part of the motion is brought about by mixed gliding and rocking; and *third,* because a transverse rotation is also allowed, such rotation being most marked when the knee is flexed. The knee joint, therefore, has *two degrees of freedom of motion* consisting of flexion and extension, and transverse rotation.

AXES FOR FLEXION AND EXTENSION. The axis of motion is located a distance above the joint surfaces, passing transversely through the femoral condyles. The curve of the condyles presents a changing radius which is smallest when the knee is flexed and increases with extension (Fig. 90).

We owe much of our present knowledge of the mechanics of the knee to investigations by Otto Fischer (quoted by Fick, 1911, pp. 533, 534). He marked successive points of contact between the joint surfaces on a series of x-ray pictures showing the profile of the

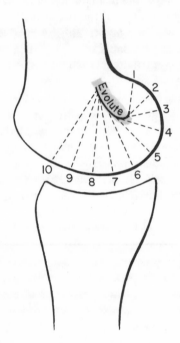

FIG. 90. Changing radius of curves of femoral condyles. Axis of motion for flexion and extension moves along *evolute*. (Redrawn from Fick, 1911, p. 538.)

femoral condyles at various knee angles, and for each point he determined the center for the curve of the condyle. By connecting these centers, a curved line (the *evolute*) was obtained, representing the path of the moving axis (Fig. 90).

AXES FOR "ROCKING" AT THE KNEE. During pure rocking, successive points of the articular surfaces contact each other, much like the rockers of a rocking chair change their position in relation to the floor. In pure rocking, *the instant axis of motion passes through the contact point between the two bones.* Rocking occurs mainly

Clinical Kinesiology

during the last 20 degrees of extension. As the terminal phase of extension approaches, the lateral condyle rocks while the medial still glides, and this results in internal rotation of the femur with respect to the tibia. This movement is referred to as *terminal rotation,* sometimes as the *locking mechanism* of the knee.

AXES FOR TRANSVERSE ROTATION. When the knee is fully extended, the tibial and fibular collateral ligaments are relatively tense, which contributes materially to the stability of the joint. These ligaments slacken when the joint flexes, and this is one of the reasons why a considerable amount of transverse rotation may take place in the flexed position.

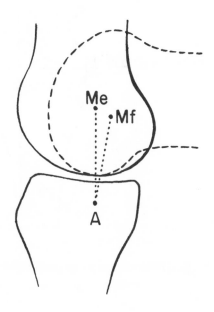

FIG. 91. Slackening of tibial collateral ligament in flexion of knee. Me—Medial epicondyle in extension; Mf —Medial epicondyle in flexion; A—Point of attachment of collateral ligament. (Redrawn from Fick, 1911, p. 542.)

In Figure 91 the position of the medial epicondyle when the knee is extended (Me) is shown as compared to its position when the knee is flexed (Mf), and it is seen that the distance from the medial epicondyle to point A (representing the attachment of the tibial collateral ligament) is less in flexion than in extension.

During knee flexion more slack is produced in the fibular than in the tibial collateral ligament, hence the movement between the femoral and tibial condyles is more extensive laterally than medially. Transverse rotation takes place about a longitudinal axis located medial to the intercondylar ridge of the tibia so that, roughly, it may be stated that the lateral condyle rotates around the medial one. (Actually, the medial condyle rotates somewhat posteriorly as the lateral condyle moves forward). The location of the axis of rotation varies somewhat at different knee angles. The instant axis of rotation when the knee is nearly extended is seen in Figure 92.

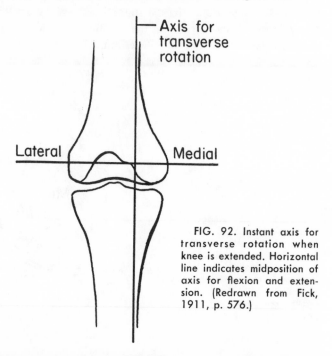

FIG. 92. Instant axis for transverse rotation when knee is extended. Horizontal line indicates midposition of axis for flexion and extension. (Redrawn from Fick, 1911, p. 576.)

EXCURSION OF TRANSVERSE ROTATION. According to Fick (1911, p. 582) when the knee is flexed to 90 degrees, normal transverse rotation amounts to about 50 degrees, at an acute knee angle to about 70 degrees. As the knee angle becomes obtuse, less and less excursion is allowed so that in the nearly extended position only 10 degrees or less is possible.

VOLUNTARY CONTROL OF TRANSVERSE ROTATION. Much of the rotary motion at the knee occurs automatically, that is, we are not aware of, nor do we have control of, such rotation. For example, in walking or in performing knee bends, we are well aware of flexion and extension, but are unable to determine whether rotation takes place. However, if the knee is flexed to 90 degrees, as in the sitting

Clinical Kinesiology

position, voluntary rotation meets with no difficulty. If the toes are turned in and out while the prominent part of the lateral tibial condyle and the lateral epicondyle of the femur are palpated simultaneously, it is easy to ascertain that a transverse rotation of the tibia with respect to the femur takes place. It may be observed that, from the neutral position, the excursion of the tibia in external rotation is larger than in internal rotation. Note that the angle of the foot to the tibia cannot be used as an indicator of the amount of rotation taking place, since the joints of the foot also participate as the toes are turned in and out.

When the knee is extended, no active rotation and very little, if any, passive rotation is allowed. This is advantageous in erect standing since it contributes to knee stability. In the extended knee position, a toeing in and out is achieved by rotation at the hip.

COMBINED AXIS. When two of the three movements of gliding, rocking and transverse rotation occur simultaneously, or all three together, a combined instant axis of motion may be constructed— its location and direction is determined by the components of the movement at each specific knee angle.

PASSIVE RESISTANCE TO KNEE EXTENSION

In subjects investigated by Smith (1956), a passive resistance to extension, supplied by extra-articular tissues (fascia and skin), was found to be present at knee angles of 160 to 180 degrees. Beyond 180 degrees, the total resistance encountered had extra-articular and articular components. The resistance torque curve rose from zero at an angle of 160 degrees to about seven ft. lb. at 190 degrees.

PATELLA (Knee Cap)

POSITION AND MOVEMENT OF PATELLA. The patella, a large sesamoid bone imbedded in the quadriceps tendon, is anchored to the tibia by means of the patellar tendon, a broad and strong tendon which does not allow any appreciable amount of elongation by the contraction of the quadriceps muscle. The result is that during flexion and extension the knee cap remains at a constant distance from the tibia. The change of position of the patella, proximally during extension and distally during flexion, occurs in relation to the femur. The patella slides up and down over a saddle-shaped area on the femur, this being divided into two surfaces by a groove. The up and down movement of the patella is accompanied by a small amount of lateral motion during flexion and medial motion during extension. The knee cap has two articular surfaces, a medial and a lateral, separated by a vertical ridge which corresponds to the groove of the femur. The patella is thus guided in its motion by the shape of the articular surfaces and it is secured in place by capsular reinforcements.

FUNCTION OF THE PATELLA. The patella plays an important role in the mechanics of the knee joint because it lifts the tendon of insertion of the quadriceps muscle away from the axis of motion of the joint, thus increasing the leverage of this muscle considerably. The effect is obtained in all positions of the joint but it is most marked when the knee is extended. At a 90-degree knee angle the knee cap has slid in between the two condyles of the femur, and at an acute angle it lies even further down and is firmly pressed to the femur.

PLACEMENT OF KNEE HINGES IN ARTIFICIAL APPLIANCES

Because of the shifting axis of motion of the human knee, it becomes somewhat of a problem to determine the correct placement of the knee hinges in long leg braces and in below-knee prostheses. Ideally, for free and unobstructed motions and for prevention of discomfort and abrasions, the axis of motion of the appliance should coincide with that of the human knee joint throughout the range. Since this cannot very well be accomplished, a compromise is necessary.

In long leg braces, if used with knee locks, no motion is desired in standing and walking, but when the braces are unlocked for sitting they will be uncomfortable unless the hinges are aligned with the axis of the flexed human knee.

A clinical method of determining the placement of the knee hinges in below-knee prostheses was suggested by Gocht, quoted by Schede (1941, p. 29). The amputee's knee is viewed from the side, and a horizontal line is drawn from front to back approximately 2.5 cm. above the joint line, which can best be palpated medially. The hinges are placed at this height, at the junction of the middle and posterior third of the before-mentioned line (Fig. 93). This point is said to represent the midposition of the knee axis. (The distance of 2.5 cm. applies to the average male adult.) Recently, a more detailed method was described. It is based on analysis of x-ray data which showed relative alignments of posterior femoral and posterior tibial condyles and the posterior border of the head of the fibula throughout 110 degrees of knee flexion (Gardner and Clippinger, 1969). The method devised a reference table to be used in conjunction with surface anatomical measurements related to the tibial tubercle and the posterior border of the fibular head.

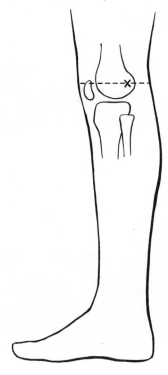

FIG. 93. Placement of knee hinges in braces and below-knee prostheses. Viewing subject from the side, hinges are placed at junction of middle and posterior third of anteroposterior line at height of epicondyles.

KNEE DEFORMITIES

DEVIATIONS IN THE FRONTAL PLANE. As previously stated, the angle between the shafts of the femur and the tibia, open laterally, normally amounts to about 170 degrees and this angulation is best observed from the front or the back. There are considerable varia-

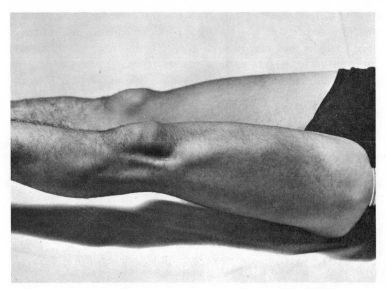

FIG. 94. Vastus lateralis in contraction. Subject maintains knee extended while lifting heel off the floor. The iliotibial tract is seen as it approaches its insertion on the tibia.

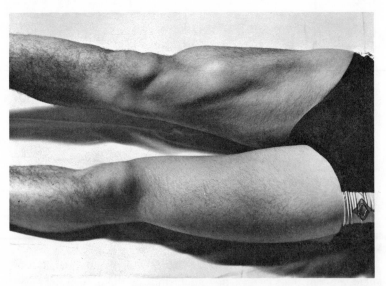

FIG. 95. Vastus medialis in contraction. Subject's right knee is held extended while the heel is raised off the floor. Note the bulk of this muscle near the knee.

tions of this angle within normal limits, but when the angle becomes much smaller than 170 degrees, the condition is referred to as *genu valgum* (knock knee). A larger angle approaching 180 degrees or an angle which opens medially is called *genu varum* (bowleg).

DEVIATIONS IN THE SAGITTAL PLANE. Normally, a subject may stand with the knees extended, slightly flexed, or somewhat hyperextended. The amount of hyperextension permitted depends upon the looseness of the capsule and the ligaments which check this motion. *Genu recurvatum* is an excessive hyperextension which develops from weight-bearing on an unstable knee, usually as a result of paralysis of certain muscles.

MUSCLES

KNEE EXTENSORS

The quadriceps, the main extensor of the knee, is made up of four parts: *rectus femoris, vastus lateralis, vastus medialis* and *vastus intermedius.* In well-developed subjects where little adipose tissue is present, the rectus femoris, the vastus medialis and the vastus lateralis may be observed as separate units (Figs. 94 and 95), while in other subjects the boundaries of these muscles are less distinct. The vastus intermedius is deeply located and cannot be observed from the surface.

The *rectus femoris* occupies the middle of the thigh, is superficial, and takes a straight course down the thigh. *Origin:* By two tendons: (1) the anterior or "straight" tendon, from the anterior inferior spine of the ilium; (2) the posterior or "reflected" tendon from just above the brim of the acetabulum; as this tendon swings forward it courses close to the hip joint and is blended with the capsule. The two tendons unite, covering part of the capsule anteriorly. *Insertion:* The muscle fibers attach to a deep aponeurosis narrowing to a broad tendon which inserts into the superior border of the patella and, by means of the patellar tendon, into the tuberosity of the tibia. *Innervation:* Two branches of the femoral nerve. *Inspection and palpation:* When the hip is flexed, the tendon of origin may be observed and palpated in the V-shaped area between the sartorius and the tensor fasciae latae as seen in Figure 114. The muscular portion is superficial and may be followed down the thigh to its insertion on the patella (Figs. 94 and 95).

The *vastus lateralis* is located on the lateral side of the rectus femoris. *Origin:* Lateral and posterior aspects of the femur, as high up as the greater trochanter and as far posterior as the linea aspera. *Insertion:* Superior border of the patella, lateral side, and, by means of the patellar tendon, the tuberosity of the tibia; also the lateral condyle of the tibia and the fascia of the leg. *Innervation:* Branches of the femoral nerve. *Inspection and palpation:* The muscle may be seen and palpated from just below the greater trochanter down to the patella (Fig. 94).

The *vastus medialis* lies in a position medial to the rectus. *Origin:* Medial and posterior aspects of the femur, as high up as the inter-trochanteric line and as far posterior as the linea aspera. *Insertion:* Medial portion of superior border of patella and, by means of the patellar tendon, the tuberosity of the tibia; also the medial condyle of the tibia and the fascia of the leg. *Innervation:* Branches of the femoral nerve. *Inspection and palpation:* The distal portion of the muscle is quite bulky and is palpated in the lower third of the thigh medially (Fig. 95).

Vastus intermedius, located underneath the rectus, is partially fused with the two other vasti muscles. *Origin:* The anterior and lateral surfaces of the femur, as high up as the lesser trochanter and as far posterior as the linea aspera. *Insertion:* Superior border of the patella, fused with the tendons of the two other vasti muscles, and directly into the capsule of the knee joint. *Innervation:* Branches of the femoral nerve. *Palpation:* If the rectus is grasped and lifted somewhat, the vastus intermedius may be palpated underneath the rectus if approached from the medial or lateral side of the rectus.

The patella lies within the *common tendon of the quadriceps* which extends above and on the sides of the patella as well as being attached to it. From the apex of the patella, the patellar ligament, the continuation of the quadriceps tendon, extends to the tuberosity of the tibia. On the sides of the patella, tendinous fibers spread out to form the *medial and lateral retinacula* which attach to the condyles of the tibia.

The *articularis genu* (subcrureus) is a small flat muscle which originates on the anterior lower portion of the shaft of the femur and inserts into the capsule of the knee joint or into the superior edge of the patella. The muscle lies beneath the vastus intermedius and is sometimes blended with it.

KNEE FLEXORS

A number of muscles pass posterior to the axis for flexion and extension of the knee, contributing to a variable extent to knee flexion. The muscles are: the three hamstrings, the gastrocnemius, the plantaris, the popliteus, the adductor gracilis and the sartorius.

The *biceps femoris* is a muscle of the posterior thigh, also known as the "lateral hamstring." *Origin:* By two heads: (1) The long head, from the tuberosity of the ischium, having a common tendon of origin with the semitendinosus; (2) the short head, from the lower portion of the shaft of the femur and from the lateral intermuscular septum. *Insertion:* The two heads unite to be inserted into the head of the fibula, into the lateral condyle of the tibia and into the fascia of the leg. *Innervation:* Branches of the sciatic nerve. The short head receives its innervation from the common peroneal portion of the sciatic nerve; the long head is supplied by the tibial portion of the sciatic nerve.

Inspection and palpation: When knee flexion is resisted (subject prone) the long head of the biceps femoris may be observed and palpated from its origin all the way down to its insertion (Fig. 96). The short head is covered largely by the long head and is, therefore,

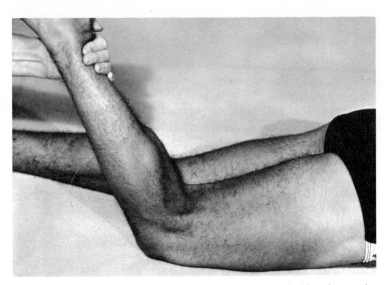

FIG. 96. Tendon of biceps femoris is seen on lateral side of posterior knee region when knee flexion is resisted. Note also the two heads of the gastrocnemius.

difficult to identify. The common tendon of the two heads also is seen in Figure 102 as it approaches its insertion on the head of the fibula. The biceps tendon is also easily palpated with the subject in the sitting position if the leg is externally rotated with respect to the femur.

The *semitendinosus* is one of the medial hamstrings, the muscular portion of which lies adjacent to that of the long head of the biceps in the posterior thigh. *Origin:* Tuberosity of the ischium, having a common tendon of origin with the long head of the biceps. *Insertion:* The medial aspect of the tibia near the knee joint, distal to the insertion of the gracilis. *Innervation:* Branches of the sciatic nerve.

Inspection and palpation: With the subject prone, the tendon may be observed and palpated posteriorly on the medial side of the knee when knee flexion is resisted (Fig. 97). Palpation of the tendon may also be done with the subject in the sitting position. The palpating fingers are placed in the "fold" of the knee, medially, where several relaxed tendons may be distinguished. If the muscles of this region are then tightened without joint movement, the tendon of the semitendinosus rises markedly from the underlying tissue, it being the most

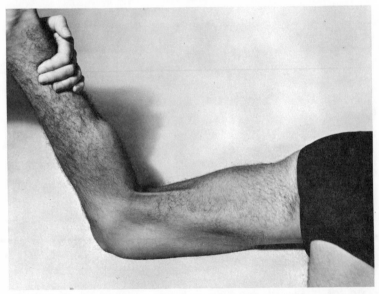

FIG. 97. The prominent tendon of the semitendinosus is seen on the medial side of the posterior knee region when knee flexion is resisted.

prominent tendon in the back of the knee. The tendon may be followed halfway up the thigh. Once the tendon of the semitendinosus has been identified, another small, firm, and round tendon may be palpated medial to the semitendinosus. This is the *tendon of the adductor gracilis* which becomes tense if the knees are pressed together. By sliding transversely over the tendon of the gracilis with the nail of one of the palpating fingers, a vibration is set up causing a sensation in the crotch in the region of the origin of the gracilis, and this identifies the gracilis with certainty. In the sitting position, internal rotation of the leg with respect to the thigh also brings out the tendons of both the semitendinosus and the gracilis.

The *semimembranosus originates* on the tuberosity of the ischium and *inserts* into the medial condyle of the tibia. *Innervation:* Branches of the sciatic nerve.

Palpation: Although this muscle has the largest cross section of the hamstrings (see Table VIII) it is not well palpable as an individual muscle because it is to a large extent covered by the semitendinosus and, proximally also, by the adductor magnus. Together with these muscles the semimembranosus makes up the large muscular mass of the medial and posterior thigh. The muscular portion of the semimembranosus extends further distally than that of the semitendinosus; therefore, its lower portion may be palpated on both sides of the semitendinosus. As the semimembranosus approaches its insertion, its tendon lies deep and can only be palpated with difficulty.

The two heads of the *gastrocnemius* (Gr. *gaster,* belly, and *kneme,* leg) originate above the femoral condyles and span the knee joint on the flexor side, and therefore belong to this region as well as to the ankle region. The muscular portion of the gastrocnemius may be seen contracting in resisted flexion of the knee (Figs. 96 and 97). Since the gastrocnemius is more important as a plantar flexor of the ankle than as a knee flexor, it is discussed in more detail in Chapter 7.

The *plantaris,* a small muscle in the posterior knee region, *originates* above the lateral condyle of the femur where it lies between the lateral head of the gastrocnemius and the popliteus close to, and partially blended with, the capsule. Following the medial border of the soleus it joins the Achilles' tendon, to be inserted into the calcaneus. *Innervation:* Tibial nerve.

The *popliteus* is the most deeply located muscle in the back of the knee. It lies close to the capsule, covered by the plantaris and the lateral head of the gastrocnemius. *Origin:* By a strong tendon from the lateral condyle of the femur. The muscle fibers take a downward-medial course and are *inserted* into the medial portion of the tibia. The insertion is widespread in a proximal-distal direction, giving the muscle a somewhat triangular shape. The location of the popliteus and the direction of its fibers are indicated in Figure 98. *Innervation:* Tibial nerve.

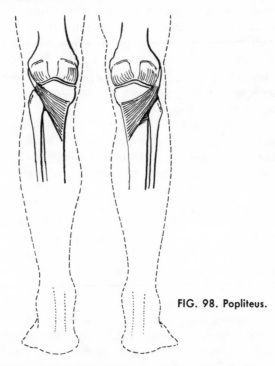

FIG. 98. Popliteus.

The tendon of insertion of the *sartorius* passes on the medial side of the knee and on the flexor side of the axis of motion. Since its action is more important at the hip than at the knee, it is further discussed in Chapter 8.

ROTATORS

The muscles which act in *internal rotation* of the tibia with respect to the femur are the two medial hamstrings, the adductor gracilis and the popliteus.

External rotation of the tibia with respect to the femur is accomplished by the biceps femoris, possibly aided by the tensor fasciae

Clinical Kinesiology

latae. That the biceps femoris is a strong external rotator may be ascertained by applying resistance to the motion with the subject in the sitting position. In certain polio cases a permanent externally rotated position of the tibia with respect to the femur results if the biceps has retained good strength while the internal rotators are paralyzed.

Discussion of Function of Muscles of Knee

WEIGHT-BEARING AND NONWEIGHT-BEARING FUNCTION

The lower extremities are concerned mainly with weight-bearing because they support the body in standing and propel the body forward in locomotion. The muscles of the knee as well as those of the ankle and hip must therefore be studied both in weight-bearing and nonweight-bearing situations. The former aspects of their function are discussed in Chapters 10 and 11.

ONE-JOINT AND TWO-JOINT MUSCLES ACTING AT THE KNEE

The muscles which control the knee are either one-joint muscles passing the knee only, or two-joint muscles passing the hip and knee, or ankle and knee.

The two-joint muscles exert their action over both joints simultaneously and the result of their contraction, in terms of movement, depends greatly upon the leverage conditions at the two joints. If the leverage is poor at one joint and is favorable over the other, the latter joint will be the principal one moving or, under certain conditions, the only one moving, subject of course to the influence of the resistance encountered at each joint.

Under ordinary conditions of use, two-joint muscles are seldom utilized to move both joints simultaneously. More often, the action of two-joint muscles at one joint is prevented by resistance due to gravity or to the contraction of other muscles. If the muscles were to shorten over both joints simultaneously and to complete the range at both joints, they would have to shorten a long distance and would rapidly lose tension as the shortening progressed. In natural motions, however, the muscles are seldom, if ever, required to go through such extreme excursion. The two joints usually move in such directions that the muscle is gradually elongated over one joint while producing movement at the other joint. The result is that favorable length-tension relations are maintained.

ONE-JOINT MUSCLES OF THE KNEE. The three vasti muscles act at the knee only, while the rectus acts at the knee and hip. The short head of the biceps and the popliteus muscle belong in the one-joint category. The other knee flexors are two-joint muscles.

TWO-JOINT MUSCLES OF THE KNEE. The action of the two-joint muscles will be considered in the following movement combinations:

Knee flexion combined with hip extension: If the subject is lying prone or standing erect and flexes the knee while extending the hip, the hamstring muscles must shorten over both joints simultaneously and difficulty is experienced in completing knee flexion. Some subjects complain of a cramp in the muscles of the posterior thigh when performing this motion. All subjects lose strength rapidly as knee flexion proceeds while the hip is extended. The range of useful excursion becomes almost exhausted.* Another factor that often limits full excursion of the hamstrings is the inability of the rectus femoris, which is being stretched over the hip and knee simultaneously, to elongate sufficiently. When spasticity of the rectus femoris is present, the interference of this muscle becomes marked, resulting in a forward tilting of the pelvis; in the prone position the buttocks then become elevated in an awkward manner.

Knee extension combined with hip flexion: In a supine or standing position, straight leg raising—consisting of hip flexion with the knee maintained extended—may be performed. The movement proceeds without strain throughout a certain range, then difficulty arises mainly from the inability of the hamstrings to elongate sufficiently and, to a lesser extent, from the decrease in strength of the rectus, which muscle has to shorten over the hip and knee simultaneously.* By performing a passive movement of hip flexion, first with the knee extended and then with the knee flexed, the effect of hamstring interference in hip flexion becomes obvious.

Knee flexion combined with hip flexion: This combination provides for elongation of the hamstrings over the hip while knee flexion is carried out, resulting in favorable length-tension relations. During hip-knee flexion the hip flexors and the hamstrings act synergically to provide a functionally useful movement, while in other movement combinations these two muscle groups may act as antagonists.

Knee extension combined with hip extension: This is a most useful combination that occurs in activities such as rising from the

*Compare page 36, "muscles of short action" (Haines, 1934).

Clinical Kinesiology

sitting position, climbing stairs, running, and jumping. The hamstrings then act as hip extensors, while the quadriceps extends the knee and, by doing so, elongates the hamstrings over the knee. In this movement, as in the previous one, an effective portion of the length-tension curve is utilized.

Knee flexion combined with plantar flexion of the ankle: The gastrocnemius is capable of performing these two motions simultaneously, but if full range at both joints is attempted, the muscle has to shorten a long distance and tension falls rapidly. It is not a very useful movement.

Knee extension combined with plantar flexion of the ankle: The quadriceps extends the knee while the gastrocnemius (and soleus) plantar-flex the ankle. As the quadriceps extends the knee the gastrocnemius becomes elongated over the knee, and optimal conditions for plantar flexion of the ankle result. This functional combination is commonly seen, as, for example, in rising on tiptoes, running and jumping.

LEVERAGE OF MUSCLES ACTING AT THE KNEE

A study of the anatomical relationship of the knee muscles reveals that the leverage of the individual flexor muscles varies considerably and that the leverage also is influenced importantly by the position of the knee joint whether in flexion or extension.

The deepest of the muscles in the posterior knee region, the popliteus muscle, lies so close to the axis of motion of the knee joint that its leverage for knee flexion is extremely poor; consequently its action as a flexor is negligible. Its leverage for internal rotation of the tibia is better. The tendons of the hamstrings lie further away from the joint axis so that these muscles have better leverage.

In the extended position of the knee, the hamstring tendons lie closer to the knee axis (and are more difficult to palpate) than when the knee is flexed. As these muscles contract in knee flexion their tendons rise to the surface, away from the joint axis, thus improving their leverage. This applies particularly to the semitendinosus and the biceps femoris. The tendon of the semimembranosus appears to be held down more firmly than that of the other two muscles.

Because the patella lifts the tendon of insertion of the quadriceps away from the joint axis, the quadriceps has comparatively good leverage for extension, a leverage which remains favorable throughout joint range but is best when the knee is extended (see p. 180).

CROSS SECTION OF KNEE MUSCLES

The cross section of the quadriceps (Table VIII) is much larger than that of the knee flexors (hamstrings, gracilis and sartorius), an indication of the greater demands placed on the extensors. In weight-bearing situations when the knee is flexed, as in squatting and climbing stairs, the extensors have to act against the superimposed body weight. In contrast, the knee flexors are required to act only on a small body segment. In the upper extremity, it may be recalled, the situation is reversed: the elbow flexors are more active and have a larger cross section than the elbow extensors, which latter muscles have ceased to be antigravity muscles in the human biped posture. In making the before-mentioned comparison between the cross section of the flexors and extensors of the knee, the gastrocnemius is disregarded as a knee flexor because it has very poor leverage as a knee flexor compared to its leverage as a plantar flexor. Furthermore, in functional activities the gastrocnemius works together with the quadriceps, not with the knee flexors.

TORQUE OF MUSCLES ACTING AT THE KNEE

Torque curves for flexors and extensors of the knee have been investigated by Williams and Stutzman (1959). As would be expected, the torque exerted by the extensors was found to be much higher throughout the range than that of the flexors. In this investigation and in subsequent studies (Mendler, 1963, 1967), peak torque values for extensors was at approximately the 60 degree position of the knee (complete extension is at 0 degree). The shape of the flexor curve indicates that in knee flexion the length-tension factor predominates over the leverage factor, a fact that is in contrast to elbow flexion where leverage has a decided influence. The highest torque values were obtained at about 30 degrees of flexion (obtuse knee angle of 150 degrees) when the muscles were relatively elongated. The effect of the position of the hip on the torque of the knee flexors was also demonstrated. In accordance with the length-tension diagram, lower values were obtained when the hip was extended than when it was flexed.

TERMINAL ROTATION ("LOCKING MECHANISM") OF THE KNEE

The term *terminal rotation* is applied to the external rotation of the tibia with respect to the femur that occurs during the last few degrees of knee extension. Since this rotation is particularly significant in the weight-bearing position when the femur is freer to move than the tibia, it is perhaps more descriptive to speak about an *internal rotation of the femur with respect to the tibia.*

H. Meyer (1853) described terminal rotation as part of the so-called "locking mechanism" of the knee, occurring when the hip and knee extend simultaneously. He points out that the iliofemoral ligament ("ligamentum superius"), because of its oblique direction, is looser when the hip is externally rotated than when the hip is internally rotated. Consequently, in complete hip extension when the iliofemoral ligament becomes tensed, this ligament causes the femur to internally rotate with respect to the pelvis (and with respect to the tibia). This internal rotation of the femur at the knee constitutes a locking mechanism, since the shape of the femoral condyle is such that flexion can take place only if the femur first externally rotates somewhat with respect to the tibia. Meyer furthermore points out that stability of the knee is also effected by the iliotibial tract which is attached to the anterior surface of the lateral condyle of the tibia. As the hip extends fully, the iliotibial tract is put on a stretch and thus stabilizes the knee against flexion.

If this theory is correct, the locking mechanism requires complete hip extension, a posture which is commonly assumed when an individual has to stand for any length of time but which is not a characteristic of erect posture under all circumstances (see Chapter 10). It can be observed that, in prolonged standing, there is a tendency to incline the trunk backward resulting in complete hip extension, and simultaneously to hyperextend the knee somewhat, a knee position which increases knee stability mechanically. For "unlocking" this posture, slight hip flexion and some external rotation of the femur are required. The former is accomplished by a forward movement of the trunk (hip flexion), and the latter requires muscle action. The popliteus muscle is considered to be the principal muscle to effect external rotation of the femur for unlocking purposes, since in the extended knee position the muscle has better leverage for rotation than the inner hamstrings.

ACTIONS OF TENSOR FASCIAE LATAE AND SARTORIUS AT THE KNEE

The *tensor fasciae latae,* which is attached to the iliotibial tract, is capable of tensing this tract and thereby may aid in maintaining the knee in extension. This muscle cannot be considered an extensor as such because the muscle has little or no leverage for extension in the flexed knee position. Fick lists it as a knee extensor but found that its work capacity as a knee extensor was extremely small (Table VIII). The main action of the tensor takes place at the hip.

The tendon of the *sartorius* courses on the flexor side of the knee but its leverage at the hip is much better than at the knee. It is therefore more important as a hip muscle than as a knee muscle. Its work capacity at the knee is very small (Table VIII).

DIFFERENTIAL ACTIONS OF COMPONENTS OF THE QUADRICEPS

While the entire quadriceps acts as a knee extensor, its component parts have some functional characteristics of their own.

The *rectus femoris* is mechanically capable of flexing the hip—its two tendons of origin course on the flexor side of the center of rotation of the hip. However, these tendons lie close to the capsule of the hip joint and their leverage is poor. Recruitment of the rectus femoris as a flexor of the hip probably does not take place as long as those hip flexors which have better leverage can perform the motion with ease. But when considerable resistance has to be overcome, the rectus femoris comes to the aid of the other hip flexors, and its contraction can then be felt by palpation. Simultaneously, a tensing of the hamstring tendons occurs and it may be assumed that these muscles become activated to prevent the rectus femoris from extending the knee when hip flexion without knee extension is willed.

It has been demonstrated by electromyography that in the supine position, with the hip extended and the legs pendent over the edge of the table, the rectus contracts synchronous with the vasti in extension of the knee. But when the knee is extended in the sitting position, electrical activity of the vasti in most subjects investigated preceded that of the rectus femoris whose activity was delayed until the range of knee extension was almost complete (Close, 1964).

In seeking an explanation for the above electromyographic findings, one may reason as follows. In the supine position, length-tension relations of the rectus femoris are favorable, hence the muscle is called upon to contract at once. When the subject is seated, the muscle is in a shortened state, unfavorable for producing tension; the vasti muscles are then more effective in producing knee extension. But toward the end of the motion when the torque required to complete extension is much greater than in the earlier range and some passive tension of the hamstring muscles may have to be overcome as well, the rectus femoris is called upon to join the vasti.

The *vastus medialis* is important in completing knee extension because it furnishes the medial traction on the patella required in this joint range. If the vastus medialis is paralyzed or much weakened, the vastus lateralis tends to pull the patella upward and laterally and the patella may then slide partially away from its articular surface on the femur. Hence the importance of strengthening the vastus medialis following injuries to the knee must be kept in mind.

DIFFERENTIAL ACTIONS OF UPPER AND LOWER PORTIONS OF TWO-JOINT MUSCLES OF THIGH

Markee and associates (1955) demonstrated on cadavers that two-joint muscles of the thigh do not extend directly from their origins above the hip to their insertions below the knee but are interrupted in their courses by strong attachments to fascia or to intermuscular tendons or to both. This interruption would enable the upper and lower portions of such muscles to act as separate units more or less, even though the intervening stabilization is only relative. Markee and co-workers state that the semitendinosus, as an example, should be considered as "two muscles attached to an intervening tendinous inscription," this inscription serving as insertion for the proximal muscle fibers and as origin for the distal fibers. From the standpoint of innervation, independent action of the two portions is feasible since they are supplied by separate nerve branches. If this hypothesis is correct, the distal portion of the muscle may act as a flexor of the knee and the proximal portion as an extensor of the hip with little or no effect on the second joint.

FUNCTION OF THE POPLITEUS IN WEIGHT-BEARING ON THE FLEXED KNEE

While the popliteus is unimportant as a knee flexor because of its poor leverage for flexion, it has long been considered important in its rotary action for unlocking the knee. An additional action of this muscle has been investigated electromyographically by Barnett and Richardson (1953). These investigators recorded strong action potentials from the popliteus when "knee bends" were performed in the standing position. When the knee approached a right angle, action potentials appeared in the popliteus and the activity persisted as long as a crouching posture was maintained. The investigators point out that when the knee is bent, the weight of the body from above tends to cause the femoral condyle to slide forward on the tibial plateau, and "although the posterior cruciate ligament is generally credited with resisting this subluxation, it appears, in fact, that it has active support of the popliteus to stabilize the knee in this position."

The posterior cruciate ligament attaches to the medial condyle of the femur, while the popliteus—by means of its strong tendon of origin—attaches to the lateral condyle. The action of the popliteus therefore, is an important complement to that of the posterior cruciate ligament in preventing a forward sliding of the condyles in weight-bearing on flexed knees.

CHAPTER 7

Ankle and Foot

BONES

PALPABLE STRUCTURES

The malleoli of the ankle, like the epicondyles of the knee, serve as landmarks for their respective regions. The *medial malleolus* (L. diminutive of *malleus,* hammer) is a strong process on the enlarged distal portion of the tibia on the inner side of the ankle. The *lateral malleolus* is found on the outer side of the ankle. It is the most distal portion of the fibula.

By palpating the malleoli, it will be noticed that the lateral malleolus projects further distally than the medial one. If the subject stands with the knee cap pointing straight forward (knee axis in frontal plane) it may also be determined by palpation that the lateral malleolus has a more posterior location than the medial one.

PALPATION ON THE MEDIAL SIDE OF THE FOOT. The tuberosity of the *navicular bone* (L. *navicula,* diminutive of *navis,* ship) is palpated at a point anterior and distal to the medial malleolus. It is a variable prominence but, in most subjects, easily identified. If some uncertainty about its location arises, it may be found as follows: With the ankle plantar-flexed, the tip of the medial malleolus and the medial aspect of the head of the first metatarsal bone (the prominence at the base of the big toe) are identified. A line connecting these two points is divided into three equal parts, and the tuberosity of the navicular bone is found at the junction of the posterior and middle thirds. On the same line, distal to the navicular bone, the *base of the first metatarsal bone* is felt, leading distally to its shaft and head. Between the base of the first metatarsal bone and the navicular tuberosity a part of the *medial cuneiform bone* may be palpated.

Beginning again at the medial malleolus, a protruding portion of the calcaneus, the *sustentaculum talare* (L. *sustentaculum,* a prop) is located a short distance below the tip of the melleolus, in a direction toward the sole of the heel. This process lies well posterior to the navicular tuberosity. Its name indicates its function, which is to support the talus—it forms a shelf on which part of the talus rests. The medial surface of the *calcaneus* (L. relating to *calx,* heel) is well palpable. This bone may be followed posteriorly to the Achilles' tendon, anteriorly to the navicular bone and downward toward the sole.

PALPATION ON THE LATERAL SIDE OF THE FOOT. A large area of the lateral surface of the calcaneus may be palpated. The posterior portion feels relatively smooth, but below and slightly anterior to the tip of the lateral malleolus a small process may be felt, which process separates the tendons of the peroneus longus and brevis. More anteriorly, near its articulation with the cuboid bone, another prominence may be felt. The *tuberosity at the base of the fifth metatarsal bone* is a large, easily identified prominence on the lateral side of the foot near the sole. The *cuboid bone* may be palpated between the calcaneus and the tuberosity of the fifth metatarsal bone and may be followed dorsally toward its articulations with the lateral cuneiform and with the navicular bones. The cuboid extends dorsally to about the middle of the foot, but this area is covered by ligaments and tendons and the various bones cannot be distinctly recognized.

The three *cuneiform bones* (L. *cuneus,* wedge), lying across the instep of the foot, form the arched part of the dorsum of the foot. The height of this arched portion varies considerably in different individuals. The *medial cuneiform bone* is identified in its medial portion between the tuberosity of the navicular bone and the base of the first metatarsal bone. The *intermediate and lateral cuneiform bones* lie in line with the second and third metatarsal bones, respectively, articulating proximally with the navicular bone.

The *heads of the metatarsal bones* are felt both on the dorsal and the plantar sides of the foot. By manipulating the toes in flexion and extension, the heads of the metatarsal bones are particularly well palpated from the plantar side. Their plantar surfaces constitute the ball of the foot on which weight is carried when standing on tiptoes. In the region of the head of the first metatarsal bone, the sesamoid bones, which are imbedded in the tendon of the flexor hallucis brevis, can sometimes be palpated and moved slightly from side to side. The *shafts of the metatarsal bones* are best palpated on the dorsum of the foot. The *phalanges* of the toes are easily recognized. The *interphalangeal joints* should be palpated and manipulated.

The *talus* (astragalus), articulating with the tibia and the fibula above, with the calcaneus below, and with the navicular bone in front, has only small palpable areas. When the ankle is fully plantar-flexed, it may be approached from its anterior side, best medially, where it may be palpated distal to the medial malleolus but proximal to the tuberosity of the navicular bone. The palpable area becomes smaller when the ankle is dorsiflexed.

NONPALPABLE STRUCTURES

Because of the joint capsules and the many ligaments (short, long, transverse, longitudinal and oblique) which cross the various joints of the foot, the shape of each individual bone cannot be palpated in detail nor can the exact location of the joints be ascertained.

It is of interest to note that several of the bones of the foot have grooves to accommodate tendons. A groove on the inferior surface of the cuboid bone contains the tendon of the peroneus longus; the tendon of the flexor hallucis longus is lodged in a groove on the talus, then courses below the sustentaculum talare of the calcaneus; the same tendon, nearing its insertion on the distal phalanx, passes through an osteofibrous groove on the plantar surface of the big toe.

In general, for palpation of bony structures, an approach from the dorsum of the foot, or laterally and medially, proves more successful than from the plantar side where an abundance of soft tissue—fatty and muscular—hampers palpation. The palpable portions of the bones, as described above, serve as landmarks for finding adjacent parts, should such detailed localization be desired.

JOINTS

TALOCRURAL JOINT (Upper Ankle Joint)

TYPE OF JOINT. The talocrural joint, between the talus and the *crus* (L. leg), is a hinge joint with one degree of freedom of motion. The talocrural joint is usually referred to as the "ankle joint," although "upper ankle joint" is more specific. The trochlea of the talus possesses a weight-bearing articular surface which apposes the distal extremity of the tibia, and medial and lateral surfaces which articulate with the malleoli. Three bones, therefore, are involved in formation of this joint: tibia, fibula and talus.

The shape of the articulating portion of the talus should be noticed it is narrower posteriorly and widens anteriorly. Mechanically, this means that when the leg-foot angle is 90 degrees or less, the malleoli fit snugly around the sides of the talus and the joint is quite stable. But when the leg-foot angle is obtuse, as in shoes with high heels, the posterior and narrower portion of the talus lies between the malleoli, and consequently there is more play in the joint. This is one reason why wearing shoes with high heels causes relative instability of the ankle joint.

AXIS OF MOTION. The axis of motion of the upper ankle joint is transverse and passes through the trochlea of the talus (Fig. 99). A line connecting the two malleoli indicates its approximate direction. Since the lateral malleolus extends further posteriorly than the medial one, this axis is not parallel to the axis for flexion and extension of the knee. The amount of deviation of the axis of the upper ankle joint from the knee axis may be determined grossly as follows.

The subject stands with the knee caps pointing straight forward so that the knee axes come to lie in the frontal plane. An outline of the feet is traced on a paper on which the subject stands, and the vertical projections of the malleoli are marked on the paper. By connecting the floor projections of the malleoli, a line indicating the direction of the axis of the upper ankle joint is obtained. The amount of devia-

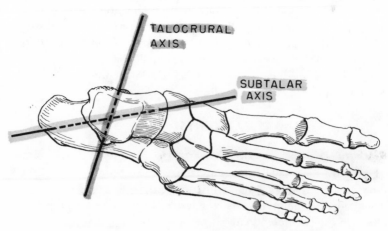

FIG. 99. Axes of upper ankle joint (talocrural) and lower ankle joint (subtalar). (Redrawn from Elftman, 1960.)

tion of this line from the frontal plane may be measured with a goniometer. Individual variations of this angle are considerable.

MOVEMENTS OF THE UPPER ANKLE JOINT. These movements are best described as *dorsiflexion*, toward the dorsal side of the foot, and *plantar flexion*, toward the plantar side of the foot. If the terms flexion and extension are used, misunderstandings may arise. Functionally, plantar flexion of the ankle may be called extension, since it is part of a general extension movement of hip, knee and ankle. From the anatomical standpoint, dorsiflexion may claim the name extension, since the movement occurs toward the extensor side of the limb. To avoid this dilemma, it is customary to use the terms dorsiflexion and plantar flexion, which terms are descriptive and cannot be misunderstood.

SUBTALAR JOINT (Lower Ankle Joint)

The inferior surface of the talus presents three articular facets which rest on corresponding areas of the calcaneus to form the subtalar joint, or lower ankle joint. Anteriorly, the talus articulates with the navicular bone. This complex set of articulations allows movements about an oblique axis, allowing the foot to be turned in (*inversion*) and turned out (*eversion*).

AXIS OF MOTION. The axis of motion for inversion and eversion is represented by a line which begins on the lateral-posterior aspect of the heel and proceeds in a forward-upward-medial direction, as seen in Figure 99 (Manter, 1941; Hicks, 1953; Elftman, 1960; Isman and Inman, 1969).

TRANSVERSE TARSAL JOINT

The transverse tarsal joint is also called the *midtarsal joint*. A disarticulation at the transverse tarsal joint is known as *Chopart's amputation* (after the French surgeon, François Chopart), and the joint itself is sometimes referred to as *Chopart's joint*. The bones which go into the formation of this joint are the *talus* and *calcaneus* proximally, and the *navicular* and *cuboid* distally. Functionally, with respect to this joint, the navicular and cuboid bones may be considered as one segment since very little movement is permitted between them.

The *talonavicular joint* is of the condyloid type, the convex head of the talus fitting into the concave surface of the navicular bone. The *calcaneocuboid joint* is saddle-shaped. When the foot skeleton is viewed from above, the joint line of the transverse tarsal articula-

---

Ankle and Foot   **201**

tion has the shape of an S (Fig. 99). The character of this rather complicated joint with its shifting axes of motion, its relation to the upper and the lower ankle joints, and its muscular control has been discussed by Elftman (1960).

MOVEMENTS OF THE TRANSVERSE TARSAL JOINT. This joint permits movement of the front part of the foot in relation to the back part, called *pronation* when the arch of the foot becomes lowered, *supination* when the arch is raised (Elftman, 1960).

The tarsometatarsal joints allow some flexion and extension; the first and fifth also allow slight abduction-adduction.

Biomechanical considerations and the complicated movements of these three joints (talocrural, subtalar, transverse tarsal) continue to receive considerable investigation particularly with reference to any clinical implications for prosthetic and orthotic problems and for surgical stabilization of the foot and ankle (Inman, 1969a; Inman, 1969b; Isman and Inman, 1969).

METATARSOPHALANGEAL JOINTS

These joints correspond to the metacarpophalangeal joints of the hand, and, like the latter, they permit a considerable range of motion. In the hand, motions toward the palmar side of the hand are of larger range than toward the dorsal side. In the foot, the reverse is true: range in extension is more pronounced than in flexion. This fact is related to the weight-bearing function of the foot, for in rising on tiptoes and in walking, range in extension is more important than range in flexion.

TYPE OF JOINT AND AXES OF MOTION. The metatarsophalangeal joints, like their counterparts in the upper extremity, are of the *condyloid* type, possessing two degrees of freedom of motion and permitting flexion-extension and abduction-adduction movements, the latter being less important and less well under control than in the hand. The *axes of motion* for these movements pass through the center of the head of the metatarsal bone, that for flexion-extension in a transverse direction, the one for abduction-adduction in a dorsal-plantar direction. Orientation for abduction-adduction is a line through the second toe, while the corresponding line in the hand goes through the third finger.

INTERPHALANGEAL JOINTS

The interphalangeal joints of the toes are similar to those of the fingers, the great toe possessing one such joint, the four lesser toes two joints each.

DEFORMITIES OF THE FOOT

Foot deformities may develop from various causes, such as congenital malformations of bones, muscular paralysis, stresses and strains in weight-bearing, and poorly fitting shoes, or from a combination of several of these as follows:

Pes valgus: A more or less permanent pronation-eversion of the foot, the body weight acting to depress the arch. Several stages may be recognized, the last stage being known as *pes planus* or structural, rigid, flat foot.

Pes varus (club foot): A more or less permanent supination-inversion of the foot so that the weight is transferred to the outside of the foot and the medial border of the foot is off the ground.

Pes calcaneus: Subject walks on heel. The front part of the foot does not touch the ground.

Pes equinus (L. *equinus,* relating to a horse): Subject walks on ball of foot with the heel off the ground.

Pes cavus: Exaggerated high arch, or hollowness of the foot.

Combination of two of the above deviations also occurs, such as *calcaneovalgus, equinovarus,* and *equinocavus.*

Hallux valgus: A lateral deviation of the great toe at the metatarsophalangeal joint. This condition is often accompanied by a *bunion,* or inflammation of the bursa on the medial side of the toe joint.

MUSCLES OF THE ANKLE AND FOOT

The muscles, which pass over the ankle joints, originate on the tibia and the fibula, except for the gastrocnemius and the plantaris which take their origins on the femur. Since no muscles attach to the talus, the muscles passing from leg to foot act simultaneously on both the upper and the lower ankle joints. The toes are activated both by *long muscles,* that is, those which originate above the ankle joints, and by *short muscles,* originating below these joints.

The muscles which act on the ankle, or on the ankle and the toes, and which originate mainly on the shank, may be divided into three groups: posterior, lateral and anterior.

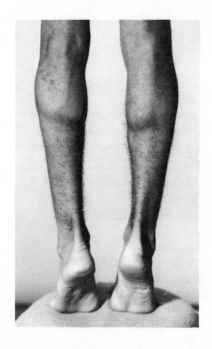

FIG. 100. Both soleus and gastrocnemius contract in rising on tiptoes. Note that the medial head of the gastrocnemius descends somewhat further than the lateral head.

POSTERIOR GROUP OF MUSCLES

The *gastrocnemius* (G. *gaster*, belly, and *kneme*, knee) makes up the major portion of the muscles of the calf. *Origin:* By two tendinous heads, the *medial* and the *lateral*, from above the condyles of the femur, these origins being partly adherent to the capsule of the knee joint. The medial head is the largest of the two and its muscular portion descends further distally than that of the lateral head (Fig. 100). The muscle fibers of the two heads converge to be *inserted* into a broad tendon-aponeurosis which begins as a septum between the two heads and which fuses with the aponeurosis over the soleus muscle. Distally, this tendon-aponeurosis narrows to form the *tendo calcaneus* (Achilles' tendon) which attaches to the calcaneus. *Innervation:* Branches of the tibial portion of the sciatic nerve.

Inspection and palpation: The gastrocnemius is responsible largely for the characteristic contour of the human calf. It is seen contracting in rising on tiptoes, walking, running, and jumping. In athletic individuals, particularly in males, the muscle bellies of the gastrocnemius when contracting are short and bulky, and the tendinous portions are comparatively long.

Clinical Kinesiology

The *soleus* (L. *soles,* sole, sandal), like the gastrocnemius, belongs to the posterior group of the leg. These two muscles together were formerly called the *triceps surae,* or three-headed muscle of the calf. *Origin:* Upper portion of the tibia and fibula. *Insertion:* A tendinous aponeurosis covering the posterior surface of the muscle, which aponeurosis narrows distally and unites with the tendon of the gastrocnemius to form the tendo calcaneus. *Innervation:* Tibial portion of sciatic nerve.

Inspection and palpation: The soleus is covered largely by the gastrocnemius, but in the lower portion of the calf it protrudes on both sides of the gastrocnemius so that it may here be observed and palpated. When the subject rises on tiptoes, both gastrocnemius and soleus contract strongly (Fig. 100). A comparatively isolated contraction of the soleus may be seen if the subject lies prone with knee flexed and plantar-flexes the ankle against slight resistance (Fig. 101). The foot should be stabilized on the dorsal side so that the subject may press lightly against the examiner's hand.

The *tibialis posterior* is the most deeply situated muscle of the calf. It lies close to the interosseous membrane between the tibia and the fibula, covered by the soleus and the gastrocnemius. *Origin:* Interosseous membrane and proximal portion of the tibia and the fibula. In the upper calf it occupies a central position between the flexor digitorum longus medially and the flexor hallucis laterally. In the lower calf it takes a more medial course. Its tendon lies in a groove on the medial malleolus and is held down by a broad ligament. It then continues to the sole of the foot to be *inserted* into the tuberosity of the navicular bone and, by means of fibrous expansions, into adjacent tarsal bones and into the bases of the metatarsals. The spreading out of its insertion provides a tendomuscular support on the plantar side of the foot.

Inspection and palpation: The tendon of the tibialis posterior is observable and well palpable both above and below the medial malleolus. It is particularly easy to identify below the medial malleolus where it lies superficially and, in most individuals, can be seen heading toward the tuberosity of the navicular bone. Above the malleolus, its tendon lies close to those of the flexor digitorum longus and the flexor hallucis longus. These tendons may be identified by alternating inversion of the ankle (which activates the tibialis posterior) with flexion of the toes (which brings out the toe flexors). For palpation of these tendons, it is suggested that the subject be seated on a chair,

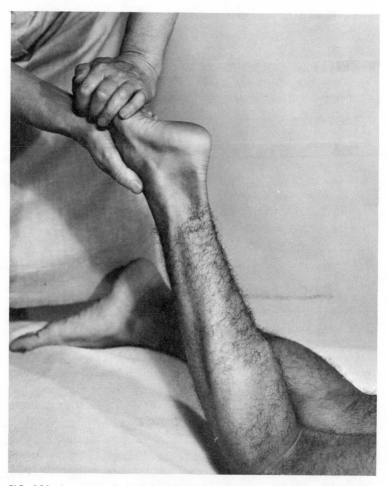

FIG. 101. A comparatively isolated contraction of the soleus is obtained when plantar flexion is performed while the knee is flexed.

the limb to be tested being crossed over the other one so that the foot is relaxed and plantar-flexed. It will be noticed that the tendon of the tibialis posterior lies closer to the medial malleolus than the other two tendons. The relationship between these three tendons just above the medial malleolus is expressed by the *Tom, Dick and Harry rule:* Tom for tibialis, Dick for digitorum, and Harry for hallucis.

The *flexor digitorum longus* is a deep muscle, lying medially in the calf, covered by the soleus and the medial head of the gastrocnemius.

Clinical Kinesiology

Origin: Tibia, below the insertion of the popliteus, and the intermuscular septum between it and the tibialis posterior. In the lower leg it crosses over the tibialis posterior so that at the malleolus it comes to lie behind the tendon of the tibialis posterior. Its tendon enters the sole of the foot near the sustentaculum talare, crosses the tendon of the flexor hallucis longus, and divides into four parts which *insert* into the bases of the distal phalanges of the second to fifth toes. On its way to its insertion, each tendon perforates the corresponding tendon of the short toe flexor, this arrangement being similar to that of the hand. *Innervation:* Tibial nerve. *Palpation* of the tendon of the flexor digitorum longus has been described with that of the tibialis posterior. Its muscular portion may, in part, be palpated on the medial side of the calf.

The *flexor hallucis longus* is located under the soleus on the lateral side of the calf. It is a rather strong muscle, its cross section being considerably larger than that of the flexor digitorum longus (Table XI). *Origin:* Posterior surface of the fibula, and intermuscular septa. Its tendon passes behind the medial malleolus, through a groove in the talus, and then under the sustentaculum talare. After entering the sole of the foot, it crosses the tendon of the flexor digitorum longus on this tendon's deep side. At the metatarsophalangeal joint it passes between the two sesamoid bones in the tendon of the flexor hallucis brevis. *Insertion:* Base of the distal phalanx of the great toe. *Innervation:* Tibial nerve. *Palpation* of its tendon may be done above the medial malleolus, as previously described, and in the region of the sustentaculum talare, by alternating flexion and extension of the great toe. Since the average individual is unable to flex the great toe without simultaneously flexing the lesser toes, its tendon is difficult to distinguish from that of the flexor digitorum longus.

LATERAL GROUP OF MUSCLES

This group is located on the lateral side of the shank, anterior to the calf group, occupying a comparatively small area and being separated from the anterior and posterior groups by intermuscular septa. There are two muscles in this group: the peroneus longus and peroneus brevis.

In its location, the *peroneus longus* (Gr. *perone,* brooch, fibula) appears as a direct continuation of the biceps femoris. The peroneus longus *originates* from the head of the fibula while the biceps femoris inserts into this head. The peroneus longus, however, has an origin other than just the head of the fibula—it takes its origin also from the neighboring area of the tibia, from the shaft of the fibula and from intermuscular septa. The muscle fibers converge to form a tendon which passes in a groove behind the lateral malleolus and then to the cuboid bone where it enters the sole of the foot. It is here lodged in a groove of the cuboid bone, which groove has an oblique direction forward and medially. *Insertion:* Plantar surface of first cuneiform bone and base of first metatarsal.

The *peroneus brevis,* as its name indicates, is shorter than the peroneus longus. *Origin:* Fibula, lower than the longus, and intermuscular septa. Its tendon passes behind the lateral malleolus, then across the calcaneus and the cuboid, to be *inserted* into the dorsal surface of the tuberosity of the fifth metatarsal bone.

The two peronei muscles are *innervated* by the superficial branch of the common peroneal nerve. (It may be recalled that the common peroneal nerve is the lateral division of the sciatic nerve and that it winds around the head of the fibula before dividing into a deep and a superficial branch).

Inspection and palpation of the two peronei muscles: The muscular portion of the peroneus longus is identified just below the head of the fibula and may be followed down the lateral side of the leg. From halfway down the leg to the ankle, the two peronei muscles are palpated together. Nearly all of the brevis is covered by the longus, but in the lower part of the leg it can be felt separately from the longus.

When eversion is resisted, as seen in Figure 102, both muscles contract. The tendon of the peroneus brevis stands out more than the tendon of the peroneus longus and can be followed to its insertion on the fifth metatarsal bone. At the malleolus it appears as if the tendons of the peronei muscles might slip over to the front side, but they are anchored firmly by retinacula. Above the malleolus, the tendon of the peroneus longus lies slightly posterior to that of the brevis, and, at least in some individuals, it is well palpable. Below the malleolus, the tendon of the peroneus longus is held down close to the bone. It lies on the plantar side of the tendon of the peroneus brevis, but is rather difficult to identify. (See also Fig. 109B).

Note that when eversion of the foot is resisted in the sitting position, as in Figure 102, external rotation of the leg with respect to the

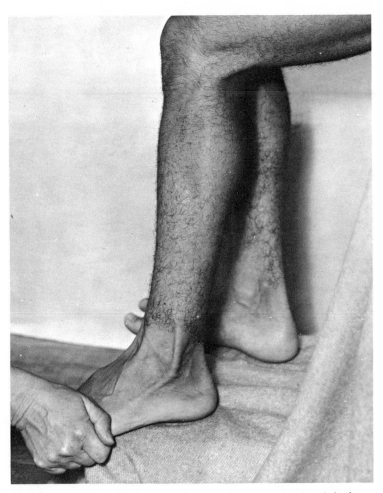

FIG. 102. The tendons of the peroneus longus and peroneus brevis both pass posterior to the lateral malleolus. The tendon of the brevis may be followed to its insertion on the fifth metatarsal bone. Note also the tendon of the biceps femoris of knee.

thigh occurs simultaneously; the prominent tendon of the biceps femoris is seen at the knee.

ANTERIOR GROUP OF MUSCLES

The anterior group is located on the lateral side of the anterior margin of the tibia, the sharp bony ridge palpable from the tuberosity

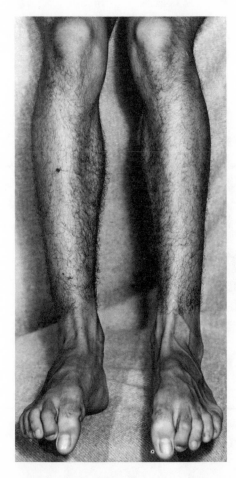

FIG. 103. The anterior tibialis is superficial and can be observed all the way from its origin to its insertion. Its tendon is strong and prominent as it passes the ankle joint.

of the tibia all the way down to the ankle. It is separated from the lateral group by an intermuscular septa but appears, on palpation, to be continuous with it. The muscles of the anterior group are the tibialis anterior, extensor hallucis longus, extensor digitorum longus and peroneus tertius.

The *anterior tibialis* is responsible for the roundness of the shank anteriorly. When this muscle is paralyzed, a flatness or even slight concavity of this region results, so that the anterior margin of the tibia becomes even more prominent than normal. *Origin:* Lateral condyle and shaft of tibia, interosseous membrane and fascia of leg. The muscle becomes tendinous well above the ankle and its tendon passes over the dorsum of the ankle, held down by the transverse and cruciate ligaments. *Insertion:* Medial aspect of the medial cuneiform bone and base of the first metatarsal bone. *Innervation:* A branch from the common peroneal nerve and a branch from the deep peroneal nerve.

Inspection and palpation: Because the muscle is superficial throughout its course, it may be observed and palpated all the way from its origin to its insertion. The muscular portion is palpated proximally, on the lateral side of the anterior margin of the tibia when the foot is dorsiflexed. Its tendon is observed and palpated as it passes over the ankle where it rises considerably when the foot is dorsiflexed (Fig. 103). In the illustration the subject flexes the toes so that the tendon of the extensor hallucis longus, which lies just lateral to that of the anterior tibialis, will not be seen. If one wishes to observe both tendons simultaneously, the ankle should be held dorsiflexed and the great toe should be flexed and extended.

In its upper portion the *extensor hallucis longus* is covered by the anterior tibialis and by the extensor digitorum longus. *Origin:* Middle portion of shaft of the fibula and interosseous membrane. Its tendon passes on the dorsum of the ankle, lateral to the tendon of the tibialis anterior, and is held down by ligaments. *Insertion:* Base of distal phalanx of great toes. *Innervation:* A branch from the deep peroneal nerve.

Inspection and palpation: By resisting dorsiflexion of the great toe, as seen in Figure 104, the course of the tendon of extensor hallucis longus over the dorsum of the foot may be observed. The muscular portion is palpated in the lower half of the leg, but since it is almost entirely covered by the anterior tibialis and the extensor digitorum longus, it cannot be easily distinguished from these muscles.

The *extensor digitorum longus and peroneus tertius* muscles are described together because they usually are not well differentiated in their upper portions. The peroneus tertius is the most lateral part of the extensor digitorum longus, but is sometimes described as a separate muscle. The extensor digitorum longus is superficial, bordering laterally to the peronei muscles, medially to the anterior tibialis. *Origin:* Upper portion of the tibia and fibula, interosseous membrane, intermuscular septa and fascia; the peroneus tertius originates from the distal portion of the fibula and from the interosseous membrane. The common tendon passes on the dorsum of the ankle, and, like the other tendon in this region, it is held down by the transverse and

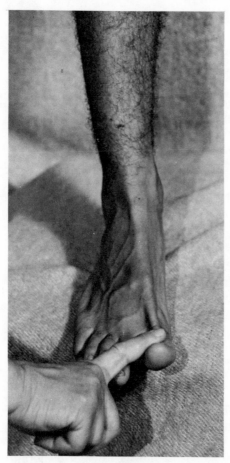

FIG. 104. The tendon of the extensor hallucis longus is observed when the great toe is dorsiflexed against resistance. It lies just lateral to the tendon of anterior tibialis at the ankle.

cruciate ligaments. The tendon divides into five slips, the most lateral one being the tendon of the peroneus tertius. *Insertion:* Four tendons go to the bases of the middle and distal phalanges of the four lesser toes; the tendon of the peroneus tertius goes to the dorsum of the fifth metatarsal bone. *Innervation:* A branch from the deep peroneal nerve.

Inspection and palpation: To bring out the tendons of the toe extensors without simultaneous contraction of the anterior tibialis, the subject sits on a chair and lifts the toes off the floor while maintaining the sole on the floor. If resistance is given to the four lesser toes, the individual tendons stand out better (Fig. 105). The tendon of the peroneus tertius, when present and observable, is seen lateral

Clinical Kinesiology

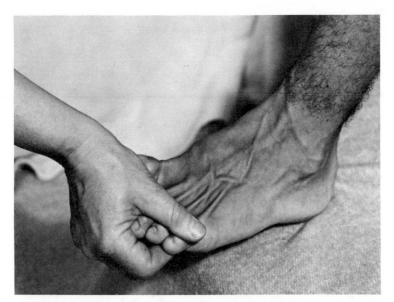

FIG. 105. The tendons of the extensor digitorum longus are seen as they pass the ankle and proceed toward the four lesser toes. Examiner resists on the dorsum of the toes. In this subject the tendon of the peroneus brevis, which passes lateral to the other tendons, could not be found.

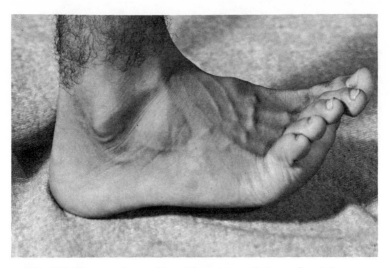

FIG. 106. The muscular portion of the extensor digitorum brevis is seen on the lateral side of the dorsum of the foot. The tendons of insertion of this short muscle are hidden under those of the long toe extensors.

to the tendon going to the fifth toe. This tendon is variable in its insertion and the muscle may be missing altogether.

The extensor digitorum longus also acts on the ankle joint, an action which can best be observed if dorsiflexion of the foot is resisted by pressure on the dorsum of the toes, as seen in Figure 105.

MUSCLES ORIGINATING BELOW THE ANKLE JOINTS

These muscles are comparable to the intrinsic muscles of the hand inasmuch as they are short muscles acting on the digits only. Some of these muscles are almost identical with corresponding muscles of the hand, while others differ considerably.

The *extensor digitorum brevis arises* on the anterolateral side of the foot. Its muscular portion which consists of four parts lies, in part, beneath the tendons of the long extensor. Of the four tendon slips, the most medial one inserts into the base of the proximal phalanx of the great toe; the other three slips join the lateral side of those tendons of the extensor digitorum longus which serve the second to fourth toes. The muscle portion serving the great toe is the largest of the four and is sometimes described as a separate muscle, the *extensor hallucis brevis. Innervation:* Branch of the deep peroneal nerve.

Inspection and palpation: The extensor digitorum brevis is variable in size. In some subjects it is rather flat and hardly palpable, and in others a round firm muscle belly may be seen and palpated on the lateral side of the foot. It is seen in Figure 106 anterior to the lateral malleolus.

Since the tendons of the extensor digitorum brevis attach on the lateral side of the tendons of the longus, the former tendons compensate for the oblique direction of the latter. When the two muscles contract together, as they tend to do, the toes are extended without deviation.

It is suggested that the muscles of the sole of the foot be studied in an atlas of anatomy and that specific attention be given to the following:

Flexor digitorum brevis is comparable to the flexor digitorum superficialis in the hand, except that it is a short muscle.

Abductor hallucis is comparable to the abductor pollicis brevis. The abductor pollicis longus has no counterpart in the foot.

Quadratus plantae (flexor accessorius) inserts into the tendon of the flexor digitorum longus and has no counterpart in the hand.

The *lumbricals* have a similar location to those of the hand.

The *interossei* are much like those in the hand, except that with respect to abduction and adduction, they are oriented to the second instead of the third digit.

Discussion of Function of Muscles Acting at Ankle Joints

PLANTAR FLEXION OF THE ANKLE (Talocrural Joint)

Plantar flexion of the ankle is performed mainly, and almost exclusively, by the *gastrocnemius and the soleus,* together known as the *triceps surae.* The attachment of the common tendon of insertion to that part of the calcaneus which protrudes posteriorly gives excellent leverage to these muscles. Their large cross section (Table X), which far exceeds that of all the other ankle muscles combined (including the cross sections of the anterior and lateral groups), is also an indication of the functional demands placed on these two muscles.

There are other muscles whose tendons pass posterior to the axis of motion of the talocrural joint but they have poor leverage and are quite ineffective as plantar flexors. These muscles do not act on the calcaneus but insert into more distal parts of the foot and have specific actions at other joints.

The marked difference in leverage between the triceps surae and the other posterior muscles in plantar flexion of the ankle may be appreciated by measuring the perpendicular distance from the axis of the talocrural joint to the line of action of the various muscles. In the case of the triceps surae, this distance in the adult is approximately two inches, while the tendons of the posterior tibialis and the peronei muscles lie so close to the malleoli that they barely pass posterior to the axis. The tendon of the flexor digitorum longus lies only slightly further back. The flexor hallucis longus has somewhat better leverage but its action as a plantar flexor of the ankle still is insignificant compared to that of the triceps surae.

DIFFERENTIATION BETWEEN THE GASTROCNEMIUS AND THE SOLEUS IN PLANTAR FLEXION OF THE ANKLE. Because the two heads of the gastrocnemius originate above the axis of the knee, this muscle is most effective as a plantar flexor when the knee is extended. The soleus, originating below the axis, is uninfluenced by the position of the knee. When the ankle is plantar-flexed while the knee is in a flexed position, the soleus is likely to be more active than the gastrocnemius. This is the case when the heel is being pushed off the floor in the sitting position and when the subject lies prone with the knee flexed and plantar-flexes the ankle (Fig. 101). In both instances it can be ascertained by palpation that the soleus acts in a relatively isolated fashion. However, if, in the positions just mentioned, great force is required, both muscles may be felt contracting simultaneously.

Function of the gastrocnemius and soleus muscles was investigated in six normal subjects (Herman and Bragin, 1967). Subjects were tested in a prone position with knees extended and tension and electromyographic activity were recorded with respect to muscle length, degree and rate of tension development in graded voluntary isometric contraction. Gastrocnemius activity was observed to be greatest when the ankle was plantar-flexed, when contractions were maximal and when tension developed rapidly. The soleus was most active in positions of ankle dorsiflexion and when contractions were minimal.

FUNCTION OF THE SOLEUS IN ERECT STANDING. Basler (1942) found that the force requirements of the plantar flexors for equilibration at the ankle in normal erect standing never exceeded one-seventh of the total strength of this muscle group. (When a load was carried, the tension would rise to one-fifth or more of the total strength.) It would seem that either the soleus or the gastrocnemius, unaided by the other, would be capable of producing sufficient tension for normal equilibration. Since the force needed is comparatively small it is difficult to ascertain by palpation the extent to which one or the other muscle is involved.

The soleus has been found to contain more "red" or "slow" muscle fibers than the gastrocnemius which possesses predominantly "pale" or "fast" fibers (Denny-Brown, 1929). This would indicate that the soleus is concerned more with stabilization at the ankle and control of postural sway than the gastrocnemius. Being composed of slow-firing motor units, the soleus operates economically, i.e., with less fatigue for sustained contraction than the gastrocnemius which contains predominantly rapid-firing motor units.

The importance of the soleus as a postural muscle has been confirmed by electromyography. Joseph (1960), in studying the activity of various muscles in the "standing-at-ease" position, found continuous electrical activity in the soleus in all of the twelve subjects investigated; activity in the gastrocnemius could be detected only in seven of the twelve subjects.

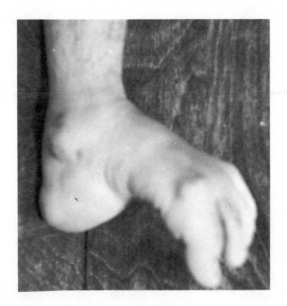

FIG. 107. Post-poliomyelitic paralysis of the triceps surae. The long toe flexors, although passing posterior to the axis of the talocrural joint, are incapable of plantar-flexing the ankle. With the triceps surae out of action, the long toe flexors are instrumental in the development of a calcaneocaval deformity.

TRICEPS SURAE IN RISING ON TIPTOES, WALKING, RUNNING, AND JUMPING. The gastrocnemius and the soleus are both involved in activities requiring forceful plantar flexion of the ankle. In rising on tiptoes both muscles are seen to contract simultaneously (Fig. 100), and their state of contraction may be ascertained by palpation. In running and jumping, the action of the gastrocnemius is indispensable since its fibers possess the quality of producing a rapid rise in tension. (The function of the triceps surae in walking is discussed in Chapter 11.)

PARALYSIS OF THE PLANTAR FLEXORS OF THE ANKLE. When the gastrocnemius-soleus group is paralyzed, the patient cannot rise on tiptoes and the gait is severely affected (see Chapter 11). The act of climbing stairs is awkward and slow, and activities such as running and jumping are all but impossible. The deep calf muscles ("Tom, Dick and Harry"), although passing posterior to the axis of the upper ankle joint, are incapable of substituting for the triceps surae.

The effect of an isolated paralysis of the triceps surae may be observed in post-poliomyelitic patients in whom the deep calf muscles

---

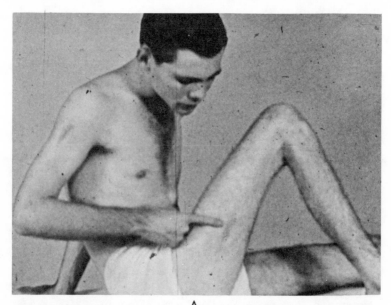

A

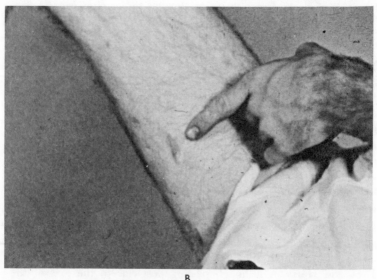

B

FIG. 108. Penetrating shrapnel injury causing a severance of the tibial portion of the sciatic nerve, leaving the common peroneal nerve intact. A, Exit of shrapnel; B, entrance of shrapnel. (Frames from a motion picture.)

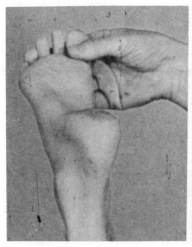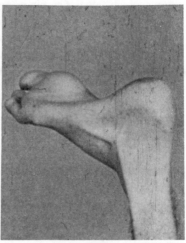

A   B

FIG. 109. Same patient as in Figure 108. A, Patient prone, knee flexed. Passive plantar flexion is performed. B, When patient attempts to plantar-flex the foot actively, the foot swings out in marked eversion. The tendons of the peroneus longus and brevis (plainly visible) course so close to the axis of the talocrural joint that their action in plantar flexion is practically nil. (Frames from a motion picture.)

have been spared. If these patients are children (whose feet are pliable) a calcaneocaval deformity tends to develop (Fig. 107). It is obvious that the tibialis posterior, the flexor hallucis longus and the flexor digitorum longus, although their tendons pass posterior to the joint axis, are incapable of plantar-flexing the ankle. These muscles have poor leverage at the upper ankle joint and, furthermore, do not attach to the calcaneus. Their tendons pass to the sole of the foot and when the muscles contract they affect more distal joints rather than the talocrural joint. The tendons of the flexor digitorum longus and flexor hallucis longus have a shortening effect on the foot in a front-to-back direction, and the calcaneus, having lost the counterbalancing effect of the triceps surae, assumes a dorsiflexed position. These elements all contribute to the development of a calcaneocaval deformity.

TIBIAL NERVE PARALYSIS. Clinically, the ineffectiveness of the peronei muscles as plantar flexors of the ankle was observed in a patient who had a complete paralysis of all the calf muscles as the result of a gunshot injury to the tibial portion of the sciatic nerve, an injury which left the common peroneal nerve intact (Fig. 108). To induce the patient to perform plantar flexion, this movement was first carried out passively several times (Fig. 109A), then the patient was asked to repeat the movement. No plantar flexion resulted but the foot swung out in marked eversion (Fig. 109B). Note in the illustration the sharp outline of the tendons of the peroneus longus above, the peroneus brevis below, the lateral malleolus. The long lever arm of the triceps surae as compared to the short leverage of the peronei muscles can be well appreciated in this illustration.

DORSIFLEXION OF THE ANKLE (Talocrural Joint)

This movement is performed by the anterior tibialis, the extensor hallucis longus, the extensor digitorum longus and the peroneus tertius. Of these muscles the tibialis anterior is by far the most important dorsiflexor—it has a straight line of pull for dorsiflexion, a comparatively large cross section (see Table X) and favorable leverage. This muscle also has the advantage of acting exclusively over the talocrural joint while the toe extensors tend to extend the toes first thus losing effectiveness at the ankle.

ISOLATED PARALYSIS OF THE ANTERIOR TIBIALIS. When the anterior tibialis is paralyzed and the toe extensors are intact, dorsiflexion of limited range can be performed. The extensor hallucis longus is then seen contracting strongly with the result that the great toe extends full range but comparatively little dorsiflexion of the ankle occurs. Extensor digitorum longus also participates in dorsiflexion and, if acting in an isolated fashion, will simultaneously produce strong eversion of the subtalar joint. Such eversion, however, when unwanted, can be compensated for by the tibialis posterior.

INVERSION OF THE ANKLE (Subtalar Joint)

Inversion is performed by the posterior tibialis, the gastrocnemius-soleus combination and the long toe flexors, which muscles all course on the inversion side of the axis of the subtalar joint. The tibialis posterior is the inverter *par excellence* while the others can invert in limited range only. The tibialis posterior, as previously stated, has extremely poor leverage as a plantar flexor, although its leverage for inversion is excellent. It controls this movement regardless of whether the ankle is dorsiflexed or plantar-flexed, and this can be readily ascertained by palpation.

In many textbooks the tibialis anterior is also identified with inversion. However, the insertion of this muscle is directly in line with the axis of the subtalar joint so that it is neutral with respect to inversion-eversion. Clinically, the inability of the anterior tibialis to invert the ankle was demonstrated by the patient (in Figure 109) whose posterior tibialis was paralyzed. When the patient was asked to turn the foot out and in alternately, he everted the foot full range, then returned it to a neutral position. It may be stated that the anterior tibialis is capable of inversion from the fully everted position to the neutral position, but not beyond this point. (The anterior tibialis is also capable of everting the foot from the fully inverted position to the neutral position.) Fick lists the tibialis anterior both with the inverters and the everters (but last on each list), and its work capacity in these movements is very small (Table XI).

EVERSION OF THE ANKLE (Subtalar Joint)

This movement is performed by the peroneus longus and brevis, the extensor digitorum longus, and the peroneus tertius. The tendon of the extensor hallucis longus, although slightly on the eversion side of the foot courses so close to the axis of inversion-eversion that it has little effect on eversion. The peronei muscles are the main everters and they act in this capacity regardless of the position of the talocrural joint, whether this joint is dorsiflexed or plantar-flexed. The tendons of the peronei muscles may be palpated behind or below the lateral malleolus in all eversion movements. Figure 109 illustrates the strong eversion action of these muscles.

PRONATION-SUPINATION OF TRANSVERSE TARSAL JOINT

During standing (weight is carried on the foot) and particularly during walking (the body weight shifts from heel to toe), the transverse tarsal joint *pronates,* that is, the arch is lowered, this motion being caused mainly by the superimposed body weight. When the body weight shifts forward to the ball of the foot, the *plantar aponeurosis,* acting as a bowstring, is instrumental in raising the arch (Hicks, 1954). The tightness of the plantar aponeurosis may be palpated on passive dorsiflexion of the toes, whether performed in a nonweight-bearing position, or in weight-bearing, as in rising on tiptoes.

A moderate amount of pronation-supination is characteristic of normal walking. In some individuals the arch becomes almost obliterated during weight-bearing, but this must not be considered a "flat foot" as long as the condition reverses itself toward the end of stance phase. The amplitude of the pronation-supination movement which varies considerably in individuals appears to depend mainly upon the condition of the ligamentous apparatus of the foot, less upon the condition of the muscles. For example, a ballet dancer was seen in the clinic because she was worrying about getting flat feet. All of the muscles passing from her leg to her foot and the muscles in the sole of her foot were tested and found to be strong and under excellent control. Yet, in the standing position and on each step in walking, her feet pronated markedly. In this patient, the ligaments ordinarily responsible for arresting the motion probably had been excessively stretched during ballet practice. The muscles, although capable of preventing excessive pronation when attention was focused on the foot, did not do so automatically.

TARSOMETATARSAL MOVEMENTS

The term *supination* has been applied above to a motion of the posterior part of the foot which causes the arch to rise. Simultaneously, however, a twist in the opposite direction ("pronation twist") of the anterior portion of the foot is required if the first metatarsal head is to be kept on the ground during weight-bearing. This motion is made possible mainly by motions occurring at the three medial tarsometatarsal joints. Investigations by Hicks (1953) revealed that during supination approximately ten degrees of *plantar flexion of the first tarsometatarsal joint* occurs, lesser range of motion in plantar flexion taking place at the second and third joints. Conversely, pronation (lowering of the arch) is accompanied by *extension* of the tarsometatarsal joints.

INTERDEPENDENCE OF MOVEMENTS OF THE VARIOUS JOINTS

An attempt has been made above to describe motions at some of the joints of the foot separately, but these joints do not function in an isolated fashion—they are all interdependent. Note that the anterior talocalcaneal joint has a common capsule with the talonavicular joint; that the subtalar and the transverse tarsal joints are controlled by the same muscles; and that tarsometatarsal joints participate in raising and lowering the arch.

CLINICAL NOMENCLATURE

Clinically, a distinction between the movements of the various joints of the foot is not always made, the terms *everted feet* and *pronated feet* being used interchangeably by many workers. Both terms describe a foot condition characterized by a lowering of the arch.

EXERCISES FOR "FALLEN ARCHES"

The physical therapist is often asked to give exercises for "correction of fallen arches," and it is then important to realize, first, that the ligamentous mechanisms of the foot are all-important in maintaining the arch and that, therefore, undue strain of the ligamentous structures by faulty weight-bearing must be avoided; second, that the height of the arch (within normal limits) varies among individuals; and third, that many joints interact in determining the foot posture. The common practice of having an individual with "weak arches" or "fallen arches" walk on a tilt-board or externally rotate the femur (and the tibia) in standing raises the inner border of the foot but does not actually tackle the problem, inasmuch as it does not bring the first metatarsal head into correct position.

MUSCLE ACTION IN STANDING AND IN TOE-STANDING

One might be inclined to assume that the intrinsic muscles of the foot, and particularly those which course longitudinally on the medial side of the foot, are primarily responsible for the maintenance of the arch. Such assumption, however, has been proven erroneous by electromyographic studies which showed no consistent activity in the intrinsic muscles in ordinary standing (Basmajian, 1967). Investigators did record strong electrical activity of the intrinsic muscles in toe-standing, an activity which coincided with that of the gastrocnemius muscle. (Phasic action of the intrinsic muscles of the foot in walking is discussed in Chapter 11.)

Gray (1969) studied the electrical activity of four leg muscles in erect standing (soleus, tibialis anterior, tibialis posterior, peroneus longus). Results of the investigation substantiate findings of earlier authors that in subjects with normal arches muscles play no role in the support of the arches in standing. Such support is provided by osseous and ligamentous structures. The investigation further indicates that in subjects with flat feet the four leg muscles became

---

activated to provide relative static stability of the subtalar and transverse tarsal joints to prevent further flattening of the arch.

FLEXION AND EXTENSION OF METATARSOPHALANGEAL JOINTS

If the metatarsophalangeal joints are compared to their counterparts in the hand, it will be seen that range in flexion predominates in the hand while the range in extension is freer in the foot, corresponding to the grasping function of the hand and the weight-bearing function of the foot.

When, in walking, the body weight is transferred from heel to toe and the foot deploys itself from the ground, a considerable range in extension of the metatarsophalangeal joints is required. This extension movement is effected by the superimposed body weight, but excessive movement is checked by the toe flexors. Since these muscles are being passively stretched, they are physiologically well prepared to produce tension, as they are first engaged in a lengthening contraction and then in a shortening contraction, the latter contributing to the "push-off," a particularly important action in running.

ABDUCTION AND ADDUCTION OF METATARSOPHALANGEAL JOINTS

These movements, like those in the hand, are performed by the interossei muscles, supplemented by the special abductors of the great and little toes. Infants move their toes freely in abduction and adduction while adults have more difficulty. The first and the fifth toes are usually the easiest ones to move, but sometimes the ability of controlling the toes in these movements is altogether lost.

MOVEMENTS AT INTERPHALANGEAL JOINTS

Flexion and extension of these joints tend to occur as mass movements, it being difficult to move one toe without the others.

USE OF TOES FOR SKILLED ACTIVITIES

Potentially, movements performed by the human hand are also present in the foot, except for opposition of the thumb which is not represented in the foot. The ability of developing the foot as an effective grasp organ and for use in skilled activities is demonstrated by children with congenital amputations of the upper extremities, particularly if the entire limbs are missing. These children learn to use their feet in an extraordinarily skilled manner and are capable of doing practically everything with their feet that normal children do with their hands.

CHAPTER 8

Hip and Pelvic Region

BONES

PALPABLE STRUCTURES

Palpation may conveniently begin by placing the thumbs laterally on the *crests of the ilia,* one on the right and one on the left side. Under normal conditions, these two points are level in the standing position. Clinically, a lateral tilt of the pelvis is discovered by checking the height of the crests of the ilia. The symmetry of the pelvis may also be checked from the front by placing the thumbs on the *anterior superior spines of the ilia* which, in most individuals, are easily located, often being visible under the skin. In obese individuals, it may be best to start palpation on the crests of the ilia laterally, and to follow the downward curve of the crests anteriorly until the anterior superior spines are located.

If the crests are followed in a posterior direction, the *posterior superior spines of the ilia* are located. The subject in Figure 110 is palpating them with his thumbs. These prominences are broader and sturdier than the anterior spines and feel rough under the palpating fingers. Below each posterior spine is a depression, which is the posterior landmark for the *sacroiliac joint.*

To locate the *greater trochanter of the femur,* the subject places his thumb on the crest of the ilium laterally and reaches down on the thigh as far as possible with his middle finger. The greater trochanter is a large bony prominence over which the fingers may slide from side to side and upward and downward.

Other points on the pelvis, such as the pubic symphysis, the rami of the pubic bones, and the rami of the ischia, may also be palpated, at least in part. The *tuberosities of the ischia* (the "sit bones") are

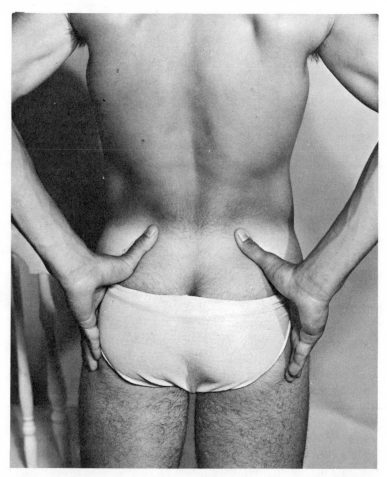

FIG. 110. The subject's thumbs are palpating the posterior superior spines of the ilia. The spines are best located by following the crests of the ilia in a posterior direction.

easy to locate when the subject is sitting on a hard chair. Once located in the sitting position, the tuberosities should also be palpated in the standing position. They are then approached below the gluteal fold and are best palpated when the gluteus maximus and the hamstrings are relaxed. Such relaxation is achieved by having the subject lean slightly backward from the waist, which transfers the center of gravity of the upper part of the body well behind the axis of the hip joint.

NONPALPABLE STRUCTURES

These include: the *sacroiliac joint* (see p. 257); the *acetabulum* (L. a shallow vinegar vessel or cup), the socket of the hip joint, into which the head of the femur fits; the *posterior anterior and inferior gluteal lines* on the outer surface of the ilium, which separate the areas of origin of the three gluteal muscles; the *anterior inferior iliac spine,* located below the superior spine and separated from it by a notch; the *posterior inferior iliac spine;* the *greater sciatic notch;* the *spine of the ischium;* the *head and neck of the femur;* and the *lesser trochanter of the femur.*

SHAPE OF FEMUR—DEVIATIONS IN THREE PLANES

In order to appreciate the shape of the femur, one must view this bone from the front, from the side and from above or below.

A *front view* reveals an oblique direction of the *anatomical axis of the femur,* which is represented by a line through the femoral shaft (Fig. 111). The *mechanical axis of the femur* is a line connecting the centers of the hip and knee joints. In the erect position this line is vertical or nearly vertical. The neck of the femur forms an angle with its shaft which, in the normal adult, is approximately 125 degrees.

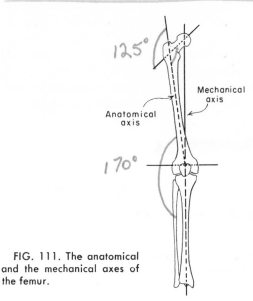

FIG. 111. The anatomical and the mechanical axes of the femur.

This angle, however, varies considerably in different individuals, being usually less than 125 degrees in women. Differences in the size of this angle are related to the greater width of the pelvis in females. Note that the neck-shaft angle is not strictly in the frontal plane, but that the greater trochanter lies somewhat posterior to the head of the femur (see below).

A *side view* of the femur shows a bowing of the shaft of the femur in the sagittal plane, the convexity being directed forward.

In viewing the femur *from above or from below,* the deviations in the horizontal plane may be observed consisting of an *anterior torsion of the head and the neck of the femur with respect to its shaft.* In erect standing, when the femoral condyles are in a neutral position (the transverse knee axis in the frontal plane), the center of the head of the femur is located anterior to the tip of the greater trochanter.

PLACEMENT OF HIP HINGES IN ARTIFICIAL APPLIANCES

When a pelvic belt is used for a patient who wears long leg braces or who uses an above-knee prosthesis, the hinges which connect the pelvic belt with the rest of the appliance should be placed in line with the transverse axis of the hip joint, so that there is no inter-ference with the free forward swing of the limb or with hip flexion in sitting. The height of the axis of the hinges is determined by locating the tip of the greater trochanter which is approximately level with the center of the femoral head. Because of the anterior torsion of the head and the neck of the femur, the hinges are placed slightly ante-rior to the tip of the greater trochanter (provided of course that the femur is neutral with respect to internal-external rotation).

DEFORMITIES OF FEMUR AT THE HIP

Coxa vara is a pathological condition characterized by a decrease in the neck-shaft angle of the femur so that this angle becomes smaller than 125 degrees, that is, approaches 90 degrees. As a result, there is an over-all *shortening of the limb.*

Coxa valga presents the opposite changes, that is, an increase in the size of the neck-shaft angle which becomes larger than 125 degrees, resulting in a *lengthening of the limb.*

Coxa plana is caused by a pathological condition (osteochondritis) resulting in a flattening of the spherical surface of the femoral head, a deformity which occurs mainly in children.

HIP JOINT (ARTICULATIO COXAE)

The hip joint is perhaps the best example of a ball-and-socket joint in the human body. The joint surfaces of the head of the femur and the acetabulum correspond better to each other and have firmer connections than the joint surfaces of the shoulder joint. This promotes stability but limits range of motion. The hip joint has three degrees of freedom of motion: *flexion-extension, abduction-adduction* and *internal-external rotation.* In most activities, combinations of these three types of movements occur.

AXES OF MOTION

At the hip joint, movement may take place about any number of axes, all passing through the center of the femoral head, but for descriptive purposes, three axes perpendicular to each other are usually chosen.

In standing, the *axis for flexion and extension* is transverse (horizontal, in a side-to-side direction). A line connecting the centers of the two femoral heads is called the *common hip axis.* Movement about the common hip axis takes place when, for example, the pelvis rocks forward and backward in standing or when, in back-lying position, both knees are pulled up toward the chest.

The *axis for abduction and adduction* (in standing) is horizontal, in a front-to-back direction. The limb may move in relation to the pelvis, as in lifting the limb laterally, or the pelvis may move in relation to the limb, as in inclining the trunk to the side of the stance leg or as in lowering the pelvis on the side opposite the stance leg. In each instance, whether the limb or the pelvis moves, the correct term to use is abduction or adduction of the hip.

The *axis for internal and external rotation* (in standing) is vertical and this axis is identical with the mechanical axis of the femur (Fig. 111). In internal rotation, the greater trochanter moves forward in relation to the front part of the pelvis or, conversely, the front part of the pelvis moves toward the greater trochanter. External rotation is a movement in the opposite direction.

MUSCLES

The posterior muscles are the gluteus maximus, the hamstrings and the posterior portion of the adductor magnus. In addition, there is a deeply located group consisting of six small muscles, all external rotators of the hip.

The *gluteus maximus* (Gr. *gloutos,* buttock) is the large, superficial muscle which is responsible for the roundness of the buttock region. *Origin:* Posterior portion of the crest of the ilium, lumbodorsal fascia, parts of the sacrum and coccyx, and sacrotuberous ligament. The fibers take a downward and lateral course and are *inserted* (1) into the iliotibial tract and (2) into the gluteal tuberosity of the shaft of the femur, on the posterior aspect of the femur. *Innervation:* Inferior gluteal nerve.

Inspection and palpation: The gluteus maximus may be observed when the subject is prone or standing erect. Like the quadriceps,

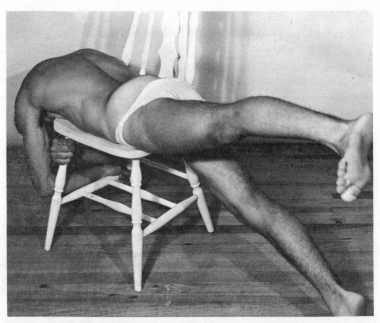

FIG. 112. The gluteus maximus is strongly activated when the hip is extended and externally rotated.

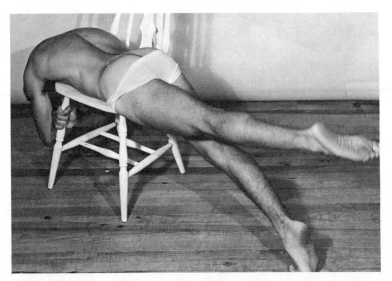

FIG. 113. When the hip is extended and internally rotated, the inner extensor group of muscles contracts while the gluteus maximus markedly decreases its contraction.

it can be tightened by simply "setting" it without any joint motion being carried out. For stronger activation of the muscle, the hip is extended and externally rotated (Fig. 112), in which case the muscle acts in its two functions simultaneously. If palpated when the limb is in this position the muscle feels very firm. Strong contraction of the gluteus maximus may also be observed in stair walking and in running and jumping.

The *hamstrings* have been discussed in Chapter 6. They should now be observed and palpated in their function as hip extensors.

Palpation in prone position: If the hip is extended and simultaneously internally rotated (Fig. 113), the hamstrings and part of the adductor magnus, all originating from the tuberosity of the ischium, may be felt contracting while the gluteus maximus, at least in part, ceases contracting. Note that this inner extensor group of muscles cannot raise the limb as high as when the gluteus maximus participates in the movement. The shift from one muscle group to the other should be observed by maintaining the hip extended while alternating internal rotation with external rotation.

Palpation in standing erect: In standing, the hamstrings may be palpated close to their origins on the ischial tuberosity. First, the subject inclines the trunk somewhat backward so that the center-of-gravity line of the upper part of the body falls well behind the axis of the hip joint. This secures relaxation of the hip extensors, and the ischial tuberosities may then be palpated more easily. The finger tips are placed below the tuberosities, but close to them, and as deeply as the tissue will allow. The subject now reverses the trunk movement, that is, inclines the trunk slightly forward. The instant the center-of-gravity line passes anterior to the common hip axis a contraction of the hamstrings, acting as hip extensors, is felt. By swaying the trunk slightly forward and backward, alternating contraction and relaxation of these muscles is brought about.

When the same trunk movements are repeated while the buttocks are being palpated, very little, if any, contraction of the gluteus maximus can be detected. The hamstrings, rather than the gluteus maximus, appear to be utilized in small-range anteroposterior balance of the pelvis. On the other hand, if a large range of hip flexion is performed by inclining the trunk forward and then quickly returning the trunk to the erect position, a strong contraction of the gluteus maximus may be felt. These clinical observations have been substantiated by electromyography (Joseph, 1960).

The *six external rotators* are small muscles, located in the posterior gluteal region and covered by the gluteus maximus. They originate from both inside and outside the pelvis, have a more or less horizontal direction, and insert into the region of the greater trochanter in such a fashion that they have an external rotary action at the hip.

The uppermost of the six external rotators is the *piriformis,* the lowermost is the *quadratus femoris,* and these two can be palpated with fair accuracy. Palpation of the piriformis will be described with that of the lateral group with which this muscle is closely associated. The quadratus femoris is palpated in the area between the tuberosity of the ischium and the greater trochanter and it may be felt contracting when the hip is externally rotated. The other four, the *gemellus superior,* the *gemellus inferior,* the *obturator internus* and *obturator externus* are located between the piriformis and the quadratus femoris. They can be palpated as a group but not very well individually.

ANTERIOR MUSCLES

This group of muscles includes the *rectus femoris,* the *sartorius,* the *tensor fasciae latae,* the *iliopsoas,* and the *pectineus.* The tensor has

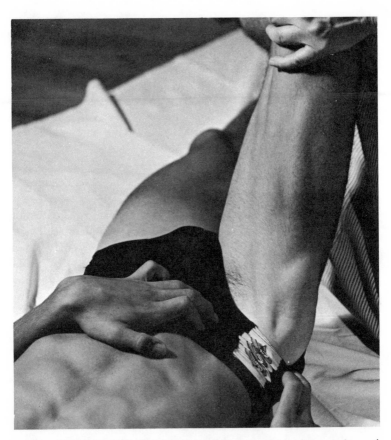

FIG. 114. Near the hip (flexed and externally rotated), the sartorius and the tensor form a V, the sartorius taking a medial direction, the tensor a lateral direction. The tendon of the rectus femoris may be palpated in the V between the other two muscles. The muscular portion of the rectus is seen further down the thigh.

an anterolateral location, and the pectineus has an anteromedial location.

The *rectus femoris* has been described in Chapter 6. *Palpation* of its tendon of origin as the muscle acts in flexion of the hip will be described under the tensor fasciae latae (page 234). The work capacity of the rectus in knee extension is greater than in hip flexion (Tables VIII and XIII).

The *sartorius* (L. *sartor*, a tailor) is a superficial band-like muscle extending obliquely down the thigh from the anterior to the medial side of the thigh. *Origin:* Anterior superior spine of the ilium. *Insertion:* Medial surface of the tibia at the height of the tuberosity of the tibia, and fascia of the leg. *Innervation:* Femoral nerve.

Inspection and palpation: When the hip is flexed and externally rotated, the sartorius may be observed and palpated from its origin down almost to its insertion (Fig. 114). In many subjects the lower portion of the muscle cannot be well observed but may be followed by palpation if the subject alternately contracts and relaxes the muscle. This is best accomplished if the examiner carries the weight of the limb with the hip flexed and externally rotated and the knee flexed (muscle relaxed), then asks the subject to hold the limb in position actively (muscle contracts).

The perpendicular distance from the axis for flexion and extension of the hip to the line of action of the sartorius is considerable. Therefore, even though the muscle's cross section is relatively small, it can exert a comparatively large torque. It should be noticed that, as the muscle contracts, it rises from the underlying structures, and this mechanically enhances its action. Because of its great length, it can shorten a long distance.

The sartorius is a two-joint muscle, passing on the flexor side of the knee where it is in close relation to the tendons of the gracilis and the semitendinosus. The sartorius is more important as a hip flexor than as a knee flexor. Fick found this muscle's work capacity in hip flexion twice that in knee flexion (Tables VIII and XIII).

The *tensor fasciae latae,* like the sartorius, has effect both on the hip and the knee. *Origin:* Crest of the ilium and adjacent structures, laterally to the origin of the sartorius. *Insertion:* Iliotibial tract, about one-third of the way down the thigh. *Innervation:* Branch of the superior gluteal nerve.

Inspection and palpation: The tensor fasciae latae is palpated near the hip, but more laterally than the upper portion of the sartorius. A strong contraction is brought out by resisting flexion of the internally rotated hip (Fig. 115). The relation of the tensor to the sartorius and the rectus femoris is seen in Figure 114. The tensor forms the lateral border of the V-shaped area where the tendon of the rectus femoris is palpated. The relation of the tensor to the anterior portion of the gluteus medius should be noted—the two muscles lie side by side in the anterolateral hip region.

The *iliotibial tract* extends on the lateral side of the thigh, from the ilium above to the tibia below. The gluteus maximus and the

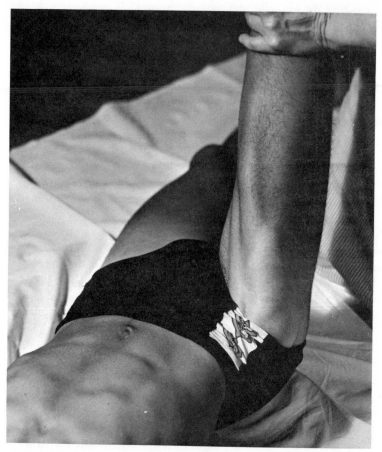

FIG. 115. The tensor fasciae latae is seen contracting as resistance is given to flexion of the internally rotated hip. The rectus femoris and the sartorius are also seen.

tensor both insert into this tract, the gluteus maximus from behind, the tensor from the front. The iliotibial tract is seen in Figure 94 as it approaches its insertion on the tibia.

The *iliopsoas* consists of two parts, the *iliacus* and the *psoas major,* which have separate *origins* but a common *insertion.* That portion of the iliopsoas which lies below the hip joint is located medial to, and is partially covered by, the upper portion of the sartorius.

The *iliacus* takes its *origin* from the iliac fossa and from the inner sides of the anterior spines of the ilium. The muscle covers the anterior side of the hip joint and the femoral neck. It winds around the neck in a medial and posterior direction to be *inserted* into the lesser trochanter of the femur. *Innervation:* Branches of the femoral nerve.

The *psoas major* (Gr. *psoa,* the loins) is located in the posterior wall of the abdominal cavity, close to the lumbar vertebrae and the ilium. *Origin:* Vertebral bodies, intervertebral disks and transverse processes of T12 to L5. The muscle fibers form a round, rather long belly which lies medial to the iliacus. *Insertion:* Lesser trochanter of the femur. *Innervation:* By branches directly from the lumbar plexus.

Palpation of the iliacus and psoas major: The *iliacus* is difficult to palpate since it lies behind the abdominal viscera and is rather flat. It follows, and partly fills out, the iliac fossa.

The *psoas major,* in spite of its deep location, may be palpated as follows: In the sitting position, the subject inclines the trunk slightly forward to secure relaxation of the abdominal muscles. The palpating fingers are placed at the waist, between the lower ribs and the crest of the ilium, and with gentle pressure are made to sink in as deeply as possible toward the posterior wall of the abdominal cavity, near the vertebral column. In some subjects this meets with no difficulty. The subject now flexes the hip, raising the foot just off the floor (Fig. 116) and the round firm belly of the psoas major may be felt as the muscle contracts.

It is suggested that the student first palpate the psoas major on himself before attempting to do so on another person. Palpation is best done if the bowels are fairly empty and should not be attempted if it causes discomfort.

The *pectineus* is a rather flat muscle bordering laterally to the iliopsoas and medially to the adductor longus. *Origin:* Superior ramus of the pubic bone and neighboring structures. *Insertion:* Along a line (pectineal line) on the upper posteromedial aspect of the femur, below the lesser trochanter. The area of insertion of this muscle is approximately as wide as its origin, giving the muscle a quadrangular shape. *Innervation:* Femoral nerve.

The pectineus belongs essentially to the adductor group of muscles, its fibers running approximately parallel to those of the adductor longus. *Palpation* of the pectineus as a separate muscle is difficult, but it may be felt contracting together with other muscles. It is suggested that the student palpate this muscle on himself, as follows: In the sitting position, the palpating fingers are placed in the crotch

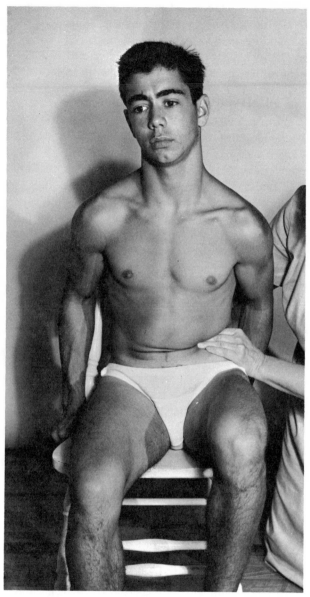

FIG. 116. Palpation of psoas major. If the subject's abdominal muscles are relaxed, the examiner may place the palpating fingers deep enough to feel the contraction of the psoas major when the subject lifts the foot off the floor, flexing the hip beyond 90 degrees.

where some of the adductor tendons can be grasped from front to back. The hip is now flexed further with adduction and external rotation, and the motion is continued until the legs are crossed. The tendon of the adductor longus is prominent and easily recognized; the pectineus lies just lateral to the adductor longus.

LATERAL MUSCLES

The muscles of this group—the *gluteus medius,* the *gluteus minimus,* the *tensor fasciae latae* and the *piriformis*—are located laterally, on the abductor side of the hip. The tensor, described with the flexors, lies anterolaterally and the piriformis posterolaterally.

The *gluteus medius* is the largest of the lateral hip muscles. It is covered, in part, by the gluteus maximus and by the tensor, but its upper middle portion is superficial, covered only by thick fascia. *Origin:* In a fan-shaped fashion from the crest of the ilium and from a large area on the outer surface of the ilium, as far down as the anterior gluteal line, a line which separates its origin from that of the gluteus minimus. From this wide origin the fibers converge to be *inserted* into the greater trochanter, near its tip. This muscle, like the deltoid in the upper limb, has anterior, middle and posterior portions, but these portions are not clearly separated from each other. The posterior portion is comparatively small and supplemented by the piriformis muscle, to be described on page 240. *Innervation:* Superior gluteal nerve.

Inspection and palpation: The *middle portion* of the gluteus medius is palpated laterally below the crest of the ilium when the hip is abducted, either in the side-lying position (subject lying on the side opposite to the muscle palpated), or in the standing position (Fig. 117). In the illustration, the subject is standing on the left foot while abducting the right hip by raising the limb laterally.

The *anterior portion* is palpated when the hip is internally rotated either in the supine position or in standing. This portion lies close to the tensor fasciae latae and acts together with the tensor in internal rotation. If the posterior margin of the tensor is first identified by the tests previously described, the gluteus medius may be palpated posterior to the tensor. The two muscles may also be identified by making them alternately contract and relax and by following the palpated muscle distally. If the muscle takes a direction toward the greater trochanter, it is the anterior portion of the gluteus medius; if the muscle takes a more anterior course, it is the tensor fasciae latae.

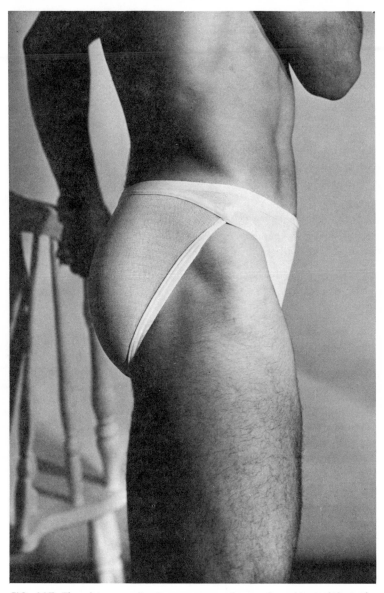

FIG. 117. The gluteus medius is seen contracting as the subject abducts the
right hip, raising the right foot off the floor.

In palpating the anterior portion of the gluteus medius, it should be remembered that the gluteus minimus, which is covered by the medius, also participates in internal rotation and that the muscle tissue palpated represents the combined contraction of the two muscles.

The *posterior portion* of the gluteus medius is palpated in back of the middle portion when the hip is abducted. A part of the posterior portion is seen in Figure 117. This portion contracts strongly if the hip is abducted and externally rotated at the same time. However, with external rotation, other muscles in this region enter, so that the gluteus medius cannot be palpated in an isolated fashion.

The entire gluteus medius may also be felt as it contracts in supporting body weight on one leg, palpation being carried out on the side of the stance leg. In this case, the gluteus medius furnishes lateral stabilization of the pelvis to prevent sagging of the pelvis on the opposite side. This is the most important function of the gluteus medius.

The *piriformis,* the pear-shaped muscle (L. *pirum,* pear), belongs to the second layer of muscles in this region as does the gluteus medius, both of which are covered here by the gluteus maximus. *Origin:* Ventral surface of the sacrum, sciatic notch and sacrotuberous ligament. The fibers take a downward-lateral course, following the posterior border of the gluteus medius to be *inserted* into the inner portion of the greater trochanter. *Innervation:* A branch derived directly from the first and second sacral nerves.

Palpation: The muscle is palpated in external rotation, especially if the gluteus maximus is relaxed as when the limb is raised slightly forward. The palpating fingers are placed posterior to the greater trochanter and moved about somewhat until the best spot for palpation is located. Once the muscle has been identified, it may also be palpated in the sitting position, by *abducting the hip* against resistance. Due to the changed position of the greater trochanter in relation to the pelvis in sitting, the piriformis changes its action from principally that of an external rotator to that of an abductor.

In palpating the piriformis, its close association with the posterior portion of the gluteus medius, in regard to location and action, should be kept in mind. The two muscles are likely to be felt contracting simultaneously.

The *gluteus minimus* belongs to the third and deepest layer of the muscles in the gluteal region. It lies close to the capsule of the hip joint and is covered by the gluteus medius. *Origin:* Fan-shaped, from the outer surface of the ilium, between the anterior and inferior gluteal lines, and from the septum between it and the medius. *Insertion:* Anterior border of the greater trochanter of the femur. *Innervation:* Superior gluteal nerve.

Palpation: The muscle cannot be very well differentiated from the medius since both muscles contract simultaneously in abduction and internal rotation. The anterior portion of the muscle is the thickest part and is felt, together with the medius, when the hip is internally rotated.

MEDIAL MUSCLES (Adductor Group)

The adductor group is identified as the large muscular mass of the medial thigh, bordering anteriorly to the vastus medialis and the sartorius (Fig. 114), posteriorly to the hamstrings. This group comprises the following muscles: *adductor magnus, adductor longus, adductor gracilis, adductor brevis,* and *pectineus.* The obturator externus, the quadratus femoris and the lower portion of the gluteus maximus also are capable of adducting the hip but do not belong to the adductor group proper.

From the functional standpoint, it is not necessary to study the exact *origin and insertion* of individual muscles of the adductor group. In general, these muscles arise from the rami of the pubes and the rami of the ischia and insert into the shaft of the femur. Part of the adductor group lies anterior and part posterior to the axis of flexion and extension of the hip joint. The line of action of these muscles in relation to the axis changes when the hip flexes, so that each muscle's action can be determined only for a specific position of the joint. This applies equally to the rotary action of the adductor muscles.

The *nerve supply* to the adductor group is mainly from the obturator nerve. The adductor magnus, however, is innervated by a branch from the sciatic nerve as well as by a branch from the obturator nerve, and the pectineus is supplied by the femoral nerve.

Discussion of Function of Muscles Acting at the Hip

WEIGHT-BEARING AND NONWEIGHT-BEARING FUNCTIONS OF HIP MUSCLES

In erect standing with weight on both legs, the pelvis is in unstable equilibrium over the common hip axis so that the pelvis, which serves as origin for most of the muscles spanning the hip joint, is more movable than the segments which serve as distal attachments of the muscles, these segments being relatively stabilized by the superimposed body weight.

In standing on one leg, the pelvis is in unstable equilibrium on the femoral head of the stance limb, so that pelvic motions about all three axes of the hip joint are relatively free. The limb that is off the ground, no longer stabilized by the body weight, is free to move in relation to the pelvis.

The actions of the hip muscles, like those of the knee and ankle, must therefore be studied both in weight-bearing and in nonweight-bearing situations. The function of the muscles in weight-bearing will be considered in detail in Chapters 10 and 11, while general principles of their actions and some aspects of their function in moving the lower limb with respect to the trunk will be discussed here.

MULTIPLE ACTIONS OF HIP MUSCLES

Since the hip joint has three degrees of freedom of motion, most of the muscles spanning the joint exert action about all three axes simultaneously. The leverage of a muscle with respect to the three axes, however, usually differs considerably so that often the action about one axis predominates. For example, the iliopsoas has so much better leverage for flexion than for rotation, the latter leverage being extremely small or none, that its rotary action may be altogether disregarded. Other muscles have comparatively good leverage about two axes, as for example the gluteus maximus which is an extensor and an external rotator or the pectineus which is a flexor and an adductor, the rotary motion of the latter being relatively unimportant..

PORTIONS OF A MUSCLE MAY HAVE DIFFERENT ACTIONS. Muscles such as the *gluteus maximus* and the *gluteus medius* cover large areas so that one portion of the muscle may be capable of an action different from another portion. Each of the above muscles (the gluteus maximus and gluteus medius), however, has a main action that is shared by all portions of the muscle, which action of the gluteus maximus is extension and of the gluteus medius is abduction. The upper portion of the maximus is located so that it acts in *abduction;* the location of the lower portion permits action as an *adductor.* The anterior portion of the medius is located well for *internal rotation,* while its posterior portion acts in *external rotation.*

CHANGE OF ACTION DUE TO JOINT ANGLE. The leverage of the muscles about the three axes changes with the joint angle so that the effectiveness of a muscle, for a certain motion, may decrease as the angle changes. At a certain point, the action of the muscle may reverse itself, for example, from flexion to extension or from internal to external rotation. A detailed determination of these changes for a number of the hip muscles was made by R. Fick, and the results are found in Volume III of his publication (1911). Because it would be too lengthy to recapitulate here the findings for all the muscles, the adductor group will be used as an example:

The *pectineus* acts as an *adductor* throughout the range of flexion. It is a *flexor* in all positions of the joint but, as flexion proceeds, the leverage of this muscle as a flexor decreases to the point of no leverage in extreme flexion. Its work capacity as a flexor surpasses its work capacity as an adductor.

The *adductor longus* acts as an *adductor* in all positions of the joint. It *flexes* in the first 70 degrees of flexion but its leverage decreases continuously to the point of no leverage at 70 degrees; beyond 70 degrees of flexion the muscle becomes an *extensor.* In the extended position of the joint it is a *weak internal rotator;* in the flexed position it becomes a *weak external rotator.*

The principal action of the *adductor brevis* is *adduction.* From the hyperextended position to about 50 degrees of flexion, it is a *flexor;* beyond 50 degrees of flexion it becomes an *extensor.* In extension it is a weak external rotator, and this action increases with flexion.

The main action of *adductor magnus* is *adduction,* and this applies to its upper as well as its lower portion. In the extended position and up to about 50 degrees of flexion, the *upper portion* is a *flexor,* but in further flexion it becomes an *extensor.* The *lower portion* of the adductor magnus is already, in the erect standing position, an *extensor,* and this extension action increases as the joint flexes. The muscle also has a weak internal rotary action.

The main action of the *adductor gracilis* at the hip is *adduction.* In the extended position and up to 20 to 40 degrees of flexion, the muscle is a *flexor,* but in further flexion it becomes an *extensor.*

TWO-JOINT MUSCLES ACTING AT THE HIP

The hip muscles are either one-joint muscles acting at the hip only, or they pass two or more joints and have actions, or potential actions, over all these joints.

LENGTH-TENSION RELATIONS.   The efficiency of a two-joint muscle is substantially influenced by the positions of the two joints, in accordance with the laws governing length-tension relations of muscle. Therefore, the *rectus femoris* is more effective as a hip flexor if the knee flexes simultaneously with the hip, because this permits the muscle to contract within a favorable range. For the same reason, the rectus is more efficient as a knee extensor if the hip extends simultaneously with the knee. The *hamstrings* are more efficient as hip extensors when the knee extends simultaneously with the hip; the hamstrings are more efficient as knee flexors when the hip flexes simultaneously with the knee.

LEVERAGE OF TWO-JOINT MUSCLE OVER EACH JOINT.   A two-joint muscle usually has better leverage over one joint than the other, and better leverage means more torque. The main action of a two-joint muscle, therefore, is over the joint where it has the best leverage. The rectus femoris is more efficient as a knee extensor than as a hip flexor, and the sartorius is more important as a hip flexor than as a knee flexor. As far as the hamstrings are concerned, some of Fick's data indicate that, in general, the semimembranosus and the long head of the biceps are more important as hip extensors than as knee flexors. The effects of the semitendinosus seem to be reversed: this muscle produces more torque in knee flexion than in hip extension. However, if a valid comparison is to be made, the torque curves of each muscle over the two joints would have to be compared, but sufficient data for such comparison is not available.

HIP FLEXOR TENSION INFLUENCED BY THE POSITION OF THE PELVIS. The hip flexors, in general, become somewhat elongated, and therefore more efficient, if the pelvis is tilted backward (pubic symphysis raised, ischial tuberosities lowered) simultaneously with hip flexion. This applies to all hip flexors. The psoas major, in addition, is influenced by the position of the vertebral column, since a flattening of the physiological forward convexity of the lumbar spine, such as takes place in sitting, causes it to become elongated.

MUSCLES ACTING IN FLEXION OF THE HIP

HIP FLEXION IN ERECT STANDING. When in the standing position one hip is flexed, that is, the knee is pulled up toward the chest, it may be ascertained by palpation that the iliopsoas, the rectus femoris, the sartorius and the tensor spring into action. The internal rotary action of the tensor appears to be compensated by the external rotary action of the sartorius, and the knee extensor action of the rectus appears to be checked by gravity and perhaps also by the action of some of the knee flexors. Both internal and external rotary actions have been ascribed to the iliopsoas, but for all practical purposes this muscle should be considered as a pure flexor. The combined action of the iliopsoas, rectus femoris, sartorius and tensor muscles (in proper proportion) results in pure flexion. When flexion is combined with abduction, adduction, or rotation, additional muscles are recruited in accordance with the needs. For example, if the tendon of the adductor longus is palpated in the crotch during pure flexion, this muscle appears inactive, but as soon as adduction and/or internal rotation is combined with flexion, the tendon of the adductor longus becomes tensed.

HIP FLEXION IN SITTING POSITION. Since, in the sitting position, the hip is already flexed to about 90 degrees, additional flexion necessitates actions by the hip flexors in the shortened range of their excursion. When flexion to an acute hip angle is carried out, the sartorius and the tensor can be felt contracting strongly, but in this range these muscles have lost much of their tensile strength and are incapable of carrying out the motion without the aid of the iliopsoas. In fact, as may be concluded from observation of patients with paralysis, the iliopsoas is the only hip flexor which can produce enough tension to flex beyond 90 degrees in the sitting position.

PARALYSIS OF THE HIP FLEXORS

In post-poliomyelitis patients having a *paralysis of the sartorius* while the tensor is intact, voluntary flexion is accompanied by internal rotation—this is best observed when the patient is in the supine position. If the *tensor is paralyzed* and the sartorius is intact, voluntary hip flexion is accompanied by external rotation and some abduction. Some poliomyelitic patients, having paralysis of one of the above muscles (depending on the amount of additional involvement), are able, when concentrating on straight hip flexion, to carry out this

---

Hip and Pelvic Region   **245**

motion, but invariably display the characteristic combination when attention is not focused on the manner of execution of the motion.

A patient with *bilateral paralysis of the iliopsoas* of unknown etiology provided an opportunity for evaluating the functional importance of this muscle. As far as could be determined, no other muscles were involved. The hip could be flexed with comparative ease to about 90 degrees, although the strength of this motion was reduced, but flexion beyond this point in the sitting position did not succeed. The main disadvantage of the loss of the iliopsoas, however, was the subject's inability to sit erect on a stool. The posture assumed was one of forward inclination of the trunk (hip flexion), a position which shifts the responsibility of balancing the trunk from the flexors to the extensors of the hip. If the examiner brought the trunk back to a vertical position, the subject quickly grasped the sides of the stool to avoid falling backward. In palpating the sartorius, this muscle was found to contract to the best of its ability but it could not produce enough tension to balance the trunk. This is understandable because, in the sitting position, both hip and knee are flexed so that the sartorius contracts in an unfavorable range, apparently coming close to active insufficiency. In the sitting position, the length-tension relations of the iliopsoas are more favorable. This applies particularly to the psoas major which, owing to its origin on the lumbar spine, becomes relatively elongated as the lumbar spine straightens out in sitting.

In the case cited, the iliopsoas paralysis also affected the subject's standing and walking posture, which was characterized by a forward tilt of the pelvis (hip flexion), accompanied by a lumbar lordosis. The walk also lacked in speed and in smoothness, and there was some external rotation of the hip both during swing phase and stance phase.

A general principle, which may be derived from the postural adjustment seen in the patient with bilateral paralysis of the iliopsoas, is that in the erect position—sitting or standing—*the trunk tends to incline toward the weak or paralyzed muscles.* As will be seen later, this principle applies equally to other muscles engaged in balancing the body or body segments in the erect position.

A study of the actions of the hip flexors must also include an analysis of muscle action in sit-ups, and in single and double leg raising in the supine position. In these activities, the abdominal muscles act synergically with the hip flexors to furnish the necessary fixation to the pelvis.

MUSCLES ACTING IN EXTENSION OF THE HIP

Five important muscles pass behind the axis for flexion and extension of the hip and serve as extensors in all positions of the joint, namely the *gluteus maximus*, the *biceps femoris* (long head), the *semimembranosus*, the *semitendinosus*, and the *adductor magnus* (posterior portion). When the hip is flexed, as when the trunk is inclined forward in standing, the ischial tuberosities are carried backward in relation to the hip axis, and this improves the leverage of those extensor muscles which originate on the tuberosities.

The hip extensors should be observed and palpated both when the lower extremities move in relation to the trunk and when the trunk moves in relation to the lower extremities. In many activities, both segments move simultaneously.

PRONE-LYING UNILATERAL HIP EXTENSION WITH KNEE EXTENDED. Palpation of the gluteus maximus and the inner extensor group in the prone position has already been described. To obtain a larger range of motion than seen in Figures 112 and 113, the subject should be prone on a table with the hips flexed over the edge of the table. A range of about 90 degrees in hip extension may then be observed. The changing muscular requirements when external or internal rotation is carried out simultaneously should again be observed: increased activity of the gluteus maximus in external rotation, decreased activity of the gluteus maximus in internal rotation, and increased activity of the inner extensor group in internal rotation.

PRONE-LYING UNILATERAL HIP EXTENSION WITH KNEE FLEXED. When the hamstrings are palpated in hip extension while the knee is flexed, they can be felt "bunching up," that is, they become short and thick. In this movement combination, length-tension relations are most unfavorable and the muscles may come close to, or arrive at, the point of active insufficiency. Subjectively, an uncomfortable cramplike feeling is experienced in the posterior thigh region when full range hip extension is attempted while the knee is maintained flexed to an acute angle. Children and young adults may not complain about discomfort, but in older subjects this movement is extremely uncomfortable and may produce a cramp, and therefore should be used with caution or avoided.

Since very little tension can be produced by the hamstrings when they contract in their shortened range, hip extension with the knee flexed requires strong action of the gluteus maximus. This movement combination has been advocated as an isolated test for the gluteus

Hip and Pelvic Region   **247**

maximus. While it is true that, in hip extension with the knee flexed, the gluteus maximus must be credited with doing most of the work, the hamstrings still contract to the best of their ability and the adductor magnus contributes its part, so that an isolated action of the gluteus maximus is by no means achieved.

PRONE-LYING BILATERAL HIP EXTENSION, KNEES EXTENDED. In unilateral hip extension in the prone position, the pelvis remains comparatively stable, yet some synergic contraction of the extensors of the vertebral column is required and may be observed and palpated. But when both limbs are raised simultaneously, the leverage action on the pelvis, due to the contracting hip extensors and to the weight of the limbs, becomes marked. Therefore, the demand on the extensors of the vertebral column, and in particular on the lumbar extensors, is much increased. The strong tension in these muscles should be observed and palpated.

The action of the hamstrings and the gluteus maximus as extensors of the pelvis with respect to the thighs in erect standing has already been mentioned in connection with the palpation of these muscles. Further discussion of their functions will be found in Chapters 10 and 11.

MUSCLES ACTING IN ABDUCTION OF THE HIP

SUPINE, UNILATERAL ABDUCTION.   If in the back-lying position the hip is abducted by moving the limb sideward, the abductors on that side, mainly the *gluteus medius and gluteus minimus,* are activated. Synergic action of the hip-hikers on the same side occurs automatically, so that the crest of the ilium moves upward in a direction toward the rib cage. If these muscles were idle, contraction of the abductors would approximate the crest of the ilium and the greater trochanter by moving origin and insertion simultaneously, and hip abduction, as far as side motion of the limb were concerned, would become rather ineffective. Owing to the action of the hip-hikers, the abductors are kept at a favorable length during abduction. The lateral tilt of the pelvis, which is produced by the hip-hikers, directly aids the side movement of the limb by rotating the acetabulum outward. Although this motion of the pelvis is only slight, the hip-hikers may be likened to the serratus anterior in the upper limb which rotates the glenoid cavity in a direction favorable for abduction.

SUPINE, BILATERAL ABDUCTION.   In bilateral abduction the traction exerted on the ilium by the abductors on one side is counterbalanced by an equal traction on the opposite side; hence, the pelvis remains level and stable.

SUPINE, HIP-HIKING. If the hip-hikers are utilized first on one side and then on the other, without simultaneous contraction of the abductors, a lateral tilt of the pelvis to alternate sides takes place. The muscles of the extremities remain inactive, but the entire limb follows the motion of the pelvis, and the result is a shortening of the limb on alternate sides. When the hip-hikers on the right side contract, they cause *adduction* of the right hip and *abduction* of the left hip as the pelvis moves in relation to the limbs.

Electromyographic studies by Close (1964) have revealed that electrical activity is present in the iliopsoas muscle in the last range of abduction of the hip. As pointed out by the above investigator, in the neutral position of the hip the distal portion of the iliopsoas muscle courses anteriorly and directly over the femoral head, but as abduction proceeds the muscle slides over to the lateral side of the center of rotation of the hip joint and thus becomes mechanically capable of abduction. When the tendon of the iliopsoas muscle is transplanted to the greater trochanter (Mustard, 1952; Close, 1964) the muscle comes to lie lateral to the center of rotation of the hip joint in all positions of the joint. The transplant has been found efficient in assisting or replacing weak or paralyzed gluteal muscles not only in voluntary abduction of the thigh with respect to the pelvis, but also in lateral stabilization of the pelvis in automatic activities such as walking.

MUSCLES ACTING IN ADDUCTION OF THE HIP

When adduction of the hip is carried out against resistance and with the thigh in a neutral position with respect to flexion, extension and rotation, the five main adductors previously enumerated contract as a group. Their individual functional characteristics in various degrees of hip flexion have been described. Since some of these muscles, or parts of the same muscle, have opposite secondary actions, these actions counterbalance each other when pure adduction is carried out.

The total cross section of the adductors far surpasses that of the abductors. At first glance, it would perhaps appear illogical that this is the case, since in the erect position the hip abductors have to work against gravity while gravity does the work for the adductors (see Chapter 10). Activities such as squeezing an object between the knees and climbing a rope, which require force in adduction, are relatively rare and hardly warrant such large cross section. The explanation of the adductors' large bulk is found in their functions as flexors, extensors and rotators and, in general, in their stabilizing action as co-contractors with the abductors. The electrical activities of these muscles in walking are illustrated in Chapter 11.

MUSCLES ACTING IN ROTATION OF THE HIP

From previous discussions it is obvious that many muscles about the hip joint have rotary actions. Which of these muscles are utilized for rotation depends on the position of the joint with respect to flexion, extension, abduction, and adduction; for example, the gluteus maximus, when extending the hip fully, also externally rotates the hip. The *six small external rotators* (piriformis, gemellus superior, gemellus inferior, obturator internus, obturator externus and quadratus femoris) have a good angle of pull for external rotation, but the external rotary components of these muscles decrease in flexion of the hip, and at 90 degrees of hip flexion they possess a considerable abductor component.

The anterior portions of the *gluteus medius and minimus* are the main *internal rotators,* and when the hip is flexed they are aided by the *tensor.* With the hip in extension, some of the *adductors* also aid in internal rotation. By palpation on a supine-lying subject, it may be ascertained that the adductor tendons in the crotch become tense when the subject internally rotates the hip.

CHAPTER 9

Head, Neck and Trunk

BONES

PALPABLE STRUCTURES OF THE SKULL

If the fingers are placed behind the ear lobes, the mastoid portion of the temporal bone can be palpated, its lowest part being the *mastoid process* (Gr. *mastos,* breast, and *eidos,* resemblance). In the erect position, this process is best felt if the head is bent forward slightly so that the sternocleidomastoid muscle, which attaches to it, is relaxed. When the head is tipped backward, the muscle tightens and only part of the process may be reached for palpation.

By moving the fingers in a posterior direction from the mastoid process, the *occipital bone* with its *superior nuchal line* is reached. The lateral portion of this ridge serves, in part, as attachment to the sternocleidomastoid muscle, and its medial portion, in part, as attachment to the trapezius.

At the point where the two superior nuchal lines of the right and the left sides meet in the median line is a small eminence, the *external occipital protuberance;* the external occipital crest extends from the protuberance to the foramen magnum, also in the median line. These bony eminences, which are not too well palpable, serve as attachment to the *ligamentum nuchae,* a strong ligamentous band extending from the seventh cervical vertebra to the skull. This ligament gives attachment to the trapezius muscle and to a number of posterior neck muscles. It is best palpated when it is slack—when the head is tilted backward.

NONPALPABLE STRUCTURES OF THE SKULL

Among these nonpalpable structures are the following: the *inferior nuchal line of the occipital bone* which is almost parallel with the superior nuchal line but is hidden from palpation by muscles; the *occipital condyles,* one on each side, which go into the formation of the atlanto-occipital joints; the *jugular processes* of the occipital bone, which are located lateral to the occipital condyles, serve as attachment to one of the short posterior neck muscles (rectus capitis lateralis): and the *foramen magnum* of the occipital bone which transmits the medulla oblongata.

On the anterior side of the foramen magnum is the *basilar part of the occipital bone.* This portion of the bone lies on the anterior side of the axis of motion of the atlanto-occipital joints and serves as insertion for the deep flexor muscles of the head (longus capitis, rectus capitis anterior).

PALPABLE STRUCTURES OF THE NECK AND VERTEBRAL COLUMN

FIRST AND SECOND CERVICAL VERTEBRAE. The first cervical verte-bra, the *atlas,* has a *transverse process* which protrudes more lat-erally than do those of the other vertebrae in this region. This process may be palpated, and is found just below the tip of the mastoid proc-ess. This region is rather sensitive to pressure and it is suggested that the student identify it on himself before doing so on another person. The *posterior tubercle of the atlas* (its rudimentary spinous process) lies deep but may be found in its relation to the second cervical verte-bra. The *spinous process of the axis,* the second cervical vertebra, is strong and prominent and is therefore easy to identify.

THIRD TO SIXTH CERVICAL VERTEBRAE. The lateral portions of these vertebrae present a number of processes and tubercles which may be palpated, although each one may not be identified accurately. These vertebrae have short and perforated transverse processes and their articular processes protrude laterally; therefore, the palpable areas of these vertebrae feel very uneven. Their short bifid spinous processes may be felt in the median line though they are covered by ligamentum nuchae.

VERTEBRA PROMINENS (C7). Because of the prominence of its spinous process which is longer and sturdier than those of the other cervical vertebrae and not bifid, the vertebra prominens can be identified easily in most individuals. Often, however, the spinous process of the first thoracic vertebra is equally prominent. If the sub-ject bends the head forward, identification of these processes are facilitated. If two processes in this region seem to be equal in size, they are identified as those of C7 and T1.

THORACIC AND LUMBAR VERTEBRAE. When the subject bends forward, flexing the entire spine, the spinous processes of the vertebral column become somewhat separated from each other and may be palpated throughout the thoracic and lumbar regions. The vertebra prominens is used as a starting point for counting the vertebrae, which can be done accurately in most subjects, particularly if the subject is told to "make the back round." Vertebral columns, however, present a great deal of individual variations. One or the other spinous process may be less developed and more difficult to locate, and minor lateral deviations of the processes are also common.

In the thoracic region, the spinous processes are directed downward and overlap each other, so that the spinous process of one vertebra is located approximately at the height of the body of the next lower one. In the lumbar region, the spinous processes are large and directed horizontally, so that the height of the spinous process more nearly represents the height of its body. The change from one type to another is a gradual one. The two lowest thoracic vertebrae resemble the lumbar ones, having rather horizontally directed spinous processes which are approximately at the height of the intervertebral disk between its own body and the body of the next lower vertebra.

NONPALPABLE STRUCTURES OF THE VERTEBRAL COLUMN

Since the vertebral column is imbedded in muscles posteriorly and laterally and not available for palpation anteriorly, its general structure and the characteristics of its individual parts should be studied on the skeleton with the aid of a good textbook of anatomy. An anatomical orientation must precede clinical palpation. It is suggested that the preliminary study include: (1) The *physiological curves* of the vertebral column: cervical, thoracic, lumbar and sacrococcygeal (Fig. 126). (2) The *general structure of a vertebra:* body and arch, enclosing the vertebral foramen; laminae; transverse, articular and spinous processes; *specific characteristics* of the 7 cervical, 12 thoracic and 5 lumbar vertebrae; the intervertebral disks (see also p. 256). (3) *Ligaments* which bind the vertebrae together: anterior and posterior longitudinal ligaments, extending the entire length of the column; ligamenta flava (L. *flavus,* yellow), between the laminae of adjacent vertebrae; ligamenta intertransversaria, interspinalia and supraspinalia; and ligamentum nuchae.

For clinical orientation, the following *landmarks* may be used to determine the height of specific vertebrae: *C6*—level with the arch of the cricoid cartilage which is identified in the lower anterior neck region; *body of T4*—height of junction of the manubrium and the body of the sternum; *body of T10*—level with the tip of the xiphoid process; *spinous process of L4*—level with highest portion of crest of ilium; *S2*—height of posterior superior iliac spines.

SACRUM AND COCCYX. The exterior surface of the sacrum is palpated as a direct continuation of the lumbar spine. The *medial sacral crest* represents the rudimentary spinous processes of the sacral vertebrae, the processes being fused with the rest of the bone. On both sides of the crest are rough areas serving as attachments to ligaments, fascia, and muscles. The approximate boundaries of the sacrum may be determined by following the crests of the ilia in a posterior direction, where the sacrum is interposed between the two ilia. The "dimples" medial to the posterior superior spines of the ilia indicate the posterior approach to the sacroiliac joints.

Caudally, the sacrum is continuous with the coccyx, and the two bones form a marked posterior convexity so that the tip of the coccyx has a deep location between the two gluteal eminences. If a subject sits on the front portion of a hard chair and then leans against the back of the chair, the coccyx may be felt contacting the chair.

THORAX, OR RIB CAGE. This consists of the 12 thoracic vertebrae in back, the sternum in front, and the 12 ribs. Most of the external surfaces of the thorax may be palpated. Some difficulty arises in palpating the upper ribs which are hidden by structures of the neck and by the clavicle. In obese individuals, palpation of the last two, or "floating," ribs may be difficult also. Those portions of the ribs which lie close to the vertebral column are covered by muscles but, beginning at their angles, the ribs may be palpated in their lateral, forward and downward courses. It should be recalled that the first to seventh ribs attach to the sternum, the eighth to tenth ribs join with each other by means of cartilage, and the eleventh and twelfth ribs have free ends.

When the ribs on the left side are being palpated, it is suggested that the subject place his left hand on top of his head and that he stretch the left side so that the ribs become somewhat separated from each other. In stretching the side of the thorax, the distance between the lowest part of the rib cage laterally and the crest of the ilium increases, permitting the floating ribs to be more or less easily located. In the ordinary erect position, this distance is very short. In pathological conditions, as in advanced states of lateral curvature of the spine, the ribs may actually come to rest on the ilium and nerves may become pinched, causing pain.

STERNUM. This may be palpated from the xiphoid process below, to the manubrium and the sternoclavicular joints above.

JOINTS

ATLANTO-OCCIPITAL JOINTS

TYPE OF JOINTS. The atlanto-occipital joints are of the condyloid type, with two degrees of freedom of motion. The two joints work in unison to provide movements between the head and the vertebral column. The shallow concave joint surfaces on the atlas, one on each side of the vertebral canal, support the two convex condyles of the occipital bone. The problem of supporting the head from below without interfering with the passage of the medulla oblongata into the vertebral canal, yet provide needed mobility of the head, has thus been solved excellently.

AXIS OF MOTION. The movement of the head at the atlanto-occipital joints is mainly a nodding movement in the sagittal plane, about a transverse axis through the two condyles. The approximate location of this axis is demonstrated by placing the tips of the two index fingers pointing toward each other on the mastoid processes. Small lateral bending movements are also permitted but these are quite limited. For all practical purposes, the two condyloid joints, acting together and restricting each other, have one degree of freedom of motion, which permits flexion and extension.

ATLANTO-AXIAL JOINTS

The two upper vertebrae articulate with each other by means of one centrally located and two laterally located joints. Centrally, the *dens of the axis* (odontoid process) fits into a ring formed by the arch of the atlas anteriorly and its transverse ligament posteriorly, so that a pivoting movement of the atlas around the dens can take place. Laterally, the nearly horizontal but somewhat-curved joint surfaces of the atlas above and the axis below take part in the movement.

Head, Neck and Trunk

AXIS OF MOTION. The axis of motion for the centrally located joint is a vertical one, through the dens. The movement which takes place around the dens, however, is also determined by the shape of the joint surfaces of the lateral joints. Because of the convex shape of the joint surfaces of the axis, the *rotary movement* is not strictly in a horizontal plane, but a screwlike movement takes place. The atlanto-axial joint, therefore, is sometimes referred to as a "screw joint."

INTERVERTEBRAL JOINTS FROM C2 TO S1

The vertebral bodies from C2 to S1 are separated and flexibly bound together by intervertebral disks which allow small motions in all directions. But the nature of the motions in the various regions of the vertebral column is determined largely by the direction of the joint surfaces of the articular processes.

CERVICAL REGION. In the upper cervical region the articular surfaces are nearly horizontal, permitting mainly *rotation*. Caudally, these surfaces change their direction and become oblique, approaching the frontal plane. Some lateral bending is therefore permitted, together with a small amount of flexion and extension.

THORACIC REGION. The articular surfaces are somewhat oblique throughout, but may be said to be directed generally in the frontal plane so that *lateral flexion* can take place. This movement, however, is restricted considerably by the ten upper ribs, and, consequently, only a small amount of motion can take place between adjacent segments. In the lowest thoracic region and at the thoracolumbar junction, however, there is more freedom of motion. Here the articular surfaces have a more oblique direction, approaching the sagittal plane, and a considerable amount of movement in all directions is permitted.

LUMBAR REGION. The articular surfaces are directed in a nearly sagittal plane throughout the lumbar region, and this permits mainly movements of *flexion and extension*.

INTERVERTEBRAL DISKS. Each disk is composed of three parts, the *anulus fibrosus*, an elastic ring of fibrocartilage which encloses the *nucleus pulposus*, a substance with high water content, and two thin *cartilaginous plates* which separate the pulp from the vertebral bodies. The pressure in the pulp is high (Peters, 1933), hence a herniation of the nucleus pulposus is likely to occur in injuries or degeneration of the anulus fibrosus.

LUMBOSACRAL JUNCTION

The angulation of the vertebral column at the lumbosacral junction which is marked in standing (Fig. 127) indicates that the joint is subjected to a great deal of shearing stress by the superimposed body weight. Its ligamentous apparatus is comparable to that of other vertebral joints and is further reinforced by the strong *iliolumbar* and *sacrolumbar ligaments.* Anatomical variations which weaken the joint and an unfavorable postural alignment may cause the fifth lumbar vertebra to slide forward on the sacrum, a pathology known as *spondylolisthesis* (Gr. *spondylos,* vertebra, and *olisthesis,* a slipping or falling).

SACROILIAC JOINT

The sacrum is firmly joined to the ilia at the two sacroiliac joints. These are true joints but, under normal conditions, motions are practically absent owing to the structure of the joint and to reinforcing ligaments, of which should be noted: the *anterior and posterior sacroiliac,* the *interosseous, sacrotuberous,* and *sacrospinous ligaments.*

MUSCLES MOVING THE HEAD, NECK AND TRUNK

FLEXORS OF THE HEAD AND NECK

These muscles exert their action anterior to the axis of motion of the atlanto-occipital and the intervertebral joints. Some of these flexor muscles lie close to the anterior surface of the bodies of the cervical vertebrae, others lie further to the front.

The deepest of these muscles are the short *rectus capitis anterior,* acting on the atlanto-occipital joint only, and the *longus capitis,* acting both on head and the cervical spine. The *longus colli* acts on the neck only. Though the main action of these muscles is flexion of the head and neck, they may also have effect on lateral bending and on rotation because of their somewhat lateral location and oblique direction. In general, they aid in balancing the head and the cervical spine. The longus muscles cover portions of the anterior convexity of the cervical curve of the vertebral column and, therefore, may aid in preventing an undue increase of this curve due to the vertical pressure of the head on the spinal column. These muscles lie too deeply to be palpated or to be investigated by the electromyographic method so that objective evidence of their function is lacking. It may be assumed, however, that they are important postural muscles which aid in the maintenance of proper alignment of the cervical spine.

The *scalene muscles* (Gr. *skalenos,* uneven; triangle with uneven sides) *originate* from the transverse processes of the cervical vertebrae and *insert* into the upper ribs. Acting bilaterally, they flex the neck on the thorax or elevate the upper ribs. Because of their anterolateral location, when acting on one side, they bend the neck laterally. In the erect position, they contribute to the balance of the neck both anteriorly and laterally. With the cervical spine stabilized, they aid in elevation of the upper ribs, an action which is called upon in deep breathing. Their action as muscles of inspiration has been substantiated by electromyography (Jones and associates, 1953).

Palpation: The *scalenus anterior* and *scalenus medius* insert into the first rib, and may be palpated during forced inspiration by placing the fingertips above the clavicle and behind the sternocleidomastoid muscle. They are also felt when, in the erect position, the head is tilted backward and when, in the supine position, the head and the neck are flexed on the thorax.

The *sternocleidomastoid muscles,* one on each side, are the most superficial of the anterior neck muscles. *Origin:* By two heads: one head from the upper border of the manubrium sterni, partly covering the sternoclavicular joint, and the other from the upper border of the clavicle. *Insertion:* Mastoid process of the temporal bone and superior nuchal line of the occipital bone. *Innervation:* Spinal accessory nerve.

Inspection and palpation: The two muscles may be observed in simultaneous action when the head is raised while the subject is in the supine position. One-sided action of the sternocleidomastoid is brought out if the subject's head is rotated toward one side and resistance to lateral flexion toward the opposite side is given (Fig. 118). The left sternocleidomastoid is also seen in Figure 82 and both muscles in Figure 78.

There are a number of other muscles located in the anterior neck region which may participate to a certain extent in head and neck flexion. These muscles belong to the supra- and infrahyoid groups,

---

FIG. 118. Testing the sternocleidomastoid muscle unilaterally. A, For strong activation of the left sternocleidomastoid muscle, the head is rotated to the right and resistance is given to lateral flexion of the head to the left. Both sternal and clavicular portions are seen. B, In this patient the clavicular portion of the right sternocleidomastoid muscle is missing. The sternal portion is seen contracting. Patient also had paralysis of the right trapezius, as seen in Figure 71.

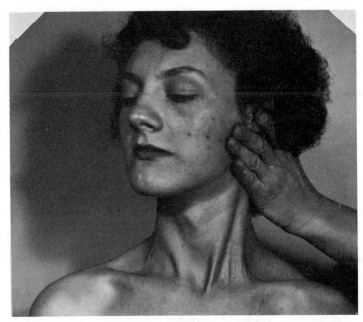

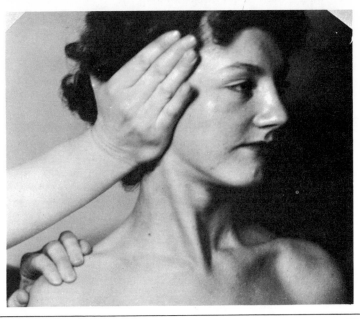

Head, Neck and Trunk

but since their main use is for purposes other than neck flexion, they will not be discussed.

EXTENSORS OF THE HEAD AND NECK

Numerous muscles are concerned with extension of the head and the neck; some muscles are deep, others are more superficial. The posterior muscles as a group are considerably bulkier than the anterior ones, indicating that greater strength is needed in extension than in flexion.

Among the deepest extensor muscles is a group of short muscles, the *suboccipital muscles,* which connect the upper two cervical vertebrae with the occipital bone and with each other. Some of these muscles are concerned mainly with extension; others are concerned with rotation.

The *longissimus capitis,* the *transversospinalis capitis* (semispinalis capitis) and the *transversospinalis cervicis* (semispinalis cervicis) are also deep muscles of the neck, acting on the head and neck. The muscles are covered by the *splenius muscle,* which in turn is covered, in part, by the trapezius and by the upper portion of the sternocleidomastoid muscle.

Palpation: Many of the neck extensors are too small and lie too deeply to be palpated; others can be palpated only as a group. Palpation of this group, with the subject in the erect position, should be done both with the head inclined backward (the muscles are relaxed), and with the head bent forward (the muscles become tense). If the head is inclined backward and then rotated left and right, some of the deeper muscles can be felt acting in their rotary capacity.

ANTERIOR AND LATERAL TRUNK MUSCLES

The anterior and lateral trunk muscles, in addition to their function as supporters of the abdominal viscera, are concerned with movements of the trunk—flexion, lateral bending and rotation. They consist of large sheaths of muscles in several layers. The fibers of the various layers run in different directions, a factor which contributes to the strength of the combined layers. A similar arrangement of fibers is seen in the thoracic region where the external and internal intercostals represent two layers corresponding to the external and internal oblique abdominal muscles.

The *linea alba is* a fibrous band in the median line of the abdominal region, extending from the xiphoid process above to the pubis below. This line unites the aponeuroses of the muscles of the right and left sides.

The *rectus abdominis* is a superficial muscle and consists of two parts, one on each side of the linea alba. *Origin:* Xiphoid process of the sternum and adjacent costal cartilages. *Insertion:* Pubic bones, near the pubic symphysis. The longitudinally arranged muscle fibers are interrupted by three *tendinous inscriptions,* the lowest one at, or slightly below, the level of the umbilicus. *Innervation:* Ventral portions of the fifth through the twelfth intercostal nerves.

Inspection and palpation: In well-developed subjects the rectus abdominis may be observed and palpated throughout its length in flexion of the trunk (Fig. 119). The tendinous inscriptions and the muscular portions between them are well recognized. In the subject shown, the lowest inscription is well below the level of the umbilicus,

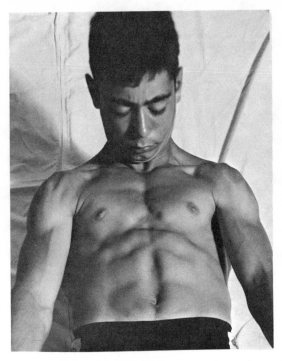

FIG. 119. Activation of the rectus abdominis. In the supine position, the head and the shoulders are raised so that the spine flexes. The three tendinous inscriptions across the muscle are seen, the lowest one slightly below the umbilicus.

Head, Neck and Trunk

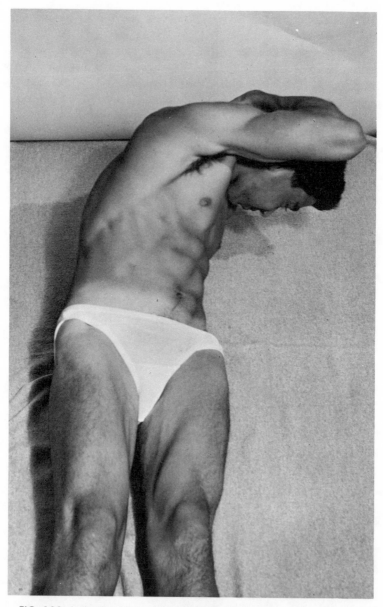

FIG. 120. Activation of the right external oblique abdominal muscle. In the supine position, head and shoulders are raised and the trunk rotated to the left. The interdigitations of the right external oblique with the latissimus dorsi and serratus anterior are seen. The rectus abdominis is also contracting.

and three "muscle hills" above this inscription can be seen. (See also Figure 120.) The widest portion of the linea alba (it is unusually wide in this subject) is found above the umbilicus. The lowest portion of the rectus is usually uninterrupted by inscriptions; in the illustration, however, the lowest portion of the rectus is hidden by the subject's shorts.

In obese individuals the tendinous inscriptions and the boundaries of the muscle cannot be recognized very well, but the tension in the muscle, when the subject raises his head while in the supine position, can always be palpated.

The *obliquus externus abdominis* (external oblique abdominal muscle) constitutes the superficial layer of the abdominal wall. It is located lateral to the rectus abdominis and covers the anterior and lateral regions of the abdomen. *Origin:* Anterolateral portions of the ribs, where it interdigitates with the serratus anterior and, at its lowest point of origin, with slips from the latissimus dorsi. *Insertion:* The upper fibers have a downward-forward direction and insert into an aponeurosis by which they are connected to the linea alba; the lower fibers are inserted into the crest of the ilium. *Innervation:* Lower intercostal nerves.

Inspection and palpation: Because of the oblique direction of the fibers of the externus, flexion of the trunk combined with rotation brings out a strong contraction of this muscle, particularly if the movement is opposed by the weight of the upper part of the body (Fig. 120). To activate the muscle on the right side, the trunk is rotated to the left; the muscle on the left side contracts in trunk rotation to the right. Bilateral action obtains in flexion of the trunk without rotation and, markedly so, in straining.

The *obliquus internus abdominis* (internal oblique abdominal muscle), being covered by the external oblique, belongs to the second layer of the abdominal wall. The muscle extends essentially over the same area as the externus, but its fibers cross those of the externus. *Origin:* Inguinal ligament and crest of ilium. From this origin the fibers fan out to be *inserted* into the pubic bone, into an aponeurosis connecting with the linea alba and into several ribs where the direction of its fibers is continuous with those of the internal intercostals. *Innervation:* Lower intercostal nerves and branches from the iliohypogastric nerve.

Inspection and palpation: In palpation the internal oblique cannot be well differentiated from the other layers of the abdominal wall.

However, the tension of the abdominal wall (seen and felt on the left side of the abdomen when the trunk is rotated to the left, as in Fig. 120) is due, at least in part, to the internal oblique. In this movement, the line of action of the external oblique on the right side and the internal oblique on the left side is a continuous one, both muscles contributing to the rotation.

The *transversus abdominis* composes the innermost layer of the abdominal wall. This muscle has been named the "corset muscle" because it encloses the abdominal cavity like a corset. The direction of its fibers is transverse. *Origin:* Lower ribs, thoracolumbar fascia, crest of ilium, inguinal ligament. *Insertion:* By means of an aponeurosis, partly fused with those of the other abdominal muscles, into the linea alba. *Innervation:* Lower intercostal nerves, iliohypogastric and ilioinguinal nerves.

Palpation: In forced expiration a tightening of the abdominal wall is felt anterolaterally between the lower ribs and the crest of the ilium. The transversus is partly responsible for this tension which involves all the layers of the abdominal wall.

The *quadratus lumborum* is a muscle of the posterior abdominal wall, having a close relation to the psoas major. *Origin:* Crest of ilium (posterior portion), transverse processes of lower lumbar vertebrae, iliolumbar ligament, and thoracolumbar fascia. *Insertion:* Transverse processes of upper lumbar vertebrae, twelfth rib, and lumbar fascia. *Innervation:* Branches from the upper lumbar nerves.

Palpation is best accomplished with the subject in a supine or standing position. The examiner grasps from front to back at the waist in the area shown in Figure 116 (where the psoas major is being palpated). The subject then hikes the hip (pulls the pelvis on that side up toward the ribs, which involves shortening of the muscle). While the psoas is palpated anteriorly near the vertebral column, the quadratus lumborum is felt laterally and posteriorly. The muscular contraction felt in this region when hiking the hip is not of the quadratus lumborum alone, but involves other lateral abdominal muscles and some of the muscles belonging to the erector spinae group.

The *external and internal intercostal muscles,* as their names indicate, are located between the ribs. They may be looked upon as the thoracic continuation of the external and internal oblique abdominal muscles. Each intercostal muscle extends between two adjacent ribs, but all of them together compose a two-layered muscle sheath enclosing the thoracic cavity. *Innervation:* Intercostal nerves.

Palpation: If an attempt is made to insert the tip of a finger between two ribs, the intercostals offer resistance. The muscles may also be felt in movements of the trunk involving a widening or narrowing of the intercostal spaces. For example, in sitting or standing, the subject reaches overhead with the left arm, then flexes the trunk to the right while spreading the ribs apart on the left side; he then returns the trunk to the upright position. The intercostals on the left side may be felt in both parts of this movement as they oppose the action of gravity, and in particular during the return movement.

POSTERIOR TRUNK MUSCLES

The posterior trunk muscles, or simply back muscles, are concerned with extension, lateral flexion and rotation of the trunk, and in general, with balance of the vertebral column. Anatomically and functionally, they have much in common with the posterior neck muscles with which they are continuous.

The entire extensor group is referred to as the *erector spinae* muscle. It is a large muscle mass which fills the space between the transverse and the spinous processes of the vertebrae and extends laterally beyond the transverse processes, partly covering the posterior portion of the thorax.

The many muscles which comprise the erector spinae group originate and insert at various levels and are named in accordance with their origin and insertion, their shape, or their action. It would serve no good purpose to discuss these muscles individually. It is suggested that the student consult an atlas of anatomy to become somewhat familiar with the following muscles: *iliocostales, longissimus, spinales, transversospinales* (including semispinalis, multifidus and rotatores), *interspinales* and *intertransversarii.* Most of these muscles are represented in all regions of the vertebral column, and their specific locations are indicated by adding *lumborum, thoracis, cervicis,* or *capitis* to their respective names, such as iliocostalis lumborum, semispinalis thoracis, semispinalis cervicis, semispinalis capitis. *Innervation:* Numerous branches of the spinal nerves from cervical, thoracic, and lumbar regions.

Inspection and palpation: The action of the erector spinae as a group may be observed best in the lumbar and lower thoracic regions when the subject, in the prone position, raises the upper part of the

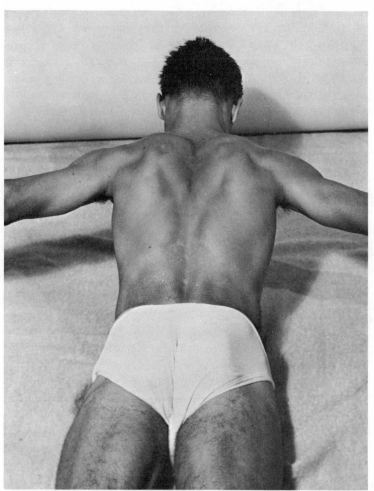

FIG. 121. The erector spinae group is best observed in the lumbar region. In the thoracic region this group is covered by the rhomboids and the trapezius. The latter muscle is seen contracting strongly.

body off the floor (Fig. 121). These muscles should also be palpated in erect standing, and the effect of swaying the upper part of the body forward and backward should be observed (during forward sway, the muscles become tense; during backward sway, the muscles are relaxed). These muscles are active also in lateral bending and in rotation of the trunk; the muscles should be palpated in these movements and their action analyzed. In walking, the erector spinae group in the lumbar region may be felt contracting on each step (see also Chapter 11).

Discussion of Function of Head, Neck and Trunk Muscles
BALANCING OF VERTEBRAL COLUMN AND HEAD

The muscles that surround the vertebral column and are located close to it provide a flexible support for the upright column, and they act to equilibrate its parts in relation to each other and in balancing the trunk as a whole in relation to the pelvis. In this action they are aided by the abdominal and intercostal muscles, which act indirectly on the vertebral column.

Many of these muscles have a function which may be compared to that of guy-ropes supporting an upright pole. As long as the pole is vertical, little or no tension in the guy-ropes is required, but as soon as there is a slight inclination of the pole, the guy-ropes opposite the side toward which the pole is inclined become tense to prevent the pole from falling over.

The "guy ropes" of the vertebral column are capable of producing tension at various lengths and, therefore, can allow deviations of the trunk or its segments in various directions while maintaining their stabilizing functions. Since some of these muscles are short (bridging two or three vertebrae only) and others are long, their actions may be adjusted to effect small or large segments of the vertebral column. For proper equilibration, a give-and-take action of the muscles on all sides of the spine is required. Among the muscles involved in such equilibration are the following:

1. *Anteriorly:* psoas major, longus colli, longus capitis, rectus capitis anterior, scalenes, sternocleidomastoid, anterior abdominal muscles, intercostals.
2. *Posteriorly:* erector spinae in lumbar, thoracic and cervical regions.
3. *Laterally:* psoas major, quadratus lumborum, scalenes, sternocleidomastoid, erector spinae, lateral abdominal muscles, intercostals.

If one of the above groups of muscles is paralyzed, the body will assume a position which eliminates the necessity of action of this group. In accordance with this rule, the vertebral column or the head will deviate toward the side of the paralyzed muscles, which throws the muscles on the opposite side into action. This rule applies to the upright position and is illustrated by examples in the next paragraph.

If the back muscles are paralyzed or weakened, the trunk tends to

---

be inclined backward so that the front muscles take over the balancing function. Paralysis of the abdominal muscles results in a forward flexion of the vertebral column. With the anterior neck muscles out of function, the subject tends to keep the head inclined slightly forward by the action of gravity while the posterior neck muscles prevent further flexion of the head and the neck.

Electromyographic Studies of Some of the Trunk Muscles

Floyd and Silver (1950), Campbell (1952), Jones and associates (1953, 1957), Koepke and associates (1955) and Taylor (1960) investigated the action of some of the trunk muscles in selected movements and during respiration. The subjects were healthy males. In most instances, the various studies yielded comparable results. These studies deserve being read in their entireties; only a few of the electromyographic findings are reported below.

MOVEMENTS

In *head raising* (supine), the rectus abdominis consistently showed strong activity; only slight activity was present in the obliques.

Bilateral leg raising (supine) activated all abdominals (rectus, obliques, and probably also the transversus).

Lateral flexion of the trunk, straining and coughing (supine) brought out the oblique abdominals but little or no activity was found in the rectus, unless the trunk simultaneously flexed.

Bending backward (standing) and returning to upright position: Strong activity was registered bilaterally in the seventh to tenth intercostals, in the scalene muscles and in the lateral abdominal muscles. In bending to the side, the same muscles were activated unilaterally.

RESPIRATION

In the past, there has been general agreement on the action of the *diaphragm* as being the most important muscle of inspiration. But the differential functions of the two layers of the intercostal muscles have been much debated. Electromyographic studies have thrown considerable light on this subject.

QUIET BREATHING. Electrical activity was essentially absent in the abdominal muscles, both during inspiration and expiration. The *scalene muscles* and the *first intercostal muscles* registered activity during inspiration and decreased their activity, or ceased to act, during expiration. Expiration appeared to occur without muscular activity.

FORCED BREATHING. During the *inspiratory phase* the *scalenes* contracted vigorously and all *intercostal muscles* investigated were recruited. Toward the end of inspiration, activity was present in the pectoralis major, sternocleidomastoid, serratus anterior, upper trapezius, pectoralis minor and abdominals. During the *expiratory phase*, activity continued in the intercostal muscles while the scalenes, pectoralis minor and sternocleidomastoid ceased to contract. The pectoralis major often became active and the *abdominal muscles*, mainly the *obliques*, contracted strongly.

Most of the investigators found it difficult or impossible to differentiate between the different layers of the abdominals and of the intercostals. Taylor, however, reports that an improved technique enabled him to lead off action potentials from the external and the internal intercostal muscles separately. He demonstrated that during vigorous respiration the two layers act in a reciprocal fashion, the *external layer during inspiration*, the *internal during expiration*.

Support of the Flexed Spine Under Conditions of Strain

The functions of the abdominals, the intercostals, and other trunk muscles in compressing the thoracic and abdominal cavities when weights are lifted or traction is applied against a firm resistance were investigated by Morris and associates (1961).

Electromyograms of the various muscle groups were recorded, and simultaneously the intrathoracic and intra-abdominal pressures were measured in both dynamic and static loading of the spine. *Dynamic loading* consisted in bending forward and lifting weights of varying heaviness while (1) flexing hips and knees and (2) flexing hips and maintaining knees extended. *Static loading* involved pulling on a strain ring while the trunk was erect and at various degrees of hip flexion.

The hypothesis of Morris and associates (1961) is, in part, as follows: The thoracic cavity, filled with air, and the abdominal cavity, filled with liquid and semisolid material, under certain circumstances, are capable of giving substantial support to the flexed spine. The contraction of the trunk muscles converts these chambers into nearly rigid-walled cylinders which resist a part of the force generated in loading the trunk, and thereby relieves the load on the spine itself.

Calculations of forces acting on the lumbosacral disk when a 170-pound man lifts a 200-pound weight (the role of the trunk is omitted) disclose that this force would amount to over 2000 pounds, much more than this region could endure without structural failure. The research data revealed that, owing to the "inflatable support," the force in the lumbosacral region was reduced by 600 pounds. Similarly, the force acting on the lower thoracic region was found to be reduced from 1568 to 791 pounds.

The often observed fact that when a heavy weight is lifted a person holds his breath and tightens the trunk muscles can thus be functionally explained as an automatic act for prevention of strain and injury to the vertebral column.

Pathological Curves of the Vertebral Column

The physiological curves of the vertebral column are discussed in Chapter 10 and illustrated in Figure 126.

KYPHOSIS. A marked increase in the posterior convexity of the thoracic curve is referred to as a *kyphosis* (Gr. *kyphosis,* a humpback). In the strict sense of the word it signifies a curvature of pathological origin, as in tuberculous spondylitis (Pott's disease), vertebral epiphysitis and ankylosing arthritis, the curves then being *structural* in nature. *Postural* or *functional* curves are flexible and are best referred to as "round back", "poor posture", or the like. *Senile kyphosis* refers to the rigid round back of old age, associated with collapse of the intervertebral disks, owing to desiccation of the nucleus pulposus.

LORDOSIS. Excessive increase in one of the forward convexities of the normal vertebral column is known as *lumbar lordosis* or *cervical lordosis.* Frequently, a lumbar lordosis may be attributed to faulty posture in general but the determining factor may also be a hip flexion contracture, or various pathologies of the osseous or neuromuscular systems may be responsible.

SCOLIOSIS (Gr. *skoliosis,* a curvature). This is a lateral deviation of the spine and may be *functional* or *structural.* A functional curve is flexible and tends to disappear when, in standing, the subject bends forward. When the curve is structural, the vertebrae deviate laterally from the midline of the body and, at the same time, are rotated about a longitudinal axis. In the thoracic region, the ribs rotate with the vertebrae so that when the patient bends forward a protuberance of the ribs on the side of the convexity of the curve is observed. For example, if there is a right thoracic curve (convexity to the right) the ribs protrude posteriorly on the right side. Deformities of the entire rib cage accompany such curves.

CHAPTER 10

Erect Posture

GENERAL PRINCIPLES OF EQUILIBRIUM AND STABILITY

CENTER OF GRAVITY

We learn in physics that the center of gravity of a body is a point about which the mass of the body is equally distributed. All bodies, regardless of shape or density, have such a central point. If one were to support the body at this point, it would be in equilibrium. *The weight of a body may be considered concentrated at its center of gravity.*

Objects, such as a brick, golf ball, and ruler, and an individual standing erect have their centers of gravity located inside their bodies. But the center of gravity of a ring, such as the rim of a wheel, is not contained within the rim but located at the center of the ring. An L-shaped homogenous object, such as an angle iron, cannot be balanced in a horizontal position by supporting it at any point along its body—its center of gravity is found *outside* its body. Similarly, the position of the segments of the human body may shift the center of gravity to the outside of the body, as when the body is in a jackknife position.

STABLE, UNSTABLE AND NEUTRAL EQUILIBRIUM

A body is in *stable equilibrium* when a vertical line through its center of gravity falls within its base of support and when tipping the body slightly causes its center of gravity to be raised. If the stable equilibrium of an upright body having a high center of gravity is sufficiently disturbed by an outside force, the body will topple over and seek a new stable equilibrium with its center of gravity lower than before, e.g., a brick stood upright and then pushed over.

Unstable equilibrium can be demonstrated by a stick balanced vertically on a finger tip. A slight tipping of the stick causes its center of gravity to be lowered and the stick will fall over. A seesaw is also in unstable equilibrium.

Neutral equilibrium is exemplified by a ball. The height of the center of gravity of a ball remains unchanged whether the ball is motionless or rolling.

RESISTANCE TO OVERTHROWING

A high slender object, such as a pencil stood upright, is less stable than a low broad object, such as a brick flat on the ground; a homogenous object leaning slightly to one side is more easily overthrown than when it is vertical. The degree of stability, that is, the resistance to overthrowing, depends upon three factors: the size of the surface of support, the height of the center of gravity above the supporting surface, and the location of the center-of-gravity line with respect to the surface of support. *The larger the supporting surface and the lower the center of gravity, the greater the stability; the closer the center-of-gravity line falls to the center of the base of support, the better the stability.*

APPLICATION OF GENERAL PRINCIPLES TO ERECT STANDING

When the first two criteria given above are applied to erect standing, it is obvious that the erect position does not offer a great deal of stability, because the surface of support is relatively small and the center of gravity lies relatively high (at about the level of S1 or S2). But, with respect to the third criterion, optimum conditions exist, since the body possesses an automatic neuromuscular mechanism which maintains the center-of-gravity line close to the center of the base of support.

BODY PROPORTIONS

Body proportions vary a great deal in individuals so that no figures of proportions can be given which apply universally. An investigation of the weights of body segments in cadavers of young adult males of average body proportions was carried out by Braune and Fischer (1889). Figure 122 illustrates segmental proportions in percentage of total body weight. The actual weights of the segments are seen next to the illustration. Dempster (1955) investigated eight

SEGMENTAL WEIGHTS (Braune and
Fischer) For limbs, means of left and
right are given.

	Kg.
Entire body	55.70
Head and neck	3.93
Trunk without limbs	23.80
Entire upper extremity	3.62
Upper arm	1.98
Forearm without hand	1.27
Hand	0.47
Entire lower extremity	10.38
Thigh	6.45
Leg without foot	2.94
Foot	1.00

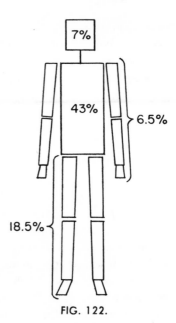

FIG. 122.

expected, the two studies yielded somewhat different results and
a report of Hanavan (1964) contains still other variations. In the
1930s, a Russian group headed by N. Bernstein (quoted by Drillis
and associates, 1964) investigated body proportions in living subjects, 76 males and 76 females, ranging in age from 12 to 75 years.
The percentage weights of the segments were found to vary but
little in the sexes. In summary, the more recent reports tended to
indicate lower proportions for the limbs. For example, Dempster's
percentage for the entire lower limb is 15.7 compared to Braune
and Fischer's figure of 18.5 per cent.

The reader is referred to Williams and Lissner (1962) for details
of the Dempster study, and to Drillis and associates (1964) for
methods now in use by the Biomechanics Group of the Research
Division of the School of Engineering and Science, New York University. The latter group is investigating volume, mass, center of
mass and mass moment of inertia of living body segments.

LOCATIONS OF CENTERS OF GRAVITY OF THE BODY

CENTER OF GRAVITY OF ENTIRE BODY

The center of gravity of one of the frozen cadavers (a male, 18
years of age) investigated by Braune and Fischer was found to be

located at the height of the inferior edge of S2, near the plane of the inlet. In a more recent study on live subjects, the center of gravity was found to lie at about the height of S1 (Åkerblom, 1948).

Hellebrandt and associates (1938) determined the percentage height of the center of gravity of the body in a group of 445 young adult women. These investigators found that the mean percentage height below the horizontal plane passing through the center of gravity was 55.

In general, it may be stated that *the center of gravity in erect standing is located in the upper sacral region, somewhat above the halfway mark between the soles of the feet and the summit of the head.*

The location of the center of gravity of the entire body has been discussed extensively in the literature, but comparatively little attention has been focused on the centers of gravity of the body segments above the weight-bearing joints. Yet, it is the location of each of the latter centers which determines the rotary forces present at each of these joints.

Braune and Fischer investigated the centers of gravity of individual body segments and then determined the centers of gravity of various combinations of segments. When the masses of two adjacent segments and their individual centers of gravity are known, their combined center of gravity can be computed. The two centers are connected by a straight line and the combined center of gravity is found on this line at a point which divides the line in inverse proportions to the masses.

CENTERS OF GRAVITY OF INDIVIDUAL LIMB SEGMENTS

The centers of gravity of limb segments were found to lie on a line connecting the joints adjacent to the segment, at a point which divided the line in approximate proportions 4:5 (four proximal to five distal parts). With only minor deviations, this held true of the thigh, leg, foot, arm, forearm, and hand. For the lower extremity, the heights of the centers of gravity are indicated in Figure 123. The center of gravity of the thigh is located at Level 6, that of the leg at Level 8. The center of gravity of the entire lower limb was found to lie at Level 7, just above the flare of the femoral condyles.

A knowledge of the levels of the centers of gravity of the limb segments is of more than theoretical interest. An above-knee amputee may ask, "How much should I weigh now? I used to weigh 150 pounds before I lost my leg." Since the lower limb constitutes 18 to 20 per cent of the entire weight of the limb and since the center of gravity of the limb is at Level 7, it is safe to say that an above-knee amputee has lost about 10 per cent of his total body weight; therefore, in the patient mentioned above, the calculated weight loss of the limb would be 15 pounds, so that his body weight should be approximately 135 pounds. The figure, 10 per cent, would apply to an amputee with a fairly long thigh stump. The approximate weight loss can also be determined for other amputation sites. The question,

FIG. 123. Heights of centers of gravity of segments of lower extremity. 6, Of thigh alone; 7, Of entire lower extremity; 8, Of leg alone; 9, Of leg and foot; 10, Of foot alone. (Redrawn from Braune and Fischer.)

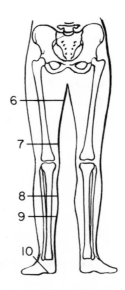

whether the prosthesis weighs more or less than the amputated portion of the limb, may be answered by using the figures given. (Usually, one finds that the prosthesis weighs less than the amputated portion.)

CENTER OF GRAVITY OF BODY MASS ABOVE THE ANKLE JOINTS

This center lies a little higher than, and has almost the same anteroposterior location as, that of the entire body; since the weight of the feet is small compared to that of the entire body, the difference in location of the center of gravity is insignificant. According to Mommsen (1927), the center of gravity of the body mass above the ankle joints lies about level with the anterior superior spines of the ilia.

CENTER OF GRAVITY OF BODY MASS ABOVE THE KNEE JOINTS

The anteroposterior location varies but little from that of the center of gravity of the entire body but, of course, lies higher, approximately level with the umbilicus.

CENTER OF GRAVITY OF BODY MASS ABOVE THE HIP JOINTS

This mass consists of head, arms, and trunk and may conveniently be referred to as HAT (Elftman, 1955). Braune and Fischer found this center to be located at the anterior border of the body of T11, which is approximately level with, or slightly below, the tip of the xiphoid process of the sternum. In ordinary standing, the anteroposterior location varies but little from that of the center of gravity of the body as a whole.

CENTER OF GRAVITY OF HEAD

Braune and Fischer found the center of gravity of the head, including the three upper vertebrae, to be located 0.7 cm. posterior to the dorsum sellae of the sella turcica ("Turkish saddle") of the sphenoid bone, that is, at the base of the skull, somewhat anterior to the foramen magnum. The center of gravity of the head alone (without the upper vertebrae) would lie a little higher. The point given by Braune and Fischer is approximately level with the upper edge of the zygomatic process of the temporal bone, which can be palpated anterior to, and above, the external meatus of the ear.

BODY BALANCE WHEN STANDING ON BOTH FEET

The locations of the various centers of gravity having been established, we may now proceed to determine where plumb lines through these centers fall in relation to the surface of support and in relation to weight-bearing joints.

BALANCE ON BASE OF SUPPORT

The surface of support is an enclosed area determined by the position of the feet (Fig. 124). The further the feet are apart, the larger is the surface of support, and the more stable the balance. The metatarsophalangeal joints may be considered the anterior limit of support, or the area of the toes may be included, but this latter area is not much utilized unless the body weight sways forward, as in preparation for rising on tiptoes.

Clinical Kinesiology

As equilibration over the surface of support is effected, the body is in continuous motion. This fact led Hellebrandt to define erect standing as "movement upon a stationary base" (1938). The magnitude of this postural sway as well as its pattern is an individual matter. The projection of the center of gravity on the surface of support has been found to oscillate around the center of the base of support and to follow an approximate figure-of-eight pattern, the anteroposterior sway usually being greater than the lateral sway (Hellebrandt and associates, 1942).

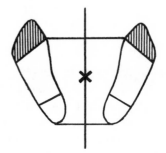

FIG. 124. Base of support of body. In ordinary standing, area posterior to metatarsophalangeal joints is mainly utilized; shaded area is utilized only during marked forward sway. X, Center of base of support.

Maintaining the center-of-gravity line near the center of the base of support secures maximum stability in erect standing and is effected by an automatic neuromuscular mechanism. If segments change their positions (e.g., when the trunk is inclined forward at the hips or the arms are moved in any direction), other segments counterbalance so that the projection of the center of gravity still remains close to the center of the base of support.

BALANCE AT ANKLE JOINT

The vertical projection of the center of gravity of the body mass above the ankle joints falls anterior to the axis of the upper ankle joint. This is inevitably so because the center-of-gravity line of the entire body remains close to the center of the base of support which lies well ahead of the ankle joints (Fig. 124). A rotary force is thus set up at the ankle which would cause the body to topple forward unless opposed by a muscular force. The calf muscles furnish this equilibrating force thereby preventing dorsiflexion of the ankle (excessive forward inclination of the shank with respect to the foot). It is believed that the soleus muscle in particular is responsible for this equilibration (Denny-Brown, 1929; Joseph, 1960). During postural sway, the body weight seldom, if ever, passes behind the axes of the ankle joints, and consequently the calf muscles remain continuously, although variably, active (Smith, 1957). The behavior of the intrinsic muscles in standing is discussed on page 223.

EFFECT OF BILATERAL CALF-MUSCLE PARALYSIS. If the calf muscles are paralyzed bilaterally the subject is forced to keep the weight in vertical alignment with the axes of the upper ankle joints, or nearly so. If the body weight passes further to the rear, the dorsiflexors of the ankle spring into action, but the safe range of backward sway is extremely limited. A subject with calf-muscle paralysis tends to keep the feet a certain distance apart or to hold on to a nearby object to feel more secure.

BALANCE AT KNEE JOINTS

The body mass above the knee joints consists of the head, arms, trunk, and thighs. A vertical line through the center of gravity of this body mass falls slightly in front of the axis for flexion and extension of the knees. During postural sway, this vertical line may occasionally, though rarely, move behind the axis of the knee joints. Most of the time, therefore, a rotary force in the sense of extension is present at the knees. What, then, prevents the knees from being extended and hyperextended?

This question was investigated by Smith (1956) who found that the counter-balancing force had three components, variable in size, depending upon the knee angle. As an example, in a subject who stood with the knees 6 degrees short of full extension (knee angle 174 degrees), the proportion of the three components were: 50 per cent, passive resistance in extra-articular tissues; 30 per cent, postural activity of the knee flexor muscles; and 20 per cent, resistance by an articular mechanism.

FUNCTION OF THE QUADRICEPS IN STANDING. Continuous quadriceps action is only required in subjects who stand in such a manner that the center-of-gravity line of the supratibial mass falls posterior to the axis of the knee joint. But such subjects are exceptions. A short burst of quadriceps activity also appears if during postural sway the center-of-gravity line momentarily passes behind the knee axis. The above has been confirmed by statography (Åkerblom, 1948) and by electromyography (Åkerblom, 1948; Joseph and Nightingale, 1954).

Hyperextension increases knee stability, but it has a delaying effect in activity situations when quick flexion of the knee is required. The "readiness position" in athletics, therefore, avoids complete knee extension. The failure of some individuals to make a quick start is due, to a great extent, to the knees being somewhat hyperextended, and "being caught flat-footed" depends as much on knee alignment as on ankle position.

STABILITY VERSUS MOBILITY. Clinically, in the rehabilitation of the disabled, the individual's requirements with respect to stability and mobility must be carefully evaluated. If *stability* is the prime requirement, as may be the case in elderly amputees, the prosthetic knee must have a large margin of safety. But a young active amputee, whose skill in controlling the prosthetic knee may develop to a remarkable extent, will prefer *mobility*, a readiness position of the prosthetic knee, for quick starting and for ease and grace in walking.

BILATERAL QUADRICEPS PARALYSIS. Because of the stabilizing effect of gravity on the knee joints, an individual with bilateral paralysis of the quadriceps muscle is capable of standing erect without braces, provided that there are not other complicating factors. In order to minimize the danger of collapse at the knee during postural sway, the individual will tend to keep the knees maximally extended, which might lead to hyperextension and *genu recurvatum*. He may also choose to incline the trunk somewhat forward, which increases the stabilizing effect of gravity.

EFFECT OF CALF-MUSCLE PARALYSIS ON KNEE STABILITY. A prerequisite for stabilization of the knee by gravity is that the body weight be kept forward as in normal erect posture, which is only possible if the calf muscles are functioning. Indirectly, therefore, these muscles are responsible for knee stability. A subject with a combination of calf-muscle and quadriceps paralysis benefits from wearing an ankle brace with dorsiflexion limited to 90 degrees or from a surgical stabilization of the ankle, because both of these measures materially improve knee stability. Similarly, a blocking of dorsiflexion of the prosthetic foot in the above-knee artificial limb improves knee stability, while allowing dorsiflexion beyond 90 degrees causes the knee to become unstable.

BALANCE AT HIP JOINTS

As previously stated, the center of gravity of HAT is located inside the thorax, approximately at the height of the xiphoid process. A vertical line through this center may fall directly through, in front of, or in back of, the common hip axis, depending upon how the individual stands. Muscle action will vary accordingly.

There has been much controversy with respect to the location of the center-of-gravity line of HAT in relation to the common hip axis in standing. The old anatomists (Meyer, 1853; Braune and Fischer, 1889; Fick, 1911) differed considerably in their opinions. Schede (1941) in his analysis of common ways of standing shows that the center-of-gravity line may fall on either side of the common hip axis, or directly above it. He stresses that *incomplete extension of the hip is essential if the knees are to be stabilized by gravity,* for when the hip is completely extended, a backward sway of the center of gravity of HAT can no longer be absorbed at the hip and, therefore, will result in flexion of the knees.

Åkerblom (1948) reports that 22 subjects out of 25 studied stood with incomplete extension at the hip, varying from 2 to 15 degrees. His subjects stood "comfortably," with the feet slightly apart and the arms hanging relaxed. Variations of the center-of-gravity line with respect to the hip axis from one measurement to the other were found, indicating equilibration at the hip as well as at the ankle. He concluded that in *comfortable symmetrical standing the upper body is usually balanced over the hip joint in unstable equilibrium.* Basmajian (1967) registered electrical activity in the iliacus in standing at ease, thus substantiating Åkerblom's findings of incomplete hip extension.

Somewhat different results were obtained by Joseph and Williams (1957) in a study of erect standing. In the 18 male subjects studied, no electrical activity was registered in the hip flexors or extensors and the investigators concluded that, in standing at ease, the hips are fully extended, further extension being checked by a passive mechanism. The subjects, however, stood with the feet about 30 cm. apart and the hands clasped behind the back, which position does not correspond to comfortable erect posture referred to by other investigators.

HIP POSTURE WHEN KNEE CONTROL IS LACKING. It is of particular importance for individuals, who have lost their ability to control the knee actively (such as above-knee amputees and patients with certain types of paralysis), to stand with the hips short of full extension so that some postural sway can be absorbed at the hip. As pointed out by Schede (1941), when an above-knee prosthesis is worn, equilibration at the hip is mandatory for knee stability. These patients tend to have some increase in the lumbar curve, but a backward tilt of the pelvis for the purpose of decreasing the lumbar curve is contraindicated, because it would cause the artificial knee to buckle.

HIP POSTURE OF PARAPLEGIC PATIENTS. The paraplegic patient, having lost control of the muscles of the ankles, knees, and hips,

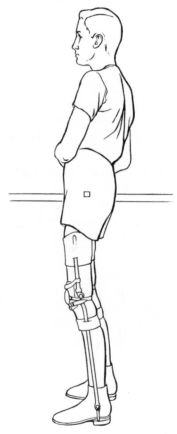

FIG. 125. Characteristic posture of paraplegic patient standing in long leg braces which stabilize knees and ankles but leave hips free. Center-of-gravity line of upper part of body falls well behind common hip axis. Square on shorts is over greater trochanter which represents approximate location of center of hip joint.

needs long leg braces to stand erect. Bracing at ankles and knees is essential, but the hips may be left free. Such a patient assumes a characteristic posture with the upper part of the body inclined backward so that the center-of-gravity line of HAT comes to fall well behind the hip axis (Fig. 125). The paraplegic hangs on the anterior ligaments of the hip joints; the ligaments may eventually stretch so that abnormal range of hip extension results.

If the paraplegic patient wishes to lean forward, as when picking up an object from the floor, he must brace himself on a firm object with one hand while picking up the object with the other hand. Otherwise, he will collapse at the hip as soon as the center of gravity of HAT moves in front of the hip axis.

BALANCE OF VERTEBRAL COLUMN

At birth the vertebral column presents one long C-curve with posterior convexity. The sacral and thoracic regions maintain posterior convexity throughout life, while the cervical and the lumbar regions develop curves in opposite directions, become convex anteriorly.

In the adult, the relationship between these physiological curves varies in individuals, so that one or the other curve may be more pronounced. According to O. Fischer, quoted by Fick (1911), in well-built young adult males assuming the so-called *Normalstellung* (perpendicular posture), the vertebral column is aligned as seen in Figure 126. A perpendicular through the center of gravity of the body passes through the common hip axis and also through the center of gravity of the upper portion of the body (at T11). With this alignment, the weight of the head and of successive portions of the vertebral column (and structures supported by this column) are favorably

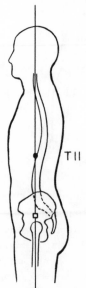

FIG. 126. Curves of vertebral column in perpendicular posture in young adult males. Center of gravity of entire body (marked by a square) as well as center of gravity of upper part of body (marked by dot at T11) are in vertical alignment with center of hip joint. A slight change in alignment occurs in comfortable posture. (After O. Fischer, redrawn from Fick, p. 494.)

distributed in relation to the anteroposterior curves. A slight change in alignment occurs in ordinary "comfortable" posture.

Abnormal curves in the thoracic and lumbar regions are discussed on page 266.

PELVIC BALANCE

The rigid sacral portion of the vertebral column, firmly connected with the ilia, is part of the pelvis. The pelvis, interposed between the lower extremities and the flexible portions of the vertebral column, possesses movements of its own. Owing to the firmness of the sacroiliac and lumbosacral junctions, however, every pelvic movement is accompanied by a realignment of the spine, most marked in the lumbar region.

PELVIC INCLINATION.   In erect standing, when the hip is flexed by a pelvic movement while the upper part of the body remains erect, the *inclination* of the pelvis is said to be *increased*—a *forward tilt* of the pelvis has occurred. When this movement takes place, the anterior superior spines of the ilia come to lie anterior to the foremost part of the pubic symphysis while these spines are normally in vertical alignment with, or lie slightly posterior to, the symphysis (Fig. 127A). The opposite movement of the pelvis (in direction of extension) is referred to as a *backward tilt of the pelvis,* and the resulting position as a *decreased pelvic inclination.*

A determination of the pelvic inclination in terms of degrees can be made by laying an oblique plane through the posterior superior spines of the ilia and the foremost portion of the pubic symphysis. The angle of this plane with the horizontal is said to be the *angle of pelvic inclination* (Fig. 127A). This method of measuring the pelvic inclination was advocated by Fick who considered an angle of 50 to 60 degrees to be normal for adult men and a somewhat larger angle to be normal for women.

Fick's method of measuring the angle of pelvic inclination has been used by many investigators, but has not been adopted universally. Sometimes, the "plane of the inlet" (inlet to the lesser pelvis) is used as a reference plane. This plane, indicated by the line a-b in the illustration, passes through the lumbosacral junction and through the foremost portion of the pubic symphysis. If this plane is used, the angle of pelvic inclination will be greater than when determined by Fick's method.

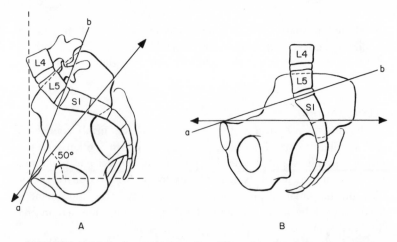

FIG. 127. Pelvic inclination in standing (A), and in sitting (B). Arrow: plane of pelvic inclination. Line a-b represents "plane of the inlet." (Redrawn from Fick, pp. 438 and 439.)

The range of backward tilt of the pelvis in the erect standing position is determined by the tension of the capsule of the hip joints and the reinforcing ligaments, noticeably, the iliofemoral or Y-ligament. If further backward tilt is attempted, this can be accomplished only by flexing the knees simultaneously with the pelvic movement, which also causes hip flexion and slackening of the ligaments.

In the sitting position, these ligaments no longer restrict the pelvic movement and the pelvis tilts backward so that the plane through the posterior superior spine of the ilia and the pubic symphysis becomes horizontal (Fig. 127B). A backward tilt of the pelvis is accompanied by a decrease in, or obliteration of, the physiological lumbar curve. Such flattening of the lumbar spine is particularly marked in sitting. A forward inclination of the pelvis is accompanied by an increase in the physiological lumbar curve.

CLINICAL EVALUATION OF PELVIC INCLINATION. It is difficult to measure the angle of pelvic inclination in the living subject. Clinically, therefore, a more practical method to determine normal or abnormal inclination of the pelvis is needed. Because the anterior superior spines of the ilia and the front part of the pubic symphysis are superficial and easily located, the alignment of these points may be observed. When the subject is viewed from the side, the pelvic inclination may be considered normal if these two points are approximately in vertical alignment, as seen in Figure 127A.

BALANCE OF HEAD AT ATLANTO-OCCIPITAL JOINTS

The center of gravity of the head is located about one inch above the transverse axis of the atlanto-occipital joints so that the head is in unstable equilibrium, much like that of a seesaw. When the head is erect, a perpendicular line through the center of gravity of the head falls somewhat anterior to the transverse axis for flexion and extension (Fig. 128A). Therefore, in ordinary standing and sitting, the posterior neck muscles are moderately active to prevent the head from dropping forward. When the head is inclined forward, as in reading, writing and sewing, the demands on these muscles increases (Fig. 128B). But when the head is allowed to drop all way forward, the ligamentum nuchae becomes tense and muscular activity is no longer needed. If the head is tipped backward, the center-of-gravity line falls posterior to the transverse axis (Fig. 128C) and the head will tip all the way back unless the flexors of the head spring into action. By palpating the anterior neck muscles (sternocleidomastoid, scalenus anterior) the point at which the center of gravity passes behind the transverse axis can be ascertained.

The effect of the changing position of the center of gravity with respect to the axis may be observed when an individual falls asleep in the sitting position. The head may drop forward or backward, depending upon the sitting posture. It is common to see both sleeping postures in a railroad coach where the backs of the seats are not high enough to accommodate the head in a comfortable position.

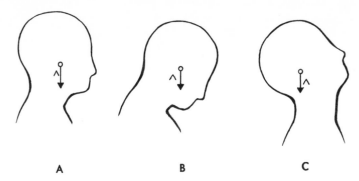

FIG. 128. Relation of center-of-gravity line of head to axis of atlanto-occipital joints in different head positions. A, Head erect, center of gravity slightly anterior to axis, posterior neck muscles moderately active. B, Head forward, increased activity of posterior neck muscles. C, Head backward, center of gravity posterior to axis, anterior neck muscles active.

COMFORTABLE (SYMMETRICAL) POSTURE

Comfortable posture is a symmetrical posture assumed in standing on both feet with the arms relaxed at the sides of the body when no attention is focused on the way the body is aligned. This corresponds approximately to the posture described by Braune and Fischer (1889) as *Bequeme Haltung*.

As previously discussed, an automatic neuromuscular mechanism is responsible for equilibration. Figure 129 illustrates comfortable symmetrical posture, although it must be added that this posture hardly deserves the term "comfortable." For if an individual has to stand for any length of time, he invariably chooses an asymmetrical posture (see below) which is less tiresome and far more comfortable.

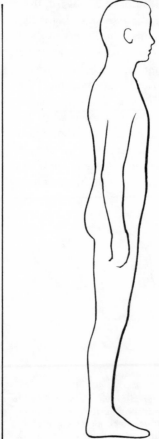

FIG. 129. Comfortable (symmetrical) posture.

PERPENDICULAR POSTURE

This posture can be assumed if the subject shifts the body weight somewhat backward until a plumb line through the center of gravity of the body falls (directly) through the axis of the talocrural joints (Fig. 126). The tip of the ear, the tip of the shoulder, and the centers of hip, knee, and ankle joints are then in vertical alignment. This body position was referred to by Braune and Fischer as *Normalstellung* but not as normal posture. It was used to facilitate measurements of body points in a three-dimensional system of coordinates.

Unfortunately, *Normalstellung* has been incorrectly translated as normal posture. This error has led to the view that perpendicular posture is a desirable posture. Obviously, perpendicular posture does not coincide with Nature's way of balancing the body and, therefore, should not be used as a standard for good posture.

Clinical applications in terms of posture training and the biomechanics of artificial limb wearers have been dealt with in other publications (Brunnstrom, 1954; Brunnstrom, 1960).

ASYMMETRICAL POSTURE

If erect standing must be maintained for any length of time, the posture of choice is to stand with the weight now on one and now on the other foot, the contralateral foot being on the ground but supporting very little weight. The hip posture is of the Trendelenburg type (see page 289) in which the abductors are relieved of action and the ligaments are relied upon. This is an energy-saving posture because there is less metabolism in ligaments than in contracting muscles. Overstretching of the ligamentous apparatus is avoided by frequent shifting from one foot to the other.

BODY BALANCE WHEN STANDING ON ONE FOOT

BALANCE ON SURFACE OF SUPPORT

Standing on one foot greatly increases the demands on the neuromuscular equilibration mechanism, since the surface of support is reduced to less than one-half, as compared to standing on both feet. The body weight must be shifted toward the side of the stance limb until the center-of-gravity line of the body comes to fall close to the center of the new base of support (Fig. 130). As this lateral shift takes place, the entire stance limb—from ankle to hip—becomes

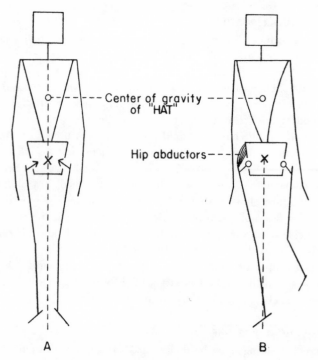

FIG. 130. Body alignment in standing on both feet and in standing on one foot. A, Standing on both feet. Pelvis is supported from both sides. Center-of-gravity line falls in the center of the base of support. B, Standing on one foot. Body weight shifts over stance limb. Hip abductors on stance side become activated to balance the pelvis.

slanted and the ankle everts to enable all parts of the sole to remain on the ground. Lateral balance becomes a major task because the safety zone for side-to-side sway is now very limited. The small incessant equilibration motions at the ankle (easily observed in a bare-footed individual standing on one foot) are evidence of the vigilance of the muscles involved in this finely coordinated balancing act which requires anteroposterior as well as lateral control.

BALANCE AT HIP

One-legged balance involves a major adjustment in the balance of the pelvis. In two-legged standing, the pelvis is supported and braced from both sides by the lower limbs (Fig. 130A). But in standing on one foot, the weight of the upper part of the body as well as of that of the contralateral limb must be supported on one femoral head, a major accomplishment indeed (Fig. 130B). Mechanically, such hip balance exemplifies leverage of the first order—the fulcrum being at the hip joint of the stance limb, and the weight and the force acting on opposite sides of the fulcrum. The combined weight of HAT and one lower limb, if unopposed, would cause the pelvis to tip laterally toward the unsupported side. If the trunk is to remain erect and the pelvis level, the abductors on the side of the stance limb must contract to counteract the weights. As may be judged from the illustration, the weights act at some distance from the fulcrum so that a considerable tension must develop in the abductors, whose leverage at the hip is less favorable than that of the weights.

HIP ABDUCTOR PARALYSIS. When the hip abductors are paralyzed, one-legged standing with the pelvis level as in Figure 130B, becomes impossible. However, the individual may still manage to balance on one foot, at least momentarily, and to do so well enough to permit walking. There are two common methods of compensating for the loss of the abductor muscles in one-legged standing and walking:

1. By skillful utilization of the weight of the upper part of the body—by inclining the trunk laterally toward the stance side until the combined center of gravity of HAT and the suspended limb comes to lie vertically over, or slightly lateral to, the hip joint. In the latter case, the adductors of the stance limb may aid in equilibration. The arms, if free to move, are also well capable of aiding in balancing. In order that the center of gravity of the entire body be maintained vertically over the base of suport, the stance limb loses its slant (Fig. 131). It should be noted that lateral trunk inclination in abductor paralysis can be modified, even eliminated, if a weight of proper size is carried in the hand on the affected side. Such a weight helps to counterbalance the weight of HAT and the unsupported limb.

2. By allowing the pelvis to sag laterally toward the unsupported side until the hip on the stance side has been maximally adducted, at which point tension in capsule, ligaments, and iliotibial tract prevents further motion (Fig. 132). This hip posture is known as *Trendelenburg sign,* a term originally employed to describe the asymmetrical position of the pelvis in congenital dislocation of the hip which renders the hip abductors ineffective. When the Trendelenburg sign is present, owing to the obliquity of the pelvis, the summit of the head comes to lie lower when the affected limb supports the body weight than when the weight is on the unaffected limb.

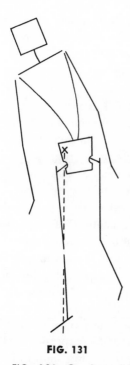
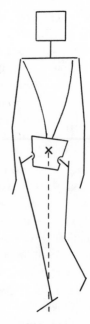

FIG. 131   **FIG. 132**

FIG. 131. One-legged balance when abductors of hip are paralyzed. Upper part of body inclines toward side of paralysis. Weight balances weight at stance hip and the abductors are relieved of their balancing function.

FIG. 132. Trendelenburg sign in paralysis or weakness of hip abductors. Stance hip is adducted. Ligamentous tension is relied upon for hip balance.

For practical illustration of the Trendelenburg sign it is suggested that the student experiment as follows:

Stand in front of a large mirror. Shift the body weight to one side and lift the opposite foot off the ground. Now allow the pelvis to sag on the side opposite the stance limb; then reverse the pelvic movement so that the pelvis again becomes level. Repeat. Observe the fall and rise of the summit of the head; also observe that when the pelvis tilts laterally, the hip on the stance side adducts; when the pelvis movement is reversed, it abducts. The latter movement is accomplished by a shortening contraction of the hip abductors on the side of the stance limb; during the former movement the hip abductors are being stretched, and, if the movement is performed slowly, these muscles contract to slow down the motion (lengthening contraction).

CHAPTER 11

Locomotion

For an analysis of the contribution of muscles to movement, a more extensive knowledge of physics than that usually included in the background requirements for students of physical therapy, occupational therapy and physical education is required. The present chapter, therefore, does not attempt such an analysis but is included mainly for orientation purposes, so that the student may become somewhat familiar with methods used in the study of locomotion, and so that he may become aware of the difficulties which arise if he is to go beyond an evaluation of muscles in static conditions to an understanding of how they control the body in motion.

When the body is stationary, the moments of force produced by the muscles about each joint must balance the moments produced by gravity, and the contribution of each muscle fiber is determined by the length-tension relationship. When the body is in motion, these factors are still present, but more difficult ones are added. The tension produced by each muscle fiber decreases with its speed of shortening and increases more the faster it is stretched (see Chapter 2). The moment of force exerted by the muscle does not move the body directly but changes its acceleration which in turn changes its velocity, which finally results in displacement. To gauge the participation of muscle in movement, one must be able to visualize the movement in terms of its acceleration, a faculty not often achieved.

HISTORICAL NOTES ON THE STUDY OF LOCOMOTION

Man has long appreciated the more apparent distinctions between activities such as walking, running and jumping, but analysis of their fundamental mechanics was not possible before the development of the science of physics. With so many other important problems awaiting physical analysis, locomotion received only sporadic attention from pioneers such as Borelli (1679) and the Weber brothers (1836). More adequate records of the sequence of changes in position were procured by Marey, the eminent French physiologist, by methods which led to the development of motion pictures (1873, 1885, 1887, 1894). The real founder of the scientific study of locomotion was Otto Fischer, a German mathematician, who was the first person to calculate the forces involved in walking (1895-1904). His work on muscles was restricted to the free swing of the leg but was a remarkable advance over previous studies. The next important step was the introduction of the force plate by Elftman (1938, 1939a), allowing the direct recording of the ground reaction and, with this as a starting point, the computation of all the muscle moments from motion picture records. Since that time the use of force plates of increasingly accurate design combined with various ingenious methods of photographic recording of body positions has been the standard method of analysis of human locomotion. Especially active in the accumulation of data has been a group of workers, headed by Eberhart and Inman, at the University of California, Berkeley. A partial summary of the early results of this work is available in Klopsteg and Wilson (1968).

Locomotion has also been studied from the standpoint of metabolic cost by measuring the amount of oxygen consumed during walking. Studies of this nature were undertaken by Benedict and Murschhauser (1915), Studer (1926), Atzler and Herbst (1927), and others.

The results achieved by these early investigators have since been added to by others, notably by Ralston and associates at the Biomechanics Laboratory at the University of California, San Francisco, by Murray and associates at the Kinesiology Research Laboratory, Veterans Administration Center, Wood, Wisconsin and by Basmajian and associates, Department of Anatomy, Queen's University, Kingston, Ontario, Canada.

GENERAL CHARACTERISTICS OF LOCOMOTION

WALKING CYCLE

During a walking cycle, the lower limbs alternate in their movements so that while one supports the body weight (stance phase), the other one swings forward (swing phase). The time during which both feet are on the ground simultaneously is referred to as *double stance*.

The swing phase begins when the toes of the rear foot leave the ground and ends as the heel contacts the ground with the limb in a forward position. This phase corresponds in time with single stance phase of the contralateral limb. The duration of double stance varies with the speed of walking. In slow walking, this period is comparatively long in relation to swing phase, but as speed increases the period becomes shorter and shorter. In running, double stance is no longer present. Instead, for a brief moment, both feet are off the ground simultaneously.

RECORDING OF THE WALKING CYCLE. A record of the duration of sole contact with the ground in walking was first accomplished by a pneumatic method (Marey, 1873); electrical contacts attached to the sole of the shoe are now commonly used. The vertical lines on the illustrations redrawn from the Berkeley study represent heel contact and toe-off positions. Scherb (1927), Mülli (1940) and Scherb and Arienti (1945) had their subjects wear a sandal into which was incorporated three electrical contacts so that separate signals were obtained from the heel, ball of great toe, and ball of little toe.

VARIATION OF WALKING SPEED

It is customary to speak of *slow, medium* and *fast* walking speeds. In the Berkeley study, cadences of 70, 95, and 120 were chosen to represent slow, medium and fast speeds. The natural manner to increase walking speed is to increase the cadence or walking rate (number of steps taken per minute) and to lengthen the stride simultaneously. If the subjects choose their own cadences and no interferences are encountered, the two components — increased cadence and increased length of stride—occur together and have a definite relationship to one another (see table).

Relations between cadence, length of stride and walking speed in two young male subjects. (After Studer, 1926.)

SUBJECT A			SUBJECT B		
Meters per min.	Steps per min.	Stride Length (meters)	Meters per min.	Steps per min.	Stride Length (meters)
16.7	46.6	0.356	15.5	39.7	0.39
24.5	54.7	0.448	20.8	48.3	0.43
28.3	57.1	0.495	24.0	51.1	0.47
35.0	66.0	0.53	27.5	55.0	0.50
41.3	79.4	0.52	31.0	57.3	0.54
48.3	84.8	0.57	36.6	67.8	0.54
57.5	88.5	0.55	41.7	74.2	0.56
66.7	101.0	0.66	45.5	79.7	0.57
74.2	107.0	0.69	52.5	87.5	0.60
84.1	105.0	0.88	55.0	87.3	0.63
101.0	112.0	0.90	66.0	100.0	0.66
116.7	126.7	0.90	83.3	108.3	0.77
			100.0	123.3	0.81
			136.7	143.8	0.95

The cadence utilized at different speeds of walking varies in individual subjects, being related to the length of the limbs, the weight distribution of body segments, etc. For example, an individual with short limbs usually takes shorter strides and more steps per minute than an individual with long limbs for a particular walking speed. When heavy boots are worn, the length of the stride tends to increase as compared to when light shoes are worn.

KINEMATICS OF LOCOMOTION

The kinematics or "geometry" of locomotion may be studied objectively by recording movements of points on the body, such as the summit of the head or the crest of the ilium, or surface landmarks representing the centers of joints or the long axes of bones. If the movement paths of these landmarks are projected on the sagittal, frontal, and horizontal planes, a three-dimensional record is obtained.

CHRONOPHOTOGRAPHY

The chronophotographic method developed by Marey (1885, 1887, 1894) consisted of making a series of exposures of a walking subject on a photographic plate. By means of a rotating shutter, exposures were made at intervals of 1/10 second. Since superimposition of several pictures on one another gave a confused record, "geometrical chronophotography" was subsequently employed. The subject was dressed in black, and brilliant metal buttons and shining bands were attached to the clothing to represent joints and bony segments. The subject, strongly illuminated by the sun, was photographed as he walked in front of a black screen. Dots and lines thus appeared on the photographic plate since the rest of the body did not show against the black background. The principles of this method of recording have since been used extensively by subsequent investigators.

INTERRUPTED LIGHTS

Eberhart and associates (1947) outfitted their subjects with small light bulbs attached to the heel and the toe of the shoe, to the crest of the ilium and to points representing the lateral projections of the centers of hip, knee and ankle joints. The subject walked in front of an open camera in a semidarkened room. A shutter which rotated

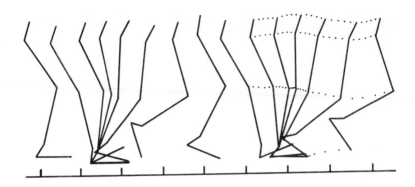

FIG. 133. Stick figures representing a normal male subject walking on level ground at a cadence of 90 steps/min. (Redrawn from Eberhart and Inman, 1947.)

at a speed of 30 revolutions per second interrupted the view of the camera so that dots instead of lines appeared on the plate. The distances between successive dots thus represent time intervals of 1/30 second. Stick figures were constructed by using every fifth frame for connecting the dots representing the crest of the ilium, the hip, knee and ankle joints, the heel and the toe (Fig. 133).

The *movement paths* of the various points may be studied on the stick figures; note that many of the dots on the original record have been omitted in Figure 133. The crest of the ilium and the hip joint show a smooth wavelike path. Two peaks occur during the walking cycle, namely at midposition of single stance of each limb. The lowest portion of the curve is seen during double stance. The movement paths of knee and ankle axes, as well as those of heel and toes, are also seen on the records.

The angular changes at the joints, as procured from the interrupted light records, are seen in Figure 134 where the angles for knee, ankle and metatarsophalangeal joints have been plotted against time. Note that when the heel strikes the ground, the curve (A) for the *knee angle* has its peak, that is, the knee is then almost fully extended. A small amount of flexion, then again extension, follows. This "double knee action" has a shock-absorbing effect. It also minimizes the vertical displacement of the center of gravity of the body and smoothens the path of the hip joint. The lowest portion of curve A, corresponding to maximal knee flexion, occurs in early swing phase, just after toe-off position. As the knee flexes, the hip flexes

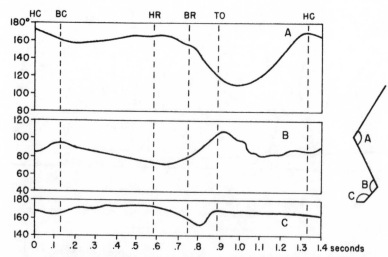

FIG. 134. Knee, ankle and foot-toe angles in level walking by normal, male subject at 90 steps/min. (Redrawn from Eberhart and associates, 1947.)

simultaneously, resulting in an over-all shortening of the limb needed for foot clearance during swing-through. The joint range at the *ankle* (curve B) is from approximately 70 to 110 degrees. The angle at the *metatarsophalangeal joints,* as could be expected, is smallest toward the end of stance phase, between ball-rise and toe-off positions (curve C).

The sagittal plane records also furnish data for the computation of *velocities* and *accelerations*. Since the distance between two successive dots represents 1/30 second, it follows that when the dots are far apart the velocity is high, while closely spaced dots represent slower motions. Figure 133 shows that velocity changes of the hip joint and the crest of the ilium are only slight, while more distal segments of the limb, such as the knee and foot, have marked velocity changes.

RECORDING OF TRANSVERSE ROTATIONS

For accurate recordings of transverse rotations of bony segments Eberhart and associates (1947) attached targets directly to the bones. This was done under local anesthesia by drilling stainless-steel pins into the ilium, the femur and the tibia at suitable locations. The targets, which consisted of small spheres mounted on light wooden rods, protruded laterally and this magnified the excursions of the segments. A camera operating above the subject recorded the top view. This study yielded information concerning the rotation of each bony segment in space as well as concerning the rotation of one segment with respect to another.

The magnitudes of the transverse rotations of the three segments (pelvis, femur and tibia) varied considerably in the subjects investigated. The composite curves for all subjects (Fig. 135) indicate that, in general,

> 1. Pelvic rotation is comparatively slight; the femur rotates more than the pelvis; and the tibia rotates more than the femur.
>
> 2. All three segments rotate inward during swing phase and this inward rotation continues through the first portion of stance phase. A sudden change from inward to outward rotation takes place at midstance and outward rotation continues until toe-off position.

The data in Figure 135 were utilized to plot the curves seen in Figure 136 which illustrates rotations of femur with respect to pelvis and rotation of tibia with respect to femur. The dip in the curve between the two peaks in the latter curve indicates an inward rotation of the femur with respect to the tibia as the knee extends fully during weight-bearing, this rotation having been described previously (page 192) as the "locking mechanism" of the knee.

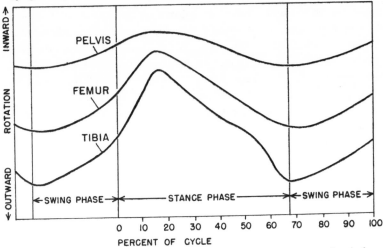

FIG. 135. Transverse rotations of bony segments of lower extremity during walking cycle. (Composite curves for all subjects.) (Redrawn from Eberhart and associates, 1947.)

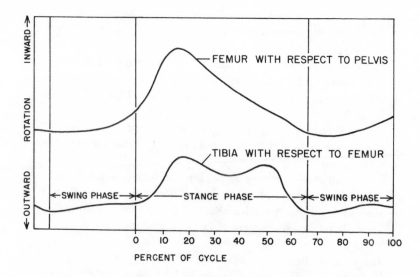

FIG. 136. Relative transverse rotations of hip and knee joints for all subjects. (Redrawn from Eberhart and Inman, 1947.)

Kinematic aspects of the classical study by Eberhart and associates have been re-examined and, in general, been substantiated by later investigators. New material and certain details of gait previously not sufficiently studied have been given special attention, notably by Murray and associates, Kinesiology Research Laboratory, Veterans Administration Center, Wood, Wisconsin, who studied the influence of age, height, sex and walking speed on walking patterns of normal persons. The practical purpose of these studies was to establish norms for walking patterns to be used in the clinic as a baseline for the evaluation of gait patterns in patients with various disabilities. For the titles of these reports, see list of references p. 323

KINETICS OF LOCOMOTION

GROUND REACTION

Results obtained by Elftman (1939a) in studying the ground reaction on the foot by means of force plates are seen in Figure 137 where three components of the ground reaction, one vertical and two horizontal ones, are illustrated. The curve for the vertical component Z rises rapidly following heel contact and presents two maxima:

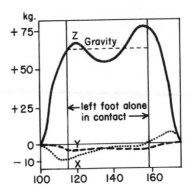

FIG. 137. Vertical and horizontal components of ground reaction on the foot, as obtained from force plate studies. (Redrawn from Elftman, 1939a.)

(1) as the supporting limb receives the full impact of the body weight, and (2) at the end of single stance phase just before the contralateral foot contacts the ground. During both of these peaks, the vertical pressure exceeds that of the individual's body weight (horizontal dotted line), while in midstance the pressure is less than the body weight. The horizontal components are labeled X and Y. The X-component (in the walking direction) has negative values following heel contact and positive values during push-off phase. The Y-component is directed laterally at right angle to the walking direction.

Figure 138 shows the path of the point of application of the ground reaction to the sole of the foot, from heel contact to toe-off position (Elftman, 1939a). The subject weighed 63 kg. and walked at a medium fast speed. Following heel contact, the path moved toward the midline of the foot and remained in the midline until the heel began to rise, then deviated medially toward the great toe. Center-of-pressure data of this kind are variable among normal subjects, and in pathological conditions marked changes are observed.

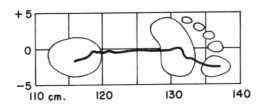

FIG. 138. Path of the point of application of the ground reaction on the foot, as obtained from force plate studies. (Redrawn from Elftman, 1939a.)

MUSCLE FORCES

In later years, the method of choice for the study of muscle action has been electromyography. The onset, duration and peaks of contraction of muscles are seen on the electromyogram, but quantitative values in terms of tension are not obtainable. Needle electrodes may be used to record the action of individual muscles during walking (Scherb and Arienti, 1945), or surface electrodes for recording muscle group action (Eberhart and Inman, 1947). The approach of the latter investigators was as follows.

Electrical activities of muscle groups were recorded as the subjects walked on level ground or ascended and descended slopes and stairs. The main muscle groups of the lower limb, with the exception of the hip flexors, were included in the study. The electromyographic signal as recorded by an oscillograph gave certain information about the activities of the muscle groups, but the wave had a complicated shape and interpretation proved difficult. A so-called integrator, a device which rectifies and filters the wave, was therefore introduced in the circuit, yielding an "integrated electromyogram."

For each muscle group studied, records of integrated electromyograms of 10 normal adult male subjects (representative steps being picked out) were superimposed upon each other, such superimposition leading to "summary curves." From the summary curves the "idealized" curves were constructed, which latter curves, in a readily understandable manner, indicate the patterns of activity of the various muscle groups during the walking cycle.

By glancing at the various curves (Fig. 139) it may be observed that muscular activity is marked at the beginning of stance, while in midstance there is little or no activity of the various muscle groups. In late stance, activity again increases. During swing phase, these records show only minor activity of the groups investigated. The sharp rise and fall of the electromyographic curves indicate a burst of activity followed by periods of inactivity. The alternation between activity and relatively long periods of recovery accounts, in part, for man's ability to walk comparatively long distances without experiencing fatigue. Furthermore, the muscles activated in walking are usually first elongated, at which time they resist a stretching force (gravity, momentum); then they may contract isometrically or reverse to a brief shortening contraction. Such a scheme, as has been discussed previously (Chapter 2), is most economical from the standpoint of expenditure of energy.

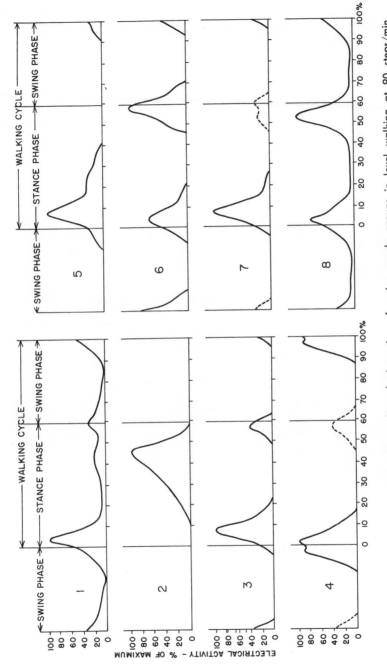

FIG. 139. Idealized summary curves representing phasic action of major muscle groups in level walking at 90 steps/min. 1, Pretibial group; 2, calf muscles; 3, quadriceps; 4, hamstrings; 5, abductors; 6, adductors; 7, gluteus maximus; 8, erector spinae. (Redrawn from Eberhart and associates, 1947.)

301

Since gravity and inertia play important roles in locomotion, the electromyograms tell only part of the story. An attempt must be made to correlate the patterns of activity of the muscles with the external forces acting on the body and on its individual segments. This may be done in part by studying the changes in potential and kinetic energy of body segments in walking. Data for the determination of such energy changes are obtainable from Fischer's investigations (1895-1904). Utilizing such data, Elftman (1955) plotted curves for changes in potential and kinetic energy of the three main units of the body, namely, the trunk (including head and arms) and the two lower limbs. The kinetic energy curve for the lower extremity shows that a muscular force is required to bring about the forward swing of the limb; the curve for the upper part of the body, on the other hand.

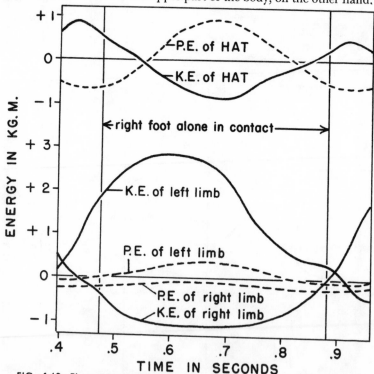

FIG. 140. Fluctuations in the kinetic energy (K.E.) and potential energy (P.E.) of the three major units of the body during one step. HAT: head, arms, trunk. (Redrawn from Elftman, 1955.)

indicates that little or no muscular activity is needed to bring about the vertical oscillations of the trunk (Fig. 140).

Rotation of the trunk and swinging of the arms are integral parts of locomotion. To the trunk muscles is assigned the double function of maintaining proper relationships between trunk segments in the erect position and of participating in bringing about accelarations and decelerations of rotations of the body about its center of gravity. As shown by Elftman (1939b), work is being performed also by the arms in walking. The swinging of the arms was found to decrease the lateral rotation of the trunk, thus facilitating a smooth reversal of rotation.

With the electromyographic records as a basis, functions of main muscle groups of the lower extremity will now be discussed.

DORSIFLEXORS OF ANKLE. The dorsiflexors of the ankle show slight activity during swing phase, at which time these muscles prevent the front part of the foot from dropping. Because the weight of the foot is comparatively small, only slight to moderate activity is needed. But following heel contact, a marked activation of the dorsiflexors is required, or the impact of the body weight on the heel would cause the foot to slap vigorously on the ground. Owing to the action of these muscles, the sole of the foot is lowered to the ground in a gradual and controlled fashion.

CALF GROUP. The activity of the calf group occurs in stance phase only, the curve rising to a maximum during the last third of stance, at a time when the opposite limb is receiving the body weight. Its peak contraction is synchronous with the maximum ground reaction on the ball of the foot, as seen on the axial load curve (Fig. 141), indicating that this group is importantly involved in the push-off.

If the proximal joints of the limb were to remain extended, plantar flexion of the ankle would exert a direct forward-upward force on the trunk. But the records show that the knee flexes rapidly as the ankle plantar-flexes and that, simultaneously, the hip is also in the process of flexing, so that the action of the calf muscles on the trunk becomes debatable. The calf muscles, however, have another important function to fulfill in late stance.

It was pointed out by Francillion (1941a and 1941b) that when in late stance after heel rise the triceps surae contracts—the soleus is said to be particularly active at this time—this contraction causes not only plantar flexion of the ankle, but also flexion of the knee, a

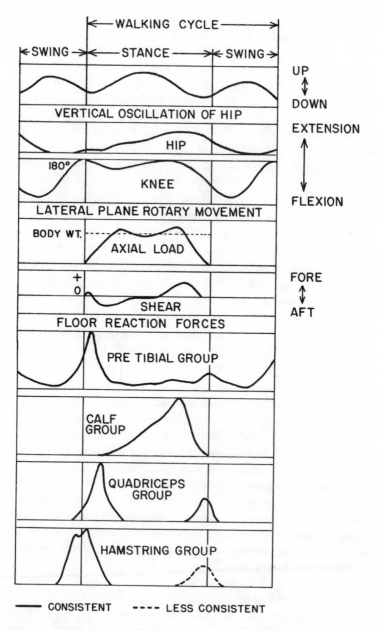

FIG. 141. Correlation of phasic muscle activity with joint displacements and floor reaction forces. (Redrawn from Eberhart and associates, 1947.)

flexion which is needed during swing phase. Eberhart and Inman (1947) state: "during the period of double support at the end of stance, ankle extension forces will go into driving the thigh forward and flexing the knee." The importance of the calf muscles for the initiation of swing has been particularly stressed by Elftman (1955): "The impulses which they (the calf muscles) provide is usually referred to as the push-off. This indeed it is, but the pushing is exerted on the limb which is preparing for its free swing and not on the trunk, as is frequently supposed."

That muscles may transmit their actions also to distant segments is exemplified by the calf muscles. When in stance phase the entire sole has reached the ground, the ankle angle becomes acute (Fig. 134) and the calf muscles are being stretched by the momentum of the body. By resisting this stretching force, the calf muscles are instrumental in slowing down the forward motion of the body and, acting through the pelvic link, in decelerating the forward swing of the opposite limb (Elftman, 1955).

QUADRICEPS GROUP. The peak of contraction of the quadriceps group occurs following heel contact, and this peak coincides with weight-bearing on a somewhat flexed knee during "double knee action," and also with the first peak of the axial load curve (Fig. 141). At this moment, the center-of-gravity line of the body falls behind the axis of the knee joint and quadriceps action is required or the knee will buckle. Note that in midstance, when the center of gravity of the body has moved in front of the axis of the knee joint, no quadriceps action is registered. The height and shape of the second quadriceps peak varies considerably in individuals.

HAMSTRINGS. The peak of the hamstring group occurs earlier than that of the quadriceps group. As the limb swings forward, these muscles are being stretched over hip and knee simultaneously, and at this time their tension builds up. It may be assumed that their function is to slow down the forward swing of the limb and to prevent, first, excessive hip flexion, and, second, an abrupt extension of the knee due to inertia. After the heel has contacted the ground and the foot is receiving the body weight, the hamstrings continue high level activity. With the foot secured on the ground by the body weight and the quadriceps acting at the knee, the hamstrings can now transfer their action to the hip. Note that at this time the quadriceps and the hamstrings act as synergists in their task to control the knee and to extend the hip, respectively.

GLUTEUS MAXIMUS. The gluteus maximus shows peak activity in early stance as the body weight is being transferred to the forward foot. It acts synchronously with the quadriceps group and partly with the hamstrings. Scherb and Arienti (1945), by leading off action potentials from various portions of the gluteus maximus, verified what had been observed earlier by palpation, namely, that the posterior fibers of the gluteus maximus start contracting first and that the contraction then moves forward in a wavelike fashion. This "fan symptom" was also found to be present in the gluteus medius.

In addition to furnishing hip control on the side of the stance limb, the gluteus maximus may also, through the pelvis link, aid in the forward swing of the contralateral limb (Elftman, 1955).

HIP FLEXORS. The Weber brothers (1836) postulated that the forward swing of the leg in walking was a pendulum motion requiring little or no muscular effort. This theory was challenged by Otto Fischer (1895-1904) who proved that a muscular force was needed, a subject which has been further elucidated by the energy studies of Elftman (1955). This still leaves unanswered the question: Which muscles are responsible for the forward swing of the limb? The calf muscles on the side of the limb which is to begin its forward swing and the hip extensors on the opposite side may supply a portion of this force, but it may be assumed also that the hip flexors become active.

During late stance and early swing phase, electrical activity has been recorded from the tensor fasciae latae by Altenburger (1933) and from the sartorius by Scherb and Arienti (1945). In using the "myokinesiographic method"—recording muscle action by palpation — the group headed by Scherb noted activity in the gracilis, sartorius, adductor longus and a portion of the adductor magnus (but found no activity in the rectus femoris). More refined methods —dual wire electrodes in the muscle—reveal that only scant electrical activity may be derived from the iliopsoas during the above period. In fact, during level walking the muscle was found to be virtually silent in many subjects (Close, 1964). This would indicate that the superficial hip flexors are mainly responsible for the initiation of swing phase. However, in paralytic cases when other hip flexors are weak the iliopsoas may become quite active prior to toe-off and during early swing phase (Close, 1964).

The *abductor group,* to fulfill its assignment as a lateral stabilizer of the pelvis (compare Fig. 132, page 290), rapidly intensifies its action after heel contact, its curve rising steeply to a maximum in early stance at a time when the impact of the body weight must be prevented from lowering the pelvis on the opposite side. The activity is maintained at a lower intensity during single stance and it fades out as double stance begins. Note that the peak of the gluteus medius is synchronous with those of the quadriceps and the gluteus maximus (Fig. 139). The gluteus medius, like the maximus, shows a wave-like contraction which starts posteriorly and proceeds anteriorly (Scherb and Arienti, 1945).

The *adductor group* has two peaks of activity which occur in early and in late stance. The early and smallest peak is almost synchronous with the peaks of the quadriceps, the hamstrings, the gluteus maximus and the abductor group. The adductors thus join the numerous muscle groups which show high activity just after heel contact. The second and higher peak is seen at or just before toe-off position.

If an attempt is made to interpret the function of the adductor group, several things must be kept in mind: first, that the adductor group is located partly anterior and partly posterior to the axis of flexion and extension of the hip and that, therefore, one portion may aid in flexion, another in extension; second, that the adductors are mechanically capable to act also in transverse rotations; and third, that muscle groups such as the abductors and adductors which are anatomical antagonists often act synergically when firm stabilization of a joint is required. The muscles of the adductor group, it may be assumed, do not limit their activities to the control of lateral oscillations of the body but may be significantly involved in the control of numerous other movements.

ERECTOR SPINAE GROUP. Two periods of activity are registered, one in early stance, the other one in late stance. Following heel contact on the *right* side, the right erector spinae has its first peak, and following heel contact on the *left* side, the right erector spinae has its second (higher) peak. Because the erector spinae on the left side acts in the same manner as the one on the right, the muscles on both sides support the vertebral column following heel contact when, owing to inertia, excessive forward motion of the trunk must be prevented. A stabilizing effect of the erector spinae muscles on the vertebral column in a lateral direction may also be inferred from the anatomical position of these muscles.

ABDOMINAL MUSCLES. Sheffield (1962) reported *inactivity of the abdominal muscles* in slow level walking at 60 steps/min. By means of fine needle electrodes the upper and lower portions of the rectus abdominus were investigated; the lateral abdominal muscles were tested at two different points at the height of the crest of the ilium, medially and laterally, but no effort was made to differentiate between the layers of the lateral abdominal muscles. None of the areas tested yielded records of electrical activity in the muscles.

INTRINSIC MUSCLES OF THE FOOT. An electromyographic study of six of the intrinsic muscles of the foot by Mann and Inman (1964) revealed that during swing phase, level walking, these muscles remained inactive. But all six muscles showed electrical activity in the last half of stance phase. In subjects with flat feet the activity of the intrinsic muscles was of longer duration, notably that of the abductor hallucis which then contracted during the entire stance phase. A study of six leg and foot muscles (tibialis anterior, tibialis posterior, flexor hallucis longus, peroneus longus, abductor hallucis, flexor digitorum brevis) (Gray and Basmajian, 1968) throws further light on the function of individual muscles in walking. Most of the muscles studied were definitely more active in flat-footed persons than in subjects with normal arches. None of the muscles contracted continuously during stance or swing phase. "Contingent arch support by muscles rather than continuous support is the rule, muscles being recruited to compensate for lax ligaments and special stresses during the walking cycle" (Gray and Basmajian, 1968).

Additional information concerning the *phasic activity of individual muscles of the lower limb,* both in normal and in paralytic subjects, has been furnished by Close (1964). For example, a muscle which is normally active during swing phase, if transplanted to take the place of a stance-phase muscle, would have to undergo "phasic conversion", and such conversion does not always materialize. By far, better results are obtained if, in the above case, a stance-phase muscle is chosen for transfer if such a muscle is available.

ARM MUSCLES. Electromyographical studies of the arms of normal subjects during gait show activity in the posterior and middle deltoid slightly before the arm starts its backward swing and this continues throughout the backward swing. During forward swing the main shoulder flexors were silent and activity was noted only in some of the medial rotators (subscapularis, latissimus dorsi, teres major) (Basmajian, 1967). In studying 12 shoulder and arm muscles, Hogue (1969) found greatest activity in the posterior deltoid. He interpreted this as activity which decelerated the forward swinging arm and extended the backward swinging arm. Posterior deltoid activity as well as that in the middle deltoid and teres major increased with increased cadence but did not show any appreciable increase as subjects ascended an incline.

ENERGY COST IN WALKING

Muscles control the energy of the body during movement partially by doing work on the body by speeding it up or raising it against gravity, but in an equally important fashion by absorbing energy from it as different parts slow down or lose potential energy as they are lowered. The details of these processes can only be studied by methods already hinted at, but the over-all metabolic cost can be assessed by measuring oxygen consumption.

The influence of speed and rate of walking on oxygen consumption was investigated by Studer (1926) and by Atzler and Herbst (1927). As would be expected, oxygen consumption per time unit was found to rise as walking speed increased (Studer, 1926). But when interest was centered on the oxygen consumption per "walking unit" (trans-

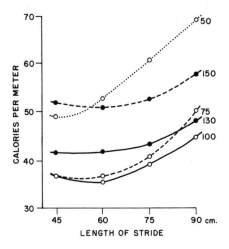

FIG. 142. Caloric consumption as related to length of stride. (Redrawn from Atzler and Herbst, 1927.)

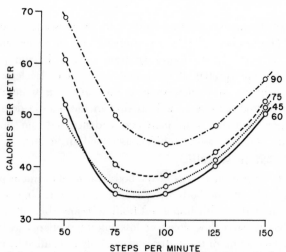

FIG. 143. Caloric consumption as related to rate of walking. (Redrawn from Atzler and Herbst, 1927.)

portation of one kilogram of body weight a distance of one meter on level surface) the picture became more complicated.

The energy cost per distance traveled when a subject walked at different speeds and with prescribed cadences of 50, 75, 100, 130 and 150 was investigated by Atzler and Herbst (1927). At each of the five cadences, the subject increased his speed by lengthening the stride. In Figure 142 the energy cost (calories per meter) is plotted against length of stride for the various cadences. With the exception of the lowest cadence, energy cost remains comparatively low at stride lengths between 45 and 75 centimeters. In Figure 143 caloric cost per meter is plotted against rate of walking for stride lengths of 45, 60, 75 and 90 centimeters. The lowest portions of the curves are found at walking rates between 75 and 100 steps per minute.

Since the lowest oxygen cost per distance traveled depends on the length of the stride as well as on the rate of walking, for each speed of walking there must be a certain length of stride and a certain cadence at which the walk can be performed with a minimum of caloric consumption. Optimal combinations for different speeds were computed by Atzler and Herbst and are seen in Figure 144. Rate of walking was first plotted against length of stride. For any point chosen, the speed of walking (product of the walking rate and the stride length) could be determined. By connecting points of equal speed, the dotted

Clinical Kinesiology

lines representing speeds of 40, 60, 80, 100 and 120 meters per minute were constructed. The caloric consumption which corresponded to each combination of length of stride and rate of walking were then plotted on lines erected perpendicular to the two-dimensional diagram previously plotted. The end points of all these lines are located on an irregularly shaped surface which represents caloric consumption as function of two variables—length of stride and cadence. In the illustrations, points which have the same heights have been connected by contour lines.

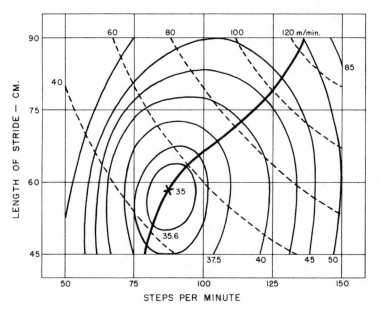

FIG. 144. Caloric consumption as function of two variables, length of stride and cadence. Dotted lines: speed in m/min. Thin solid lines (contour lines): caloric consumption. Heavy solid line: optimal combinations of cadence and length of stride for varying speeds. (Redrawn from Atzler and Herbst, 1927.)

The reading of the diagram, Figure 144, is facilitated by visualizing an irregularly shaped bowl, the deepest portion of which is found at the point indicating 35 calories, corresponding to a cadence of 87.5 and a stride length of 58.5 centimeters. The contour lines lie parallel to the two-dimensional diagram first constructed. The further these lines are from point 35 (which point indicates the lowest caloric consumption possible), the higher is the energy cost. The numbers that refer to the contour lines (35.6, 37.5, 40, 45, 50, 85) give energy cost in small calories per meter traveled, the caloric consumption in standing having been subtracted. The heavy solid line rising from point 35 toward the rim of the bowl indicates that combination of cadence and length of stride at which the highest speed is obtained with the relatively lowest energy cost.

ENERGY COST IN WALKING—HANDICAPPED SUBJECTS

Of special interest to rehabilitation personnel are studies of energy consumption of amputees and of paraplegic and hemiplegic subjects. Original studies by Ralston (1958) and more recently by Corcoran and Bengelmann (1970) on normal individuals established bases for comparison. Bard and Ralston (1959) found prosthesis and walking at "comfortable" speed used only slightly more energy than normal subjects at the same speed. When a pylon without a knee joint was used, the energy cost was higher and it rose still higher when the subject walked without prosthesis, using elbow crutches.

The walking efficiency of hemiplegic patients was found to be rather low, and the more severe the spasticity, the less the efficiency. However, the metabolic cost of these patients when they walk at a comfortable speed is not so high as to make walking hazardous if no complications are present (Bard, 1963). The energy-saving effect of wearing an ankle brace was demonstrated in the case of a moderately spastic subject (Bard and Ralston, 1959). When the subject walked with a cane but without a brace, his energy expenditure was 41 per cent greater than when he walked with a cane and wore a brace; the speed was identical in both test runs. Corcoran and associates (1970) found higher than normal (51 to 67 per cent) energy expenditures when they investigated maximum and comfortable walking speeds and the energy cost of walking at these speeds in fifteen hemiparetic patients. Also they observed lower energy costs when patients used short leg braces.

Gordon and Vanderwalde (1956) investigated energy requirements in paraplegic ambulation and found that metabolic work was at least three times the basal rate and sometimes it was five to eight times higher. The magnitude of this energy cost reflected the degree of motor loss. Their study also substantiated the fact that the ceiling for sustained paraplegic ambulation was five to six times basal metabolic rate.

Appendix

Tables I through XIII

TABLE I. Leverage factors for individual muscles flexing the elbow. Figures show force moments per unit cross section of each muscle (1 sq. cm.) and per unit of muscle force (1 kg.). Muscle force is assumed to be constant throughout range.

Flexion degrees	Pronator teres	Ext. carpi rad. long.	Brachialis	Biceps, long head	Biceps, short head	Brachioradialis
0	4.9	—5.7	11.0	11.5	12.2	9.7
10	5.7	—0.5	12.5	13.7	13.8	13.5
20	6.3	+4.5	13.8	16.8	16.4	20.5
30	6.8	8.6	15.3	21.4	20.7	30.5
40	7.3	12.3	17.0	27.0	26.3	39.8
50	8.1	16.0	19.6	32.4	31.9	48.4
60	9.3	19.5	23.0	37.4	36.9	56.4
70	10.5	22.9	26.6	40.7	40.2	64.0
80	11.4	26.4	30.0	43.5	43.0	70.3
90	12.3	29.3	33.5	45.4	45.5	75.2
100	12.9	31.4	36.5	45.5	46.1	79.8
110	12.8	32.5	35.9	42.8	43.8	81.4
120	11.8	31.9	33.4	39.2	41.0	79.9
130	10.2	28.6	31.4	35.9	37.5	72.7

(After R. Fick, 1911, pp. 318, 319.)

TABLE II. Maximal work capacities of flexors of elbow, from extension (0 degrees) to flexion (145 degrees).

Name of Muscle	Shortening (in meters)	Cross Section (in sq. cm.)	Work Capacity (in kg.m.)
FOREARM IN SUPINATION			
Brachialis	0.060	6.4	3.84
Biceps, long head	0.073	3.33	2.43
Biceps, short head	0.073	3.22	2.42
Brachioradialis	0.102	1.86	1.90
Pronator teres	0.039	3.24	1.26
Extensor carpi radialis longus	0.039	3.14	1.22
Flexor carpi radialis	0.022	2.16	0.47
Extensor carpi radialis brevis	0.015	2.22	0.33
Palmaris longus	0.010	0.93	0.09
			13.96
FOREARM IN MIDPOSITION			
Brachialis	0.060	6.4	3.84
Biceps, long head	0.070	3.33	2.33
Biceps, short head	0.070	3.22	2.25
Brachioradialis	0.119	1.86	2.21
Extensor carpi radialis longus	0.047	3.14	1.47
Pronator teres	0.043	3.24	1.39
Flexor carpi radialis	0.024	2.16	0.52
Extensor carpi radialis brevis	0.015	2.22	0.33
Palmaris longus	0.011	0.93	0.10
			14.44
FOREARM IN PRONATION			
Brachialis	0.060	6.4	3.84
Biceps, long head	0.069	3.33	2.30
Brachioradialis	0.130	1.86	2.25
Biceps, short head	0.069	3.22	2.22
Pronator teres	0.024	2.16	1.52
Extensor carpi radialis longus	0.048	3.14	1.51
Flexor carpi radialis	0.047	3.24	0.52
Extensor carpi radialis brevis	0.017	2.22	0.38
Palmaris longus	0.013	0.93	0.12
			14.66

(After R. Fick, 1911, p. 320.)

TABLE III. Maximal work capacities of extensors of elbow, from 35 degrees (elbow flexed) to 180 degrees (elbow extended).

Name of Muscle	Shortening (in meters)	Cross Section (in sq. cm.)	Work Capacity (in kg.m.)
Triceps, lateral head	0.050	6.78	3.39
Triceps, medial head	0.047	5.66	2.66
Triceps, long head	0.051	4.75	2.42
Anconeus	0.026	3.18	0.83
			9.30

(After R. Fick, 1911, p. 321.)

TABLE IV. Maximal work capacities of supinators of forearm, from complete pronation (0 degrees) to complete supination (120 degrees).

Name of Muscle	Shortening (in meters)	Cross Section (in sq. cm.)	Work Capacity (in kg.m.)
ELBOW IN EXTENSION			
Biceps brachii, short head	0.011	3.22	0.36
Supinator	0.015	2.20	0.33
Biceps, long head	0.008	3.33	0.26
Brachioradialis	0.014	1.86	0.16
Extensor carpi radialis longus	0.005	3.14	0.16
Abductor pollicis longus	0.004	1.84	0.07
Extensor pollicis brevis	0.004	1.84	0.07
Extensor pollicis longus	0.003	0.56	0.02
Extensor indicis proprius	0.003	0.37	0.01
			1.44
ELBOW AT 90 DEGREES			
Biceps brachii, short head	0.019	3.22	0.61
Biceps brachii, long head	0.016	3.33	0.53
Supinator	0.015	2.20	0.33
Abductor pollicis longus	0.004	1.84	0.07
Extensor pollicis brevis	0.004	1.84	0.07
Brachioradialis*	0.002	1.86	0.04
Extensor pollicis longus	0.003	0.56	0.02
Extensor indicis proprius	0.003	0.37	0.01
			1.68
ELBOW IN COMPLETE FLEXION			
Biceps brachii, short head	0.019	3.22	0.61
Biceps brachii, long head	0.016	3.33	0.53
Supinator	0.015	2.20	0.33
Abductor pollicis longus	0.004	1.84	0.07
Extensor pollicis brevis	0.004	1.84	0.07
Extensor pollicis longus	0.003	0.56	0.02
Extensor indicis proprius	0.003	0.37	0.01
			1.64

*To 20 degrees, starting from complete pronation.

(After R. Fick, 1911, pp. 348, 349.)

TABLE V.   Maximal work capacities of pronators of forearm from complete supination (0 degrees) to complete pronation (120 degrees).

Name of Muscle	Shortening (in meters)	Cross Section (in sq. cm.)	Work Capacity (in kg.m.)
ELBOW IN EXTENSION			
Pronator teres	0.010	3.24	0.32
Flexor carpi radialis	0.013	2.16	0.28
Pronator quadratus	0.008	2.22	0.18
Palmaris longus	0.012	0.93	0.11
			0.89
ELBOW AT 90 DEGREES			
Pronator teres	0.019	3.6	0.68
Flexor carpi radialis	0.011	2.16	0.24
Brachioradialis*	0.012	1.86	0.22
Pronator quadratus	0.008	2.22	0.18
Extensor carpi radialis longus	0.005	3.14	0.16
Palmaris longus	0.011	0.93	0.10
			1.58
ELBOW IN COMPLETE FLEXION			
Pronator teres	0.015	3.24	0.49
Brachioradialis	0.015	1.86	0.28
Flexor carpi radialis	0.010	2.16	0.22
Pronator quadratus	0.008	2.22	0.18
Extensor carpi radialis longus	0.005	3.14	0.16
Palmaris longus	0.008	0.93	0.07
			1.40

*To 105 degrees, starting from complete supination.

(After R. Fick, 1911, p. 351.)

TABLE VI. Maximal work capacities of muscles in flexion, extension, ulnar abduction and radial abduction of wrist, complete range of motion.

Name of Muscle	Shortening (in meters)	Cross Section (in sq. cm.)	Work Capacity (in kg.m.)
FLEXORS OF WRIST			
Flexor digitorum superficialis	0.045	10.7	4.815
Flexor digitorum profundus	0.042	10.8	4.536
Flexor carpi ulnaris	0.039	5.0	1.950
Flexor pollicis longus	0.041	2.9	1.189
Flexor carpi radialis	0.038	2.16	0.821
Abductor pollicis longus	0.005	1.84	0.092
All flexors:		33.40	13.403
EXTENSORS OF WRIST			
Extensor digitorum communis	0.040	4.30	1.720
Extensor carpi ulnaris	0.021	5.30	1.113
Extensor carpi radialis longus	0.034	3.14	1.068
Extensor carpi radialis brevis	0.040	2.22	0.888
Extensor indicis proprius	0.038	1.20	0.456
Extensor pollicis longus	0.025	0.56	0.140
All extensors:		16.72	5.385
ULNAR ABDUCTORS OF WRIST			
Extensor carpi ulnaris	0.020	5.30	1.060
Flexor carpi ulnaris	0.014	5.00	0.700
All ulnar abductors:		10.30	1.760
RADIAL ABDUCTORS OF WRIST			
Extensor carpi radialis longus	0.036	3.14	1.130
Abductor pollicis longus	0.021	1.84	0.386
Extensor carpi radialis brevis	0.014	2.22	0.311
Extensor indicis proprius	0.007	1.20	0.084
Extensor pollicis longus	0.014	0.56	0.078
Flexor carpi radialis	0.003	2.16	0.065
All radial abductors:		11.12	2.054

(After R. Fick, 1911, pp. 396-398.)

TABLE VII. Maximal work capacities of muscles acting on gleno-humeral joint.

Name of Muscle	Shortening (in meters)	Cross Section (in sq. cm.)	Work Capacity (in kg.m.)
IN FLEXION OF SHOULDER			
Subscapularis	0.011	25.2	2.77
Supraspinatus	0.031	7.7	2.39
Coracobrachialis	0.039	5.8	2.26
Infraspinatus & teres minor	0.014	16.5	2.21
Biceps, short head	0.048	3.2	1.54
Biceps, long head	0.030	3.3	0.99
			12.16
IN EXTENSION OF SHOULDER			
Teres major	0.101	9.8	9.90
Triceps, long head	0.054	4.7	2.54
			12.44
IN ADDUCTION OF THE SHOULDER			
Teres major	0.066	9.8	6.47
Coracobrachialis	0.052	5.8	3.01
Triceps, long head	0.041	4.7	1.92
Biceps, long head	0.019	3.2	0.61
			12.01
IN ABDUCTION OF THE SHOULDER			
Supraspinatus	0.033	7.7	2.54
Infraspinatus & teres minor	0.011	16.5	1.81
Subscapularis	0.004	25.2	1.01
Biceps, long head	0.012	3.3	0.40
			5.76
IN INWARD ROTATION OF SHOULDER			
Subscapularis	0.047	25.2	11.84
Teres major	0.023	9.8	2.25
Biceps, long head	0.021	3.3	0.69
Biceps, short head	0.003	3.2	0.10
			14.88
IN OUTWARD ROTATION OF SHOULDER			
Infraspinatus & teres minor	0.042	16.5	6.93
Coracobrachialis	0.003	5.8	0.17
			7.10

NOTE: The pectoralis major, latissimus dorsi and deltoid are missing in this table. Cross section of middle deltoid is elsewhere given as 25.3 sq. cm.

(After R. Fick, 1911, pp. 280, 281.)

TABLE VIII. Maximal work capacities of flexors and extensors of knee.

Name of Muscle	Shortening (in meters)	Cross Section (in sq. cm.)	Work Capacity (in kg.m.)
EXTENSORS			
Vasti	0.080	148.30	118.640
Rectus femoris	0.081*	28.89	23.400
Tensor fasciae latae	0.010	7.56	0.756
			142.796
FLEXORS			
Semimembranosus	0.064*	26.38	16.833
Semitendinosus	0.134	7.27	13.242
Biceps femoris	0.059	17.37	10.248
Gracilis	0.075	4.11	3.082
Sartorius	0.070	3.17	2.319
			45.774

*Muscle is "actively insufficient."

(After R. Fick, 1911, p. 585.)

NOTE: These are the figures appearing in Fick's table, but errors in calculation seem to have crept in. Furthermore, the work capacities for biarticular muscles must be re-evaluated, since these muscles are actively insufficient in a portion of the joint range.   S. B.

TABLE IX. Maximal work capacities of rotators of knee.

Name of Muscle	Shortening* (in meters)	Cross Section (in sq. cm.)	Work Capacity (in kg.m.)
EXTERNAL ROTATORS			
Tibia with respect to femur			
Biceps femoris	0.0247	19.80	4.891
Tensor fasciae	0.0077	8.40	0.647
INTERNAL ROTATORS			
Tibia with respect to femur			
Semimembranosus	0.0133	26.39	3.400
Semitendinosus	0.0109	7.65	0.834
Sartorius	0.0156	3.75	0.585
Popliteus	0.0150	5.32	0.798
Gracilis	0.0127	3.30	0.419

*Shortening by a rotation of 37.5 degrees.

(After R. Fick, 1911, p. 586.)

TABLE X. Maximal work capacities of muscles acting on talo-crural joint.

Name of Muscle	Shortening (in meters)	Cross Section (in sq. cm.)	Work Capacity (in kg.m.)
DORSIFLEXORS OF ANKLE			
Tibialis anterior	0.033	7.7	2.54
Extensor digitorum longus	0.033	2.5	0.82
Peroneus tertius*	0.031	1.7	0.49
Extensor hallucis longus	0.029	1.3	0.42
			4.27
PLANTAR FLEXORS OF ANKLE			
Gastrocnemius	0.039	23.0	8.97
Soleus	0.037	20.0	7.40
Flexor hallucis longus	0.019	4.5	0.85
Peroneus longus	0.0103	4.3	0.44
Tibialis posterior	0.007	5.8	0.41
Flexor digitorum longus	0.013	2.8	0.36
Peroneus brevis	0.0065	3.8	0.25
			18.68

*In two out of four cadavers investigated, the peroneus tertius was unusually well developed, hence the cross section given (average of 4) is quite high.
(After R. Fick, 1911, p. 610.)

TABLE XI. Maximal work capacities of muscles acting on lower ankle joint.

Name of Muscle	Shortening (in meters)	Cross Section (in sq. cm.)	Work Capacity (in kg.m.)
INVERTORS			
Gastrocnemius	0.011	23.0	2.53
Soleus	0.0116	20.0	2.32
Tibialis posterior	0.025	5.8	1.45
Flexor hallucis longus	0.015	4.5	0.67
Flexor digitorum longus	0.0205	2.8	0.57
Tibialis anterior	0.0041	7.7	0.32
		63.8	7.86
EVERTORS			
Peroneus longus	0.0245	4.3	1.05
Peroneus brevis	0.0227	3.8	0.86
Extensor digitorum longus	0.0194	2.5	0.48
Peroneus tertius	0.0226	1.7	0.38
Extensor hallucis longus	0.0090	1.35	0.12
Tibialis anterior	0.0043	7.7	0.33
		21.35	3.22

(After R. Fick, 1911, p. 629.)

TABLE XII.   Maximal work capacities of the long toe flexors and
extensors.

Name of Muscle	Shortening (in meters)	Cross Section (in sq. cm.)	Work Capacity (in kg.m.)
FLEXORS			
Flexor hallucis longus	0.0370	4.5	1.66
Flexor digitorum longus	0.0307	2.8	0.86
			2.52
EXTENSORS			
Extensor digitorum longus	0.0200	2.5	0.50
Extensor hallucis longus	0.0280	1.35	0.38
			0.88

(After R. Fick, 1911, p. 639.)

TABLE XIII.   Maximal work capacities of some of the hip muscles.

Name of Muscle	Shortening (in meters)	Cross Section (in sq. cm.)	Work Capacity (in kg.m.)
FLEXORS (sagittal plane motion of 120 degrees)			
Rectus femoris	0.060	28.89	17.33
Tensor fasciae	0.154	8.40	12.94*
Sartorius	0.133	3.75	4.99
Gracilis to 40 degrees flexion	0.013	3.3	0.43
EXTENSORS (sagittal plane motion of 120 degrees)			
Semimembranosus	0.074	26.39	19.53*
Gluteus maximus, lower portion	0.0805	22.2	17.77
Biceps, long head	0.101	14.25	14.25*
Adductor magnus, upper portion	0.1052	11.65	12.26
Adductor magnus, middle portion	0.1008	11.65	11.74
Gluteus maximus, middle portion	0.0521	22.2	11.57
Adductor magnus, lower portion	0.0695	11.65	8.10
Semitendinosus	0.074	7.65	5.66
Gluteus maximus, upper portion	0.022	22.2	4.88
Gracilis from 40 to 120 degrees	0.041	. 3.3	1.35
ABDUCTORS (frontal plane motion of 37 degrees)			
Rectus femoris	0.0115	28.89	3.32
Tensor fasciae	0.0281	8.40	2.36
Sartorius	0.0152	3.75	0.57
ADDUCTORS (frontal plane motion of 37 degrees)			
Gracilis	0.0490	3.3	1.61
Biceps, long head	0.0105	14.25	1.50
Semimembranosus	0.0030	14.55	0.44
Semitendinosus	0.0030	7.65	0.23

*The work capacity given for this muscle must be considered too large because
the muscle is actively insufficient owing to the shortness of its fibers.
(After R. Fick, 1911, p. 502.)

Clinical Kinesiology

References

ABBOTT, B. C., BIGLAND, B., AND RITCHIE, J. M.: The physiological cost of negative work. J. Physiol. 117:380-390, 1952.

ÅKERBLOM, B.: Standing and Sitting Posture. Nordiska Bokhandeln, Stockholm, 1948.

ALTENBURGER, H.: Beiträge zur Physiologie und Pathologie des Ganges. Ztschr. f.d. ges. Neurol. u. Psychiat. 148:263-271, 1933.

ATZLER, E., AND HERBST, R.: Die Geharbeit auf horizontaler Bahn. Pflueger Arch. Ges. Physiol. 215:290-364, 1927.

BACKHOUSE, K. M., AND CATTON, W. T.: An experimental study of the function of the lumbrical muscles in the human hand. J. Anat. 88: 133-141, 1954.

BARD, G.: Energy expenditure of hemiplegic subjects during walking. Arch. Phys. Med. 44:368-370, 1963.

BARD, G., AND RALSTON, H. J.: Measurement of energy expenditure during ambulation, with special reference to evaluation of assistive devices. Arch. Phys. Med. 40:415-420, 1959.

BARNETT, C. H., AND RICHARDSON, A.: The postural function of the popliteus muscle. Ann. Phys. Med. 1:177-179, 1953.

BASLER, A.: Das Gehen und seine Veränderungen durch verschiedene Unstände auf Grund experimenteller Untersuchungen. Abh. d. Med. Fakultät der Sun Yatsen University, Canton, China, 1929.

BASLER, A.: Beiträge zur Physiologie des Stehens. Arbeitsphysiol. 12: 105-119, 1942.

BASMAJIAN, J. V.: Muscles Alive. The Williams and Wilkins Co., Baltimore, 1967.

BASMAJIAN, J. V., AND LATIF, M. A.: Integrated actions and functions of the chief flexors of the elbow. J. Bone Joint Surg. [Amer.] 39A: 1106-1118, 1957.

BECK, O.: Die gesamte Kraftkurve des tetanisierten Froschgastrocnemius und ihr physiologisch ausgenutzter Anteil. Pflueger Arch. Ges. Physiol. 193:495-526, 1921-22.

BEEVOR, C.: Croonian Lectures on Muscular Movement. Delivered in 1903. Edited and reprinted for the Guarantors of "Brain." The Macmillan Company, New York, 1951.

BENEDICT, F. G., AND MURSCHHAUSER, H.: Energy Consumption during Horizontal Walking. Carnegie Institution of Washington. Publ. 231, 1915.

BETHE, A.: Beiträge zum Problem der willkürlich beweglichen Armprothesen. I. Die Kraftkurve menschlicher Muskeln und die reziproke Innervation der Antagonisten. München Med. Wschr. 65:1577-1579, 1916.

BETHE, A.: Aktive und passive Kraft menschlicher Muskeln. Ergebn. Physiol. 24:71-83, 1925.

BETHE, A., AND FRANKE, F.: Beiträge zum Problem der willkürlich beweglichen Armprothesen. IV. Die Kraftkurven der indirekten natürlichen Energiequellen. München Med. Wschr. 66:201-205, 1919.

BLIX, M.: Die Länge und die Spannung des Muskels. Skand. Arch. f. Physiol. 3:316, 1892; 4:399, 1893; 5:150, 1895; 5:175, 1895.

BORELLI, G. A.: De Motu Animalium. Lugduni Batavorum, 1679.

BRAUNE, W., AND FISCHER, O.: Ueber den Schwerpunkt des menschlichen Korpers mit Rücksicht auf die Ausrüstung des deutschen Infanteristen. Abh. d. Kgl. Sächs. Ges. d. Wissensch., Math. Phys. Klasse 26:562, 1889.

BRAUNE, W., AND FISCHER, O.: Die Rotationsmomente der Beugemuskeln am Ellbogengelenk des Menschen. Abh. d. Konigl. Sächs. Ges. d. Wissensch. Math. Phys. Klasse, Vol. 15, 1890.

BRAUNE, W., AND FISCHER, O.: Untersuchungen über die Gelenke des menschlichen Armes. Abh. Sächs. Akad. Wiss., 1887. Quoted by von Lanz, T., and Wachsmuth, W.: Praktische Anatomie, Bd. I, Teil III. Julius Springer, Berlin, 1935, p. 94.

BRUNNSTROM, S.: Muscle testing around the shoulder girdle. J. Bone Joint Surg. [Amer.] 23:263-272, 1941.

BRUNNSTROM, S.: Some observations of muscle function: With special reference to pluriarticular muscles. Physiotherapy Rev. 22:67-75, 1942.

BRUNNSTROM, S.: Comparative strength of muscles with similar function; study on peripheral nerve injuries of the upper extremity. Physiotherapy Rev. 26:59-65, 1946.

BRUNNSTROM, S.: Center of gravity line in relation to ankle joint; application to posture training and to artificial legs. Phys. Therapy Rev. 34:109-115, 1954.

BRUNNSTROM, S.: Anatomical and Physiological Considerations in the Clinical Application of Lower-extremity Prosthesis. In Orthopedic Appliances Atlas, Vol. 2, Artificial Limbs. J. W. Edwards, Ann Arbor, Mich., 1960.

BUNNELL, S.: Opposition of the thumb. J. Bone Joint Surg. 22:269-284, 1938.

BUNNELL, S.: Surgery of the intrinsic muscles of the hand other than those producing opposition of the thumb. J. Bone Joint Surg. 24:1-31, 1942.

BUNNELL, S.: Surgery of the Hand, 3rd ed. J. B. Lippincott Co., Philadelphia, 1956.

CAMPBELL, E. J. H.: An electromyographic study of the role of the abdominal muscles in breathing. J. Physiol. 117:222-233, 1952.

CLARK, D. A.: Muscle counts of motor units: A study in innervation ratios. Amer. J. Physiol. 96:296-304, 1931.

CLOSE, J. R.: Motor Function in the Lower Extremity. Analyses by Electronic Instrumentation. Charles C Thomas, Springfield, Ill., 1964.

CLOSE, J. R., AND KIDD, C.: The functions of the muscles of the thumb, the index and long fingers. J. Bone Joint Surg. 51A:1601-1620, 1969.

CORCORAN, P. J., AND BRENGELMANN, G. L.: Oxygen uptake in normal and handicapped subjects, in relation to speed of walking beside velocity-controlled cart. Arch. Phys. Med. 51:78-87, 1970.

CORCORAN, P. J., JEBSON, R. H., BRENGELMANN, G. L., AND SIMONS, B. C.: Effects of plastic and metal leg braces on speed and energy cost of hemiparetic ambulation. Arch. Phys. Med. 51:69-77, 1970.

DEMPSTER, W. T.: Space Requirements of the Seated Operator. WADC Technical Report 55-159, July 1955. Office of Technical Services, U.S. Dept. of Commerce, Washington 25, D.C.

DENNY-BROWN, D. E.: The histological features of striped muscle in relation to its functional activity. Proc. Roy. Soc. 104B:371-411, 1929.

DOODY, S. G., FREEDMAN, L., AND WATERLAND, J. C.: Shoulder movements during abduction in the scapular plane. Arch. Phys. Med. 51:595-604, 1970.

DRILLIS, R., CONTINI, R., AND BLUESTEIN, M.: Body segment parameters. Artif. Limbs 8:44-66, 1964.

DUCHENNE, G. B.: Physiologie des Mouvements. J. B. Baillière et Fils, Paris, 1867. Translated to English by E. B. Kaplan. J. B. Lippincott Co., Philadelphia, 1949.

EBERHART, H. D., AND ASSOCIATES: Fundamental Studies of Human Locomotion and Other Information Relating to Design of Artificial Limbs. Report to National Research Council, Committee on Artificial Limbs. University of California, Berkeley, 1947. (For partial summary see Klopsteg and Wilson, 1968.)

ELFTMAN, H.: The measurement of the external force in walking. Science 88:152-153, 1938.

ELFTMAN, H.: The force exerted by the ground in walking. Arbeitsphysiol. 10:485-491, 1939a.

ELFTMAN, H.: The function of the arms in walking. Hum. Biol. 11:528-535, 1939b.

ELFTMAN, H.: Knee action and locomotion. Bull. Hosp. Joint Dis. 16:103-110, 1955.

ELFTMAN, H.: The transverse tarsal joint and its control. Clin. Orthop. 16:41-45, 1960.

EYLER, D. L., AND MARKEE, J. E.: The anatomy and function of the intrinsic musculature of the fingers. J. Bone Joint Surg. [Amer.] 36-A: 1-9, 1954.

FEINSTEIN, B., LINDEGARD, B., NYMAN, E., AND WOHLFART, G.: Morphologic studies of motor units in normal human muscles. Acta Anat. 23:127-142, 1955.

FICK, A. E., JR., AND WEBER, E.: Studien über die Schultermuskeln. Würzb. Verh. 1872, 2. Abt., quoted by R. Fick in Anatomie und Mechanik der Gelenke. Teil II, p. 320.

FICK, R.: Anatomie und Mechanik der Gelenke. Teil II, Allgemeine Gelenk und Muskel Mechanik. Fischer, Jena, 1910.

FICK, R.: Anatomie und Mechanik der Gelenke. Teil III, Spezielle Gelenk und Muskelmechanik. Fischer, Jena, 1911.

FISCHER, O.: Der Gang des Menschen. Abh. Kgl. Sächs. Ges. d. Wiss., Math. Phys. Klasse. Part I, Bd. 21, 1895 (with W. Braune). Part II, Bd. 25, 1899. Part III, Bd. 26, 1900. Part IV, Bd. 26, 1900. Part V, Bd. 28, 1904. Part VI, Bd. 28, 1904.

FISCHER, O.: Kinematik organischer Gelenke. F. Vierweg, Braunschweig, 1907.

FLOYD, W. F., AND SILVER, P. H. S.: Electromyographic study of patterns of activity of the anterior wall muscles in man. J. Anat. 84:132-145, 1950.

FRANCILLION, M. R.: Zur Funktion diploneurer Muskeln im Gehakt des Menschen. Schweiz. Med. Wschr. 22:419-420, 1941a.

FRANCILLION, M. R.: Die Knieflexoren in kinetischer und phylogenetischer Betrachtung. Z. Orthop. 72:122-141, 1941b.

References   325

FRANKE, F.: Die Kraftkurve menschlicher Muskeln bei willkürlicher Innervation und die Frage der Absoluten Muskelkraft. Arch. f.d.g. Physiol. 184:300-323, 1920.

FRANKEL, V. H., AND BURSTEIN, A. H.: Orthopaedic Biomechanics. Lea and Febiger, Philadelphia, 1970.

FREEDMAN, L., AND MUNRO, R.: Abduction of the arm in the scapular plane: scapular and glenohumeral movements. J. Bone Joint Surg. 48A:1503-1510, 1966.

GARDNER, H., AND CLIPPINGER, F. W.: A method for location of prosthetic and orthotic knee joints. Artif. Limbs 13:31-35, 1969.

GORDON, E. E., AND VANDERWALDE, H.: Energy requirement in paraplegic ambulation. Arch. Phys. Med. 37:276-285, 1956.

GRANT, J. C.: An Atlas of Anatomy, 4th ed. Williams and Wilkins Company, Baltimore, 1956.

GRAY, E. G., AND BASMAJIAN, J. V.: Electromyography and cinematography of leg and foot ("normal" and flat) during walking. Anat. Rec. 161:1-16, 1968.

GRAY, E. R.: The role of leg muscles in variations of the arches in normal and flat feet. Phys. Ther. 44:1084-1088, 1969.

GRAY, H.: Anatomy of the Human Body, 24th ed. Lea & Febiger, Philadelphia, 1936.

HAINES, R. W.: On muscles of full and short action. J. Anat. 69:20-24, 1934.

HANAVAN, E. P.: A mathematical model of the human body. AMRL-TR-64-102, Aerospace Medical Research Laboratory, Wright-Patterson Airforce Base, Ohio, Oct., 1964.

HAXTON, H. A.: Absolute muscle force in ankle flexors of man. J. Physiol. 103:267-273, 1944.

HELLEBRANDT, F. A.: Standing as a geotropic reflex. Amer. J. Physiol. 121:471-474, 1938.

HELLEBRANDT, F. A., AND FRIES, E. C.: The constancy of the oscillographic stance pattern. Physiotherapy Rev. 22:17-23, 1942.

HELLEBRANDT, F. A., TEPPER, R. H., BRAUN, G., AND ELLIOTT, M. C.: The location of the cardinal anatomical orientation planes passing through the center of weight in young adult women. Amer. J. Physiol. 121:456-470, 1938.

HERMAN, R., AND BRAGIN, S. J.: Function of the gastrocnemius and soleus muscles. Phys. Ther. 47:105-113, 1967.

HICKS, J. H.: The mechanics of the foot. I. The joints. J. Anat. 87:345-357, 1953.

HICKS, J. H.: The mechanics of the foot. II. The plantar aponeurosis and the arch. J. Anat. 88:25-30, 1954.

HOGUE, R. E.: Upper extremity muscular activity at different cadences and inclines during normal gait. Phys. Ther. 49:963-972, 1969.

INMAN, V. T., AND RALSTON, H. J.: The Mechanics of Voluntary Muscle. Chapter 11, In Klopsteg, P. H., and Wilson, P. D.: Human Limbs and Their Substitutes. Hafner Publishing Co., New York, Reprinted 1968.

INMAN, V. T., SAUNDERS, J. B. DE C. M., AND ABBOTT, L. C.: Observations on function of shoulder joint. J. Bone Joint Surg. 26:1-30, 1944.

INMAN, V. T.: The influence of the foot-ankle complex on the proximal skeletal structures. Artif. Limbs 13:59-65, 1969a.

INMAN, V. T.: UC-BL dual-axis ankle-control system and UC-BL shoe insert. Bull. Pros. Res. BPR10-11:150-145, 1969b.

ISMAN, R. E., AND INMAN, V. T.: Anthropometric studies of the human foot and ankle. Bull. Pros. Res. BPR10-11:97-129, 1969.

JONES, D. S., BEARGLE, R. J., AND PAULY, J. E.: An electromyographic study of some muscles of costal respiration in man. Anat. Rec. 117: 17-24, 1953.

JONES, D. S., AND PAULY, J. E.: Further electromyographic studies on muscles of costal respiration in man. Anat. Rec. 128:733-746, 1957.

JOSEPH, J.: Man's Posture, Electromyographic Studies. Charles C Thomas, Springfield, Ill., 1960.

JOSEPH, J., AND NIGHTENGALE, A.: Electromyography of muscles of posture: thigh muscles in males. J. Physiol. 126:81-85, 1954.

JOSEPH, J., AND WILLIAMS, P. L.: Electromyography of certain hip muscles. J. Anat. 91:286-294, 1957.

KAPLAN, E. B.: Functional and Surgical Anatomy of the Hand. J. B. Lippincott Co., Philadelphia, 1953.

KLOPSTEG, P. E., AND WILSON, P. D.: Human Limbs and Their Substitutes. Hafner Publishing Co., New York, Reprinted 1968.

KOEPKE, G. H., MURPHY, A. J., RAY, J. W., AND DICKINSON, D. G.: An electromyographic study of some of the muscles used in respiration. Arch. Phys. Med. 36:217-222, 1955.

LANDSMEER, J. M. F., AND LONG, C.: The mechanism of finger control. Based on electromyograms and location analysis. Acta Anat. 60:330-347, 1965.

V. LANZ, T., IND WACHSMUTH, W.: Praktische Anatomie, Band I, Teil III, p. 94, J. Springer, Berlin, 1935.

V. LINGE, B., AND MULDER, J. D.: Function of the supraspinatus muscle and its relation to the supraspinatus syndrome. An experimental study in man. J. Bone Joint Surg. [Brit.] 45-B:750-754, 1963.

LONG, C.: Intrinsic-extrinsic control of the fingers. J. Bone Joint Surg. 50A:973-984, 1968.

LONG, C., AND BROWN, M. E.: Electromyographic kinesiology of the hand. Muscles driving the middle finger. J. Bone Joint Surg. [Amer.] 46-A:1683-1706, 1964.

MANN, R., AND INMAN, V. T.: Phasic activity of intrinsic muscles of the foot. J. Bone Joint Surg. [Amer.] 46-A:469-481, 1964.

MANTER, J. T.: Movements of the subtalar and transverse tarsal joints. Anat. Rec. 80:397-410, 1941.

MAREY, E. J.: De la locomotion terrestre chez les bipèdes et les quadrupèdes. J. Anat. et Physiol. 9:42-80, 1873.

MAREY, E. J.: Dévelopment de la méthode graphique par l'emploi de la Photographie. Paris, 1885.

MAREY, E. J.: Le Mouvement. Paris, 1894.

MAREY, E. J. ET DEMENY: Etude expérimentale de la Locomotion Humaine. Comp. rend. 105:544-552, 1887.

MARKEE, J. E., LOGUE, J. T., WILLIAMS, M., STANTON, W. B., WRENN, R. N. AND WALKER, L. B.: Two-joint muscles of the thigh. J. Bone Joint Surg. [Amer.] 37-A:125-142, 1955.

MENDLER, H. M.: Knee extensor and flexor force following injury. Phys. Ther. 47:35-45, 1967.

MENDLER, H. M.: Postoperative function of the knee joint. Phys. Ther. 43:435-441, 1963.

MEYER, H.: Das aufrechte Stehen. Arch. f. Anat. u. Physiol. 1853, pp. 2-45.

MOMMSEN, F.: Die Statik des gelähmten Bewegungsapparates. Beilageheft, Ztschr. f. Orth. Chir. 48:302-328, 1927.

MORRIS, J. M., LUCAS, D. B., AND BRESLER, B.: Role of the trunk in stability of the spine. J. Bone Joint Surg. [Amer.] 43-A:327-351, 1961.

MÜLLI, A.: Myokinesiographische Feststellung der Grenzwerte in der Automatie des physiologischen Geh-Aktes. Inaugural Dissertation, University of Zurich, 1940.

MURRAY, M. P., AND CLARKSON, B. H.: The vertical pathways of the foot during level walking. I. Range of variability in normal men. Phys. Ther. 46:585-589, 1966.

MURRAY, M. P., AND CLARKSON, B. H.: The vertical pathways of the foot during level walking. II. Clinical examples of distorted pathways. Phys. Ther. 46:590-599, 1966.

MURRAY, M. P., DROUGHT, A. B., AND KORY, R. C.: Walking patterns of normal men. J. Bone Joint Surg. 46A:335-360, 1964.

MURRAY, M. P., KORY, R. C., CLARKSON, B. H., AND SEPIC, S. B.: Comparison of free and fast walking patterns of normal men. Amer. J. Phys. Med. 45:8-24, 1966.

MURRAY, M. P., KORY, R. C., AND CLARKSON, B. H.: Walking patterns in healthy old men. J. Geront. 24:171-178, 1969.

MURRAY, M. P., KORY, R. C., AND SEPIC, S. B.: Walking patterns of normal women. Arch. Phys. Med. 51:637-650, 1970.

MURRAY, M. P., SEPIC, S. B., AND BARNARD, E. J.: Patterns of sagittal rotation of the upper limbs in walking. Phys. Ther. 47:272-284, 1967.

MURRAY, M. P., GORE, D. R., AND CLARKSON, B. H.: Walking patterns of patients with unilateral hip pain due to osteo-arthritis and avascular necrosis. J. Bone Joint Surg. 53A:259-273, 1971.

MUSTARD, W. T.: Iliopsoas transfer for weakness of the hip abductors. J. Bone Joint Surg. [Amer.] 34-A:647-650, 1952.

PETERS, C. K.: Methods of measuring the pressure of the intervertebral disk. J. Bone Joint Surg. 15:365-368, 1933.

POORE, G. V.: Nervous affections of the hand. Lancet 2:405-407, 493-496, 1881.

RALSTON, H. J.: Energy-speed relation and optimal speed during level walking. Int. Z. Angew. Physiol. 17:277-283, 1958.

RAMSEY, R. W., AND STREET, S. F.: Isometric length-tension diagram of isolated skeletal muscle fibers in frog. J. Cell. Comp. Physiol. 15: 11-34, 1940.

v. RECKLINGHAUSEN, N.: Gliedermechanik und Lähmungsprothesen. J. Springer, Berlin, 1920.

REULEAUX, F.: Theoretische Kinematik. Braunschweig, 1875.

SALTER, N., AND DARCUS, H. D.: The effect of the degree of elbow flexion on the maximum torques developed in pronation and supination of the right hand. J. Anat. 86:197-202, 1952.

SCHEDE, FRANZ: Theoretische Grundlagen für den Bau von Kunstbeinen. Ferdinand Enke Verlag, Stuttgart, 1941.

SCHERB, R.: Ein Vorschlag zur kinetischen Diagnostik in der Orthopädie. Beilageheft, Ztschr. f. orthop. Chir. 48:462-472, 1927.

SCHERB, R.: Kinetisch-Diagnostische Analyse von Gehstorungen. Technik und Resultate der Myokinesiographie. Z. Orthop. 82, Suppl., 1952.

SCHERB, R., AND ARIENTI, A.: Ist die Myokinesigraphie als Untersuchungsmethode objective zuverlässig? Schweiz. Med. Wschr. 75:1077-1079, 1945.

SCHLESINGER, G.: Der mechanische Aufbau der kuntslichen Glieder. In Ersatzglieder und Arbeitshilfen. J. Springer, Berlin, 1919.

SCHLESINGER, G.: Technische Ausnutzung der kinoplastischen Armstümpfe. Deutsch. Med. Wschr. 46:262-266, 1920.

SHEFFIELD, F. J.: Electromyographic study of the abdominal muscles in walking and other movements. Amer. J. Phys. Med. 41:142-147, 1962.

SMITH, J. W.: Observations on the postural mechanism of the human knee joint. J. Anat. 90:236-260, 1956.

SMITH, J. W.: The forces acting at the human ankle joint during standing. J. Anat. 91:545-564, 1957.

STEINDLER, A.: Kinesiology of the Human Body under Normal and Pathological Conditions. Charles C Thomas, Springfield, Ill., 1955.

STRONG, C. L., AND PERRY, J.: Function of the extensor pollicis longus and intrinsic muscles of the thumb: an electromyographic study during interphalangeal joint extension. Phys. Ther. 46:939-945, 1966.

STUDER, F.: Der Sauerstoffverbrauch beim Gehen auf horizontaler Bahn. Pflueger Arch. Ges. Physiol. 212:105-119, 1926.

SUNDERLAND, S.: The actions of the extensor digitorum communis, interosseous and lumbrical muscles. Amer. J. Anat. 77:189-209, 1945.

TAYLOR, A.: The contribution of the intercostal muscles to the effort of respiration in man. J. Physiol. 151:390-401, 1960.

TAYLOR, C. L., AND SCHWARZ, R. J.: The anatomy and mechanics of the human hand. Artif. Limbs 2:22-35, 1955.

TOURNAY, A., ET FESSARD, A.: Etude electromyographique de la Synergie entre l'Abducteur du Pouce et le Muscle Cubital Postérieur. Rev. Neurol. 80:631, 1948.

WEATHERSBY, H. T., SUTTON, L. R., AND KRUSEN, U. L.: The kinesiology of muscles of the thumb. An electromyographic study. Arch. Phys. Med. 44:321-326, 1963.

WEBER, E. F.: Ueber die Längeverhaltnisse der Muskeln im Allgemeinen. Verh. Kgl. Sächs. Ges. d. Wiss., Leipzig, 1851.

WEBER, W., AND E.: Mechanik der menschlichen Gehwerkzeuge. Gottingen, 1836.

WILKIE, D. V.: The relation between force and velocity in human muscle. J. Physiol. 110:249-280, 1950.

WILLIAMS, M., AND LISSNER, H. R.: Biomechanics of Human Motion. W. B. Saunders Co., Philadelphia, 1962.

WILLIAMS, M., AND STUTZMAN, L.: Strength variation through the range of joint motion. Phys. Ther. Rev. 39:145-152, 1959.

WILLIAMS, M., TOMBERLIN, J. A., AND ROBERTSON, K. J.: Muscle force curves of school children. J. Amer. Phys. Ther. Assoc. 45:539-549, 1965.

Index

Bone(s) (Cont.)
  humerus, 127
    epicondyles of, 53
  ilium, 225
  ischium, tuberosity of, 225
  lesser multangular, 83
  lunate, 83
  manubrium sterni, 127
  metacarpals, 83, 84
  metatarsals, 198
  navicular, 83, 197
  occipital, 251
  of skull, 251
  os magnum, 82
  patella, 174, 179
  phalanges
    of foot, 199
    of hand, 84
  pisiform, 83
  pubic, symphysis of, 225
  radius. See *Radius.*
  ribs, 127, 254
  sacrum, 254
  scaphoid, 83
  scapula, 127
  semilunar, 33
  sesamoid, 87, 179, 198
  sternum, 127, 255
  talus, 199, 200
  temporal, 251
  thorax, 254
  tibia, 200
    condyles of, 173
    tuberosity of, 173
  transverse rotation of, moment
    of force applied to, 24, 25
  trapezium, 83
  trapezoid, 83
  triangular, 83
  triquetrum, 83
  trochlea, of humerus, 54
  ulna, 81, 82
  unciform, 83
Bowleg, 183
Brace(s)
  ankle, knee stability and, 279
  for paraplegics, 281
Brachialis, 59, 61, 62, 64, 75
Brachioradialis, 58-62, 65, 66, 70,
  71, 75
Brake test, 45
Bunion, 203

CADENCE in walking, 293
Calcaneocuboid joints, 201
Calcaneus, 198
Calf, muscles of
  function of, in walking, 303-305
  paralysis of, 278, 279
Caloric consumption in walking,
  309-312
Capitatae bone, 82, 83
Capitulum of humerus, 54
Capsule of knee joint, capacity of,
  175
Carpal bones, 83
Carpal collateral ligaments, 81
Carpometacarpal joints, 86
Carrying angle, 54
Cartilage, semilunar, 175
Cartilaginous plates of intervertebral disks, 256
Cavity, glenoid, 128
Center(s) of gravity, 271
  in man, percentage height of, 274
  of body mass
    above ankle joints, 275
    above hip joints, 276
    above knee joints, 276
  of body segments, 4, 5, 274
  of entire body, 2, 3, 4, 5, 272, 273
  of head, 257, 276
  of systems of segments, 4, 5
  vertical displacement of, in
    walking, 295
Center-of-gravity line, relation of
  to ankle joints, 277
  to atlanto-occipital joints, 285
  to base of support, 277
  to hip joints, 232, 279
  to knee joints, 278
Chain segments, degrees of freedom
  of motion of, 10
Chains, kinematic, 10
Chiasma tendinum, 99
Chopart's joint, 201
Chronophotography, 294
Cineplasty, 33
Circumduction, 87, 91
Clavicle, 127
  absence of, 130
Clawhand, 104, 107, 108
"Claw" posture of hand, 104
Club foot, 203
Coccyx, 254

Clinical Kinesiology

Condyles
  occipital, 288
  of femur, 173
  of humerus, 53
  of tibia, 173
Condyloid joints, 84, 201, 202, 255
  axes of motion of, 9, 83, 87, 202
  degrees of freedom of motion of,
    9, 84, 86, 202
Contraction of muscle
  influence of speed on tension,
    42, 43, 44
  isometric, 37, 43
  isotonic, 42
  lengthening, 42, 45
    velocity of, 43, 44, 46
  shortening, 42
    velocity of, 43, 44, 46
Coraco-acromial ligament, 131, 158
Coracobrachialis, 157, 159
Coracohumeral ligament, 131, 158
Coracoid process of scapula, 63,
    128, 131, 137
Coronoid process of ulna, 54, 64, 67
Corset muscle, 264
Coxa plana, 228
Coxa valga, 228
Coxa vara, 228
Crest
  external occipital, 251
  of ilium, 254
  of sacrum, 254
Cross section
  of abductors and adductors, 249
  of anconeus, 78
  of elbow extensors, 73
  of elbow flexors, 73
  of knee muscles, 192
  of muscles. See also *Appendix*.
    anatomical, 35
    physiological, 24-25, 35
  of pronators of forearm, 74, 77
  of semimembranosus, 187
  of shoulder muscles, 171
  of subscapularis, 158
  of supinators of forearm, 74
  of triceps brachii, 78
  of triceps surae, 215
Cruciate ligament
  of ankle, 211
  of knee, 175, 195, 196
Cubitus valgus, 54
Cuboid bone, 198

Cuff muscles of shoulder, 158
Cuneiform bones, 197, 198
Curvature of spine
  kyphosis, 270
  lateral, 253
  lordosis, 270
  scoliosis, 270
Curve, Blix's, 37

DEFORMITIES
  of foot, 203, 224
  of hips, 228
  of knee, 183
Degrees of freedom of motion, 8
  of chain segments, 10
  of joints
    atlanto-occipital, 255
    ball-and-socket, 9, 132, 242
    condyloid, 9, 84, 86, 202
    elbow, 54
    hinge, 8, 54, 88, 202
    hip, 9, 238
    interphalangeal, 8, 88, 202
    knee, 175
    metacarpophalangeal, 9, 86
    metatarsophalangeal, 202
    radio-ulnar, 5, 57
    saddle, 9, 86, 114
    shoulder, 10, 132
    wrist, 9, 84
Deltoid muscle, 68, 151
  anterior and posterior, antago-
    nistic action of, 172
  paralysis of, 152, 165-166, 169
  tuberosity of, 65, 66, 151
Dens of axis, 255
Diaphragm, 268
Digits and wrist, muscles acting on,
    88
Dorsiflexors, ankle, function of,
  in walking, 303
"Double knee action," 295, 305
Dynamics, 1

ELBOW
  extensors of, cross section of, 73
  flexors of
    cross section of, 73
    electromyography of, 75, 76
    leverage curves of, 24, 46
    strength of, 78
  shoulder and, two-joint muscles
    of, 78

Elbow (Cont.)
  ulnar nerves at, 53
Elbow extension
  pectoralis major in, 79
  strength of, 78
Elbow joint, 54
  axes of motion of, 54, 55, 60
  degrees of freedom of motion of,
    54
Electromyography
  methods of, 300
  of abdominal muscles, 269
    in walking, 308
  of elbow flexors, 75, 76
  of extensor digitorum communis,
    110
  of hip extensors, 232
  of iliacus muscle in standing, 280
  of iliopsoas muscle, 249
    in walking, 306
  of intercostal muscles, 268, 269
  of interosseous muscles of hand,
    109
  of intrinsic muscles of foot, 223,
    308
  of knee extensors, 278
  of long finger flexors, 101, 110
  of lumbrical muscles, 103, 109
  of muscles used in walking, 300-
    303
  of popliteus muscle, 195
  of rectus femoris, 194
  of respiratory muscles, 268
  of sartorius muscle in walking,
    306
  of scalene muscles, 258
  of shoulder muscles, 165, 167
  of tensor fasciae latae in walking,
    306
  of thumb muscles, 120
  of triceps surae, 217
  of trunk muscles, 268
Energy
  expenditure of, in walking, 300,
    309-312
  kinetic, in walking, 302-303
  potential, in walking, 302-303
Energy changes
  in forward swing of leg, 302
  in vertical oscillations of trunk,
    302-303

Energy cost in walking, 300, 309-312
  by amputees and hemiplegic sub-
    jects, 312
Epicondyle(s)
  extensor, of humerus, 53, 70
  flexor, of humerus, 53, 70, 71
  of femur, 173, 174, 177, 181
Equilibration
  at ankle, 277, 288
  at hip, 280
    standing on one foot, 288, 289,
      290
  at knee, 278
Equilibrium, 13
  neutral, 271
  of pelvis, 283
  stable, 271
  unstable, 271
    at hip, 280
  of head, 285
  of pelvis, 242
Erector spinae, 265, 266
  function of, in walking, 307
Evolute, 176
Excitation, threshold of, of motor
  unit, 33
Excursion of muscle, 35
Extensor assembly, 106
Extensor carpi radialis brevis, 58,
  60, 61, 66, 88, 91, 98
  palmaris longus and, action of,
    121
Extensor carpi radialis longus, 58,
  60, 61, 66, 71, 88, 91, 97
Extensor carpi ulnaris, 69, 81, 88,
  92, 98, 120
Extensor digiti minimi proprius,
  88, 111, 123
Extensor digitorum brevis, 214
Extensor digitorum communis, 88,
  91, 107
  electromyography of, 110
Extensor digitorum longus, 211
Extensor hallucis longus, 211
Extensor hood, 96
Extensor indicis proprius, 70, 88
Extensor pollicis brevis, 70, 88,
  117, 118, 120
Extensor pollicis longus, 88, 117,
  118, 119
Extensor sleeve, 96

Extensors
  elbow, cross section of, 73
  hip. See *Hip, extensors of.*
  knee. See *Knee, extensors of.*
Extremity(ies)
  upper, muscles of, work done by,
    in walking, 302-303
  weight of, 273

"FAN symptom" of gluteal muscles,
  306
Femoral nerves, 183, 184, 234, 236,
  241
Femur
  adductor tubercle of, 173
  axes of, 227
  condyles of, 173
  deformities of, 227
  epicondyles of, 173
  gluteal tuberosity of, 229
  greater trochanter of, 225, 238,
    240, 241
  head of, 227
  lesser trochanter of, 227, 236
  neck of, 227
  nonpalpable structures of, 227
  shape of, 227
  tubercle adductor of, 173
Fibers, muscle. See *Muscle fibers.*
Fibula, 200
Finger extensors, wrist flexors and,
  105
Finger flexors, wrist extensors and,
  98
Fingers, dorsal aponeurosis of, 106,
  108
Flexor(s)
  elbow
    cross section of, 73
    electromyography of, 75, 76
    leverage curves of, 24, 46
  hip
    function of, in walking, 306
    function of rectus femoris as,
      244
  knee
    function of hamstrings as, 244
    leverage of, 191
Flexor accessorius, 214
Flexor carpi radialis, 71, 88, 93, 94,
  95, 105

Flexor carpi ulnaris, 88, 93, 95,
  106, 120
Flexor digiti minimi brevis, 89
Flexor digitorum brevis, 214, 308
Flexor digitorum longus, 206
Flexor digitorum profundus, 88,
  101
Flexor digitorum superficialis, 88,
  94, 95, 99
Flexor hallucis longus, 207, 308
  grooves for tendon of, 199
Flexor pollicis brevis, 89, 116, 117,
  118 .
Flexor pollicis longus, 88, 118, 119
Foot
  ankle and, 197-224
  electromyography of intrinsic
    muscles of, 223, 307
  weight of, 273
Foramen magnum, 252
Force(s)
  change of direction of, 27-28
  composition of, 14
  in lifting, 269, 270
  moment of. See *Moment of force.*
  resolution of, 15-17
  rotary component of, 15-17
Force arm, 17-18
Force couple, 26-27
Force plate, 292, 298, 299
Fossa
  antecubital, 60, 64
  iliac, 235
  infraspinous, of scapula, 128
  intercondyloid, of femur, 174
  olecranon, 54
  popliteal, 174
  supraspinous, of scapula, 128
Fovea radialis, 83
Function, muscle. See under name
  of individual muscle.
Fusiform muscles, 26

GASTROCNEMIUS, 187, 204, 216, 217,
  223
  leverage of, at ankle and knee,
    192
Gemelli, 232
Genu recurvatum, 183, 279
Genu valgum, 183
Genu varum, 183

Ginglymus joint, 54
Glenohumeral joint, 129, 131, 133-134
  axes of motion of, 132
  subluxation of, 131
Glenohumeral ligaments, 158
Glenoid cavity, 128
Gluteal lines, 227
Gluteal muscles, "fan symptom" of, 306
Gluteal nerve
  inferior, 230
  superior, 234, 238, 241
Gluteus maximus, 230
  "setting" of, 231
Gluteus medius, 238
  weight-bearing function of, 240
Gluteus minimus, 238, 241
Gravity, center(s) of. See *Center(s) of gravity.*
Grip, strength of, 36, 96, 122, 125
Groove(s)
  intertubercular, of humerus, 63, 129, 161
  for tendon
    of flexor hallucis longus, 199
    of peroneus longus, 199, 208
    of tibialis posterior, 205
Ground reaction, recording of, 292, 298

HALLUX valgus, 203
Hamate bone, 83
Hamstrings, 185, 186
  as hip extensors, 231, 232, 244
  as knee flexors, 185, 244
  hip flexors and, 190
  quadriceps and, 191, 305
Hand
  interphalangeal joints of, 87
  interosseous muscles of, 87, 104, 107, 110, 112
  intrinsic muscles of, paralysis of, 104
  lumbricales of, 87, 104, 107
  phalanges of, 84
  weight of, 273
  wrist and, 81-126
Head
  balance of, 267, 285
  center of gravity of, 276, 285
  neck and, muscles acting on, 257, 260

Head (Cont.)
  weight of, 273
High heels, effect of, 200
Hinge joints, 8, 54, 88, 199, 202
  axes of motion of, 8, 54
  degrees of freedom of motion of, 8, 54, 88, 202
Hip
  abductors of
    and hip hikers on same side, 248
    function of
    in one-legged standing, 289
    in walking, 306
    length-tension relations of, 248
    paralysis of, 289
  adductors of, function of, in walking, 307
  deformities of, 227
  equilibration at, 280
    standing on one foot, 288, 289, 290
  extension of
    knee extension and flexion and, 190
  extensors of
    electromyography of, 232
    function of, in walking, 305
    function of hamstrings as, 232, 244
    leverage of, 247
  external rotators of, 232
  flexion of
    knee extension and flexion and, 190
  flexors of
    function of, in walking, 306
    hamstrings and, 190
    paralysis of, 245
    rectus femoris as, 244
  knee and, two-joint muscles passing, 189
  leverage at, 289
  leverage of sartorius at, 234
  pelvic region and, 225-250
  rectus femoris as flexor of, 232
  two-joint muscles of, 244
Hip hikers, function of, 248
Hip hinges in leg braces, 248
Hip joint, 229
  balance at, 279
  center-of-gravity line and, 232, 279

Hip joint (Cont.)
degrees of freedom of motion of, 9, 242
movements of, 229
Hip muscles, 242
in abduction, 228
in adduction, 249
in extension, 247
in external rotation, 250
in flexion, 245
in internal rotation, 250
in weight-bearing, 242
Hip posture in paraplegia, 281
Humerus, 127
anatomical neck of, 128
intertubercular groove of, 63, 129, 161
capitulum of, 54
condyles of, 53
epicondyles of, 53
greater tubercle of, 128, 153
lesser tubercle of, 128, 157
surgical neck of, 128
trochlea of, 54
Hyperextension
of knees, 278, 279
of proximal interphalangeal joint, 102
of shoulder, 78, 132
Hypothenar, 89, 122

ILIACUS, 235
electromyography of, 280
Iliocostales, 265
Iliofemoral ligament, 193
Iliohypogastric nerve, 263
Ilioinguinal nerve, 264
Iliopsoas, 232, 235
electromyography of, 249, 306
length-tension relations of, 246
paralysis of, 245, 246
Iliotibial band, 182
as stabilizer of knee, 193
insertion of gluteus maximus into, 230
insertion of tensor fasciae latae into, 234
Ilium, 225
anterior superior spine of, 226, 234
crest of, 254
inferior spines of, 227

Ilium (Cont.)
posterior superior spine of, 221, 225, 226, 254
Ill-fitted shoes, effect of, 224
Inertia, 13
Infraglenoid tubercle, 128
Infraspinatus, 154, 172
Inguinal ligament, 263
Injury(ies)
axillary nerve, 165
median nerve, 79
musculocutaneous nerve, 79
radial nerve, 79
spinal accessory nerve, 144
tibial nerve, 218, 219
Innervation of muscles. See under individual muscles.
Innervation ratios, 33, 34
Intercarpal joints, 84
Intercostal nerves, 261, 263, 265
Intercostals, 264
electromyography of, 268, 269
Interosseous muscles
of foot, 215
of hand, 88, 104, 107, 110, 112
electromyography of, 109
Interphalangeal joints, 8, 88, 202
of hand, 88
of toes, 202
proximal hyperextension of, 102
Interspinales, 265
Intertransversarii, 265
Intervertebral disks, 256
Intervertebral joints, 256
Ischium(ia)
rami of, 241
spine of, 227
tuberosity of, 185-187, 225, 231

JOINT(s)
acromioclavicular, 129, 131
ankle. See Ankle joints.
atlanto-axial, 255
atlanto-occipital, 255, 285
ball-and-socket, 9, 131, 229
calcaneocuboid, 201
carpometacarpal, 86
Chopart's, 201
condyloid. See Condyloid joints.
degrees of freedom of motion of. See Degrees of freedom of motion.
double arthrodial, 130

Joint(s) (Cont.)
elbow. See *Elbow joint.*
ginglymus, 54
glenohumeral. See *Gleno-
humeral joint.*
hinge, 8, 54, 88, 199, 202
axes of motion of, 8, 54
hip. See *Hip joint.*
intercarpal, 84
interphalangeal. See *Interphalangeal joints.*
intervertebral, 256
knee. See *Knee joint.*
lumbosacral, 257
metacarpophalangeal, 86, 87
metatarsophalangeal, 202, 223,
224
midtarsal, 201
radiocarpal, 84
radio-ulnar, 55-59, 70
sacroiliac, 225, 254
saddle. See *Saddle joint.*
"screw joint," 256
single arthrodial, 131
spheroidal, 131
sternoclavicular, 129, 130, 255
subluxation of, 144, 145
subtalar, 201
talocrural, 199-201
talonavicular, 201
transverse tarsal, 201, 202, 221
uniaxial, 56
universal, 131
wrist. See *Wrist joint.*
Joint motion, length-tension diagrams and, 40, 46, 97
Jugular process, 252

Kinematic chains, 10
Kinematics, 1
of locomotion, 294
Kinetic energy, changes of, in
locomotion, 302
Kinetics, 13
of locomotion, 298
Knee
ankle and, two-joint muscles
passing, 189, 215
collateral ligaments of, 175, 177
cruciate ligaments of, 175, 195,
196, 211

Knee (Cont.)
deformities of, 183
equilibration at, 278
extension of
hip extension and, 190
hip flexion and, 190
plantar flexion of ankle and,
191
extensor(s) of
electromyography of, 278
function of rectus femoris as,
194
leverage of, 191
flexion of
hip extension and, 190
hip flexion and, 190
plantar flexion of ankle and,
191
flexors of, leverage of, 191
hip and, two-joint muscles passing, 189
hyperextension of, 278, 279
léverage of gastrocnemius at, 192
"locking mechanism" of, 177,
192, 297
muscles of
acting in extension, 183
acting in flexion, 185
acting in rotation, 189
cross section of, 192
length-tension relations of, 192
torque curves for, 192
prosthetic, stability of, 279
stability of
in erect standing, 278
in quadriceps paralysis, 279
terminal rotation of, 177, 192
transverse ligament of, 175
Knee bends, popliteus in, 195
Knee cap, 179
Knee hinges in leg braces, 181
Knee joint, 175-183, 200
balance at, 278
degrees of freedom of motion of,
175
"locking mechanism" of, 177,
192, 297
mechanics of, 176, 180
shifting axis of motion of, 176
transverse rotation of, 178
Knock knees, 183
Kyphosis, 270

Movement(s) (Cont.)
rotary, 12
selection of muscles in, 74
terms for, 6, 7, 8
translatory, 12
upward rotation of scapula, 130,
148
Movement synergy, 96
Multangular bones, greater and
lesser, 83
Muscle(s)
abductor digiti minimi, 89, 111
abductor hallucis, 214
abductor pollicis brevis, 89, 115,
119
abductor pollicis longus, 70, 88,
117, 118, 120
acting as guy-ropes, 267
acting in abduction
and adduction of the metatarsophalangeal joints, 224
of hip, 248
of shoulder, 164
acting in adduction
of hip, 249
of shoulder, 167
acting in dorsiflexion of ankle,
220
acting in eversion of ankle, 221
acting in extension
of head and neck, 260
of hip, 247
of knee, 183
of shoulder, 167
acting in external rotation
of hip, 250
of shoulder, 169
acting in flexion
of hip, 245
of knee, 185
of metatarsophalangeal joints,
223
of shoulder, 167
acting in inversion of ankle, 221
acting in internal rotation
of hip, 250
of shoulder, 169
acting in plantar flexion of
ankle, 215
acting in rotation of knee, 189
acting on head and neck, 257
acting on wrist and digits, 88

Muscles (Cont.)
action of, synergism and antagonism, 95
active insufficiency of, 36
activity of, patterns of, in walking, 300
adductor brevis, 241
adductor gracilis, 187, 241
adductor group, 241
adductor longus, 241
adductor magnus, 241
adductor pollicis, 89, 119
anconeus, 69, 70, 77
angle of approach of, 16
anterior tibialis, 210
antigravity, in biped posture, 192
articularis genu, 185
biceps brachii, 59, 61, 63, 70, 76,
78, 159
biceps femoris, 185
brachialis, 20, 59, 61, 62, 64, 75
brachioradialis, 58-62, 65, 66, 70,
71, 75
contractile tension curve of, 40
contraction of. See Contraction
of muscle.
coracobrachialis, 157, 159
corset, 264
cross section of. See also tables
in Appendix.
anatomical, 35
physiological, 24-25, 35
cuff of shoulder, 158
deltoid, 68, 151
diaphragm, 268
electromyography of. See Electromyography.
erector spinae, 265, 266
excursion of, 35
extensor carpi radialis brevis,
58, 60, 61, 66, 88, 91, 98
extensor carpi radialis longus,
58, 60, 61, 66, 88, 91, 97
extensor carpi ulnaris, 69, 81,
87, 92, 98
extensor digiti minimi proprius,
88, 111, 123
extensor digitorum brevis, 214
extensor digitorum communis,
88, 91, 107
extensor digitorum longus, 211
extensor hallucis longus, 211

Muscles (Cont.)
extensor indicis proprius, 70, 88
extensor pollicis brevis, 70, 88, 117, 118
extensor pollicis longus, 88, 117, 118, 119
external oblique abdominal, 262, 263
external rotators of hip, 232
fibers of
angle of approach of, to tendon, 26
line of action of, 26
number of, in muscles, 34
"pale" or "fast," 216
"red" or "slow," 216
flexor accessorius, 214
flexor carpi radialis, 71, 88, 93, 94, 95, 105
flexor carpi ulnaris, 88, 93, 95, 105, 120
flexor digiti minimi brevis, 89
flexor digitorum brevis, 214
flexor digitorum longus, 206
flexor digitorum profundus, 88, 101
flexor digitorum superficialis, 88, 94, 95, 99
flexor hallucis longus, 207
flexor pollicis brevis, 89, 116, 117, 118
flexor pollicis longus, 88, 118, 119
force-velocity curve of, 43
fusiform, 26
gastrocnemius, 187, 203, 216
gemelli, 232
gluteus maximus, 230
gluteus medius, 238
weight-bearing function, 240
gluteus minimus, 238, 241
hamstring. See *Hamstrings*.
hypothenar, 89
iliacus, 235
iliocostales, 265
iliopsoas, 232, 235
infraspinatus, 154
intercostals, 264
internal oblique abdominal, 263
interosseous
of foot, 215
of hand, 88, 104, 107, 110, 112
interspinales, 265

Muscle(s) (Cont.)
intertransversarii, 265
latissimus dorsi, 68, 151, 160
in crutch walking, 170
length-tension relations of, 35
levator scapulae, 140, 143, 151
line of action of, 23
longissimus capitis, 260
longus capitis, 252, 257, 267
longus colli, 257, 267
lumbricales
of foot, 215
of hand, 88, 104, 107
mechanical advantage of, 29, 103
metabolism in ligaments as compared to, 287
obturator externus, 232
obturator internus, 232
of hip, 242
of posterior trunk, 265
of short action, 36, 190
of shoulder region, 134
of trunk, anterior and lateral, 260
opponens digiti minimi, 89
opponens pollicis, 89, 115
palmaris brevis, 89
palmaris longus, 61, 71, 88, 93
absence of, 94, 105
passive insufficiency of, 36
passive tension curve of, 37, 38
pectineus, 232, 236, 241, 243
pectoralis major, 145, 161-163
in extension of elbow, 79
pectoralis minor, 137, 151
peroneus brevis, 208
peroneus longus, 207
peroneus tertius, 211
piriformis, 232, 238, 240
plantaris, 187
pluriarticular, 96
popliteus. See *Popliteus*.
pronator quadratus, 71-73, 77
pronator teres, 60-62, 67, 71, 77
psoas major, 236, 237, 267
quadratus femoris, 232
quadratus lumborum, 264, 267
quadratus plantae, 214
quadriceps, 183
rectus abdominis, 261
rectus capitis anterior, 252, 257, 267

Muscle(s) (Cont.)
   rectus capitis lateralis, 252
   rectus femoris. See *Rectus fe-
      moris.*
   resting length of, 37-39
   rhomboideus major, 117, 139,
      140, 147, 150
   rhomboideus minor, 137, 139,
      140, 151
   sartorius, 188, 193, 232
   scalene, 258, 267
   selection of, in movement, 74
   semimembranosus, 187
   semitendinosus, 186
   serratus anterior, 134, 145, 148
   "setting" of, of gluteus maximus,
      231
   shortening of, rate of, 42, 43
   soleus, 203, 216
   spinales, of back, 265
   splenius, 260
   sternocleidomastoid, 143, 251,
      258, 267
   subclavius, 143
   suboccipital, 260
   subscapularis, 156
   supinator, 61, 70, 71, 76
   supraspinatus, 153
   synergism and antagonism of,
      95, 171
   tendon, action of, 41, 124
   tension of
      influence of speed of shorten-
         ing on, 291
      influence of speed on stretch,
         291
   tensor fasciae latae, 193, 232, 236
   teres major, 68, 139, 158
   teres minor, 154
   thenar, 89
   tibialis anterior, 210
   tibialis posterior, 205
   transversospinales, 265
   transversospinalis capitis, 260
   transversus abdominis, 264
   trapezius, 135, 144, 147, 148
   triceps brachii, 67, 69, 77, 78, 159
   triceps surae, 205
   two-joint
      damage of, 41
      functional advantage of, 41

Muscle(s) (Cont.)
   length-tension relations of,
      189, 190, 191, 244
   of elbow and shoulder, 78
   of hip, 244
   passing knee and ankle, 189,
      215
   passing knee and hip, 189, 195
   rectus femoris, 234
   sartorius, 234
   vastus intermedius, 184
   vastus lateralis, 182, 184
   vastus medialis, 182, 184
   work capacity of, 30
   work done on, 30, 44
Musculocutaneous nerves, 63, 64,
   75, 159
   injuries to, 79
Musculospiral nerves, 69
Musculus cucullaris, 136

NAVICULAR bone, 83, 197
Neck
   head and, muscles acting on,
      257, 260
   ligament of, 251
Nerve(s)
   anterior thoracic, 138, 161
   axillary, 151, 154
      injury to, 165
   common peroneal, 208, 210
   deep peroneal, 210
   dorsal scapular, 137, 140
   femoral, 183, 184, 234, 236, 241
   iliohypogastric, 263
   ilioinguinal, 264
   inferior gluteal, 230
   intercostals, 261, 262, 265
   long thoracic, 134
   median. See *Median nerve.*
   musculocutaneous, 63, 64, 75,
      159
      injuries to, 79
   musculospiral, 69
   obturator, 241
   radial. See *Radial nerves.*
   sacral, 240
   sciatic, 185, 204, 241
   spinal, 264, 265
   spinal accessory, 136, 258
      injury to, 144
   subscapular, 157, 158
   superior gluteal, 234, 238, 241

Nerve (s) (Cont.)
suprascapular, 153, 154
thoracodorsal, 161
tibial. See *Tibial nerves*.
ulnar. See *Ulnar nerves*.
Newton's laws, 13, 21
"Normalstellung" posture, 282, 287
Nucleus pulposis of intervertebral disks, 256

OBTURATOR internus, 232
Obturator externus, 232
Obturator nerve, 241
Occipital bone, 251
Occipital condyles, 252
Odontoid process, 255
Olecranon process, 53, 69
Opponens digiti minimi, 89
Opponens pollicis, 89, 115
Opposition movements, 86, 113, 114, 115, 125
Orientation planes of body, 2, 6
Os magnum, 82
Oxygen consumption in walking, 292, 308, 309

PALMARIS brevis, 89
Palmaris longus, 61, 71, 88, 93
absence of, 94, 105
extensor carpi radialis brevis and, 121
Palpation. See under individual structures.
Paralysis
of anterior and middle deltoid, 152
of anterior tibialis, 220
of calf muscles, 281
and quadriceps, 279
of deltoid, 165
of hip abductors, 289
of hip flexors, 245
of iliopsoas, 245, 246
of intrinsic muscles of foot, 224
of intrinsic muscles of hand, 104, 105
of median nerve, 124
of plantar flexors of ankle, 217
of posterior deltoid, 169
of quadriceps, 279
of radial nerve, 121

Paralysis (Cont.)
of rhomboids, 168
of sartorius, 245
of serratus anterior, 146, 147, 149
of shoulder blade fixators, 165
of sternocleidomastoid muscle, 259
of supraspinatus, 166
of tensor fasciae latae, 245
of tibial nerve, 218, 219
of trapezius, 144, 147, 148, 149
of trunk muscles, 267
of ulnar nerve, 112, 122, 123
of vastus medialis, 195
Paraplegia, 281
Passive tension curve, 37, 103
Patella, 174, 179
leverage provided by, 180
Patterns of muscle activity in walking, 300
Pectineus, 232, 236, 241, 243
Pectoralis major, 79, 145, 161-163
Pectoralis minor, 137, 151
Pelvic balance in standing on one foot, 288, 289, 290
Pelvic inclination, 284
angle of, 283
Pelvis, 283
backward tilt of, 244, 281, 283
Peroneal nerve
common, 208, 210
deep, 210
Peroneus brevis, 208
Peroneus longus, 207, 223, 308
grooves for tendon of, 199, 208
Peroneus tertius, 211
Pes calcaneus, 203
Pes cavus, 203
Pes equinus, 203
Pes planus, 203
Pes valgus, 203
Pes varus, 203
Phalanges
of foot, 199
of hand, 84
Piriformis, 83, 232, 238, 240
Pivot point of levers, 18
Planes of body, 2, 3
orientation of movements to, 2, 6
Plantaris, 187
Plate, force. See *Force plate*.
Pluriarticular, 96

Standing (Cont.)
  pelvic inclination in, 284
  prolonged, posture in, 193
Statics, 1
Statography, 277
Sternoclavicular joint, 129, 130,
    255
  subluxation of, 144, 145
Sternocleidomastoid muscle, 143,
    251, 258, 267
  paralysis of, 259
Sternum, 127, 255
"Stick figures" illustrating locomo-
    tion, 295
Strain
  in lifting, 269
  in lumbosacral region, 270
Strength
  muscle, absolute, 30, 35
  of elbow extension, 78
  of elbow flexion, 78
  of grip, 36, 96, 122, 125
Styloid process
  of radius, 66, 81
  of ulna, 53
Subclavius, 143
Subluxation
  of glenohumeral joint, 131
  of sternoclavicular joint, 144, 145
Suboccipital muscles, 260
Subscapular nerves, 154, 157, 158
Subscapularis, 156
  cross section of, 158
  infraspinatus and, 172
Subtalar joint, 201
Supinator(s), 61, 70, 71, 76
  of forearm, cross section of, 74
Supraglenoid tubercle, 128
Suprascapular nerves, 153
Supraspinatus, 153
  paralysis of, 166
Surface of support
  in erect standing, 276
  standing on one foot, 287
Surgical neck of humerus, 128
Sustentaculum talare, 198
Sway, postural, pattern of, 277
Symphysis of pubic bones, 225
Synergic action
  of abductor digiti minimi and
    wrist muscles, 120

Synergic action (Cont.)
  of hip abductors and hip hikers
    on same side, 248
  of hip flexors and hamstrings,
    190
  of palmaris longus and extensor
    carpi radialis brevis, 121
  of quadriceps and hamstrings,
    191, 305
  of rhomboids and teres major,
    168
  of subscapularis and infra-
    spinatus, 172
  of thumb abductors and wrist
    muscles, 120
  of trapezius and other muscles,
    171
  of upward rotators of scapula and
    abductors of shoulder, 150, 164
  of wrist extensors and finger
    flexors, 98
  of wrist flexors and finger
    extensors, 105
Synergism and antagonism of
  muscles, 52, 95, 171
Synergists, 54, 95
  biceps and triceps as, 78

TALOCRURAL joint, 199-201
Talonavicular joint, 201
Talus, 199, 200
Tarsal joint, transverse, 201, 221
  movements of, 202
Temporal bone, 251
Tendon
  angle of approach of muscle
    fibers to, 26
  angle of approach of, to bone, 16
Tendinous inscriptions to rectus
  abdominis, 261
Tendon action, 124
Tension of muscle. See *Muscle
  tension.*
Tensor fasciae latae, 193, 232, 236
  electromyography of, 306
  paralysis of, 245
Teres major, 68, 139, 158
  rhomboids and, 168
Teres minor, 154
Terminal rotation of knee, 177, 192

Vertebral column (Cont.)
curves of, 253, 270, 282
intervertebral disks of, 256
landmarks for heights of vertebrae, 254
ligaments of, 253

WALKING. See also *Locomotion.*
abductors of hip in, 306
acceleration of body segments in,
291, 296
adductors of hip in, 306, 307
cadence in, 293
caloric consumption in, 309-312
expenditure of energy in, 300-302
function of calf muscles in, 303
function of dorsiflexors of ankle
in, 303
function of erector spinae in, 307
function of quadriceps in, 305
kinetic energy in, 302
movement paths in, recording of,
295, 296
muscles used in, electromyography of, 300
oxygen consumption in, 292,
309-312
patterns of muscle activity in, 300
potential energy in, 302
speed of, 293
velocities of body segments in,
296
work done by arm muscles in, 303
Walking cycle, 292
recording of, 293
"Walking unit," 309
Weber-Fick, laws of, 36
Weight
of lower extremity, 273
of prostheses, 275
of upper extremity, 273

Weight arm, definition of, 18
Weight proportions of body segments, 273
Weight-bearing, hip muscles in, 242
Work
cost of, 44, 45
done by muscles of arms in
walking, 302
done on muscles, 30, 44
formula for, 29
negative, 30, 44
units of, 29
Work capacity of muscles, 30. See
also tables in Appendix.
computation of, 30
of shoulder, 171
rectus femoris, 233
sartorius, 234
Wrist
digits and, muscles acting on, 88
hand and, 81-126
Wrist drop, 121
Wrist extensors and finger flexors,
98
Wrist flexors and finger extensors,
105
Wrist joint, 85
axes of motion of, 82, 83, 85, 86
degrees of freedom of motion of,
9, 84
Wrist muscles
abductor digiti minimi and, 120
thumb abductors and, 120

XIPHOID process, 127, 255, 276, 279

Y-LIGAMENT, 284